453 Frontenac St.
542-5502.

OUTLINE OF HISTOLOGY

**SEVENTH
EDITION**

OUTLINE OF HISTOLOGY

GERRIT BEVELANDER, Ph.D.

Department of Histology, University of Texas, Dental Branch,
Houston, Texas

SEVENTH EDITION

With 311 illustrations and 3 color plates

THE C. V. MOSBY COMPANY

Saint Louis 1971

SEVENTH EDITION

Copyright © 1971 by The C. V. Mosby Company

All rights reserved. No part of this book may be reproduced in any manner without written permission of the publisher.

Previous editions copyrighted 1942, 1948, 1955, 1959, 1963, 1967

Printed in the United States of America

Standard Book Number 8016-0680-2

Distributed in Great Britain by Henry Kimpton, London

TS/S/B   9 8 7 6 5 4 3

CONTENTS

Part I GENERAL HISTOLOGY

Part II DENTAL HISTOLOGY AND EMBRYOLOGY

Color plates

Part one
GENERAL HISTOLOGY

1
INTRODUCTION

Histology is the science that deals with the detailed structure of animals and plants and in its broader aspects correlates structural features with function. Vital functional units are called cells. Not only do different kinds of cells exhibit variations in form and structural content, but also the same cell may vary in these respects with changes in its physiological status. Our knowledge about cells and cell products has been obtained by a study of "fixed" or dead cells and by a variety of ingenious methods developed to study living cells. Each of these methods has advantages and disadvantages, but they are mutually complementary and we may conclude that all normal cells have certain attributes in common.

Cell structures and cell products are made visible by fixing these structures with suitable chemicals, followed by sectioning and staining with certain dyes. The traditional stains are hematoxylin and eosin (H & E). The basic dyes, like hematoxylin, stain the chromatin of the nucleus (basophilia), whereas the acid dyes, such as eosin, tend to stain the cytoplasm (acidophilia, oxyphilia). Although many other dyes are used, most slides utilized in routine histological and pathological studies are hematoxylin and eosin preparations. These dyes have the great advantage of relative stability, universal use, and reproducible results.

In addition to the use of stained preparations several other methods have been and are currently used to study cells. Histochemical techniques, for example, are currently being used and developed to aid in the localization of specific chemical substances within the cell. By means of these methods it is possible to localize substances such as enzymes, lipids, nucleic acids, and glycogen. Modifications of ordinary light microscopy are also utilized. Some of these are phase microscopy, which enhances contrast and is especially useful for observing living cells, and dark-field microscopy, which utilizes a special condenser producing a dark field. The latter method permits observation at a higher resolution than is possible with the usual light microscope. Ultraviolet rays, x-rays, and polarized light are also utilized for observing specimens to enhance resolution, density, or birefringence, respectively.

The most recently developed instrument used in microscopy is the electron microscope, which employs a system analogous to that of the optical microscope. It differs from the optical system, however, in that the illuminating source consists of a beam of electrons accelerated to a high velocity in a vacuum. The electron beam is projected through a specimen and focused on a fluorescent screen or photographic plate by means of electromagnetic fields, which serve as lenses. Although the electron microscope permits visualization of specimens at much greater magnification than is possible by optical methods, the important advantage of this instrument is the great increase in resolution over that afforded by other methods. Whereas the optimum resolution possible with the light microscope is of the order of 0.5μ, the electron microscope can resolve cell structure at approximately 10 Å and thus permits visualization of structures that have the dimension of macromolecules.

THE CELL

Most cells are composed of a single nucleus embedded in cytoplasm (Fig. 1-1). The term *protoplasm* is used to designate the living substance of both the nucleus and the cyto-

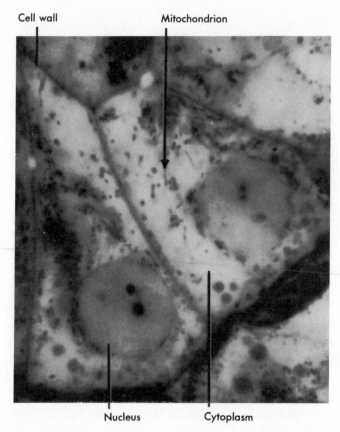

Cell wall   Mitochondrion

Nucleus   Cytoplasm

Fig. 1-1
Liver cells of turtle showing mitochondria and other cytoplasmic inclusions. (Iron hematoxylin; × 1,000.)

plasm. Protoplasm is a grayish viscous liquid (hydrosol) enclosed at all interfaces by a membrane (cell membrane). The cell membrane selectively regulates the interchange of materials between the cell and surrounding environment and upon death becomes completely permeable, or nonselective.

Cytoplasm

Cytoplasm (protoplasm) is usually considered to be a colloid and consists of approximately 60 to 75% water, part of which is free, the other part protein-bound (Fig. 1-2). Cationic salts are present as potassium, magnesium, and traces of several others; anions occur as bicarbonate and phosphate. Cytoplasmic components that are particularly concerned with the organization and structure of the cell consist of the following macromolecules: carbohydrates, proteins, and nucleic acid.

Carbohydrates of biological interest are glycogen and mucopolysaccharides. Glycogen is a storage product from which glucose is released on demand for a variety of metabolic activities. Mucopolysaccharides are frequently present as hyaluronic acid and chondroitin sulfates, components of the ground substance of connective tissue and cartilage, respectively.

Proteins responsible for the characteristic structure of the cell are molecules of high molecular weight and consist of many amino acid monomers linked in sequence by peptide bonds. They occur as structural proteins such as collagen, muscle, and keratin or as nonstructural proteins such as enzymes and some hormones.

Nucleic acids are polymers of nucleotides concerned with protein synthesis. They are remarkable in that they can exist in infinite varieties because the variation in the base pairs of the nucleic acids and the variation of the sequence of amino acids of the protein elaborated provide a code with limitless combinations.

The most important constituents of the nucleus are the nucleic acids. Two general types

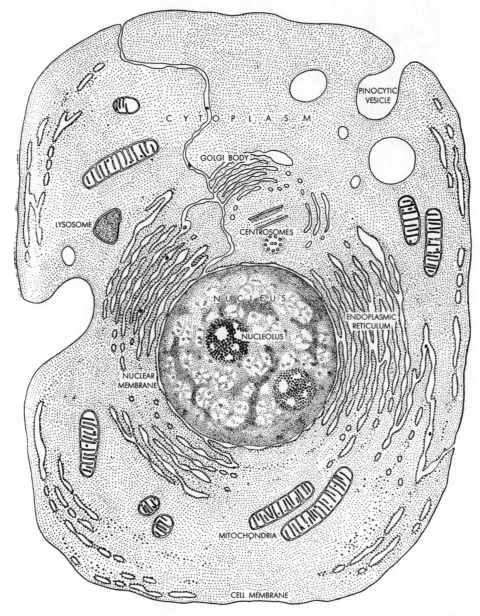

Fig. 1-2

Diagram of typical cell based on what is seen in electron photomicrographs. Mitochondria are sites of oxidative reactions that provide cell with energy. Dots that line endoplasmic reticulum are ribosomes—sites of protein synthesis. In cell division the pair of centrosomes, one shown in longitudinal section (rods) and the other in cross section (circles), part to form poles of apparatus that separate two duplicate sets of chromosomes. (From Brachet, J.: Scient. Am. **205**:51, 1961. Reprinted with permission. Copyright © 1961 by Scientific American, Inc. All rights reserved.)

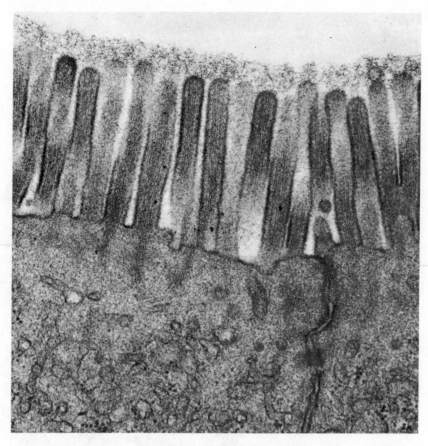

Fig. 1-3

Electron micrograph of microvilli forming striated border of small intestine of mouse and showing surface coat at periphery of microvilli. (×60,000.) (Courtesy Dr. Caramia, University of Rome.)

of nucleic acids are present—deoxyribonucleic acid (DNA) and ribonucleic acid (RNA). There is more DNA than RNA in the nucleus. DNA is a constituent of chromatin, the material in the nucleus that becomes differentiated into discrete structures known as chromosomes. Each chromosome contains as many as a thousand or more substructures, referred to as genes, which were once considered to be the smallest subunit of heredity. The chemical nature of the gene has now been determined to be the nonprotein substance DNA. The transfer of genetic information on a biochemical basis is now well established. There is excellent evidence that the DNA associated with a specific gene can transfer its information to govern the exact sequence of amino acids in specific proteins. The nuclear DNA is the molecule of heredity, and the sequence of the base pairs is the genetic code providing information and direction re-garding the specific function of the cell. This information is transferred to a class of molecules known as messenger RNA, complementary to nuclear DNA molecules, which carry genetic information from the DNA of the gene to the ribosomes, where specific protein synthesis takes place. DNA is found in every living cell and issues the orders of cell pattern and tissue organization to determine the uniqueness of a cell and its ability to duplicate itself; each type of cell contains the duplicating stencil of itself in its own DNA molecules.

Cell (plasma) membrane

The cell (plasma) membrane is visible with the light microscope in some cells as a delicate structure separating one cell from another. It serves in both an active and a passive manner to regulate the interchange of metabolites and other substances from the cell and its environ-

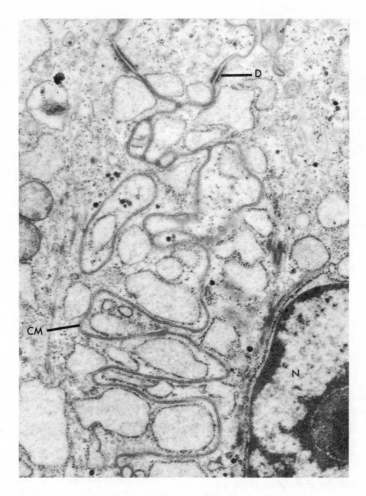

Fig. 1-4

Electron micrograph of part of an epithelial cell of mollusc mantle, showing marked folding and interdigitation of adjacent, lateral surface cell membranes. **D**, Desmosome; **CM**, cell membrane; **N**, nucleus. (×27,000.)

ment. At the electron microscope's level of resolution the plasma membrane, also known as a "unit" membrane, consists of a three-layered, polarized structure comprised of two dark layers separated by a light interval. Chemically, it is considered to be a bimolecular leaflet made up of a chain of lipid molecules, located between two protein layers.

Cell surfaces are frequently specialized. Cells specialized for absorption exhibit fingerlike projections on the free surface, called *microvilli*, which greatly increase the surface area (Fig. 1-3). Absorption or ingestion also occurs in other cells by a process known as *pinocytosis*, which is effected by the formation of small vesicles at the cell surface that ingest materials and transport them to other parts of the cell.

Phagocytosis is another method of cellular ingestion and is similar in some respects to pinocytosis.

The space between the unit membranes separating adjacent cells is approximately 100 to 200 Å. The membranes separating the cells are often parallel to one another but vary considerably in arrangement. Some, for example, exhibit a serrated or interlocking arrangement (Fig. 1-4). Toward the distal surface of certain cells the lateral cell interfaces are often specialized in the form of thickened membranes known as *terminal bars*. At the base of some cells (for example, of the kidney) prominent infoldings of the basal surface occur. This is another modification to increase surface area for transport of materials.

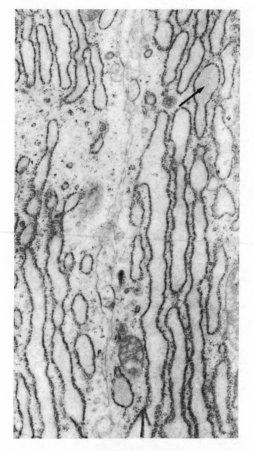

Fig. 1-5

Electron micrograph of the granular or rough endoplasmic reticulum of a young odontoblast. The lumina of the cisternae contain a dense material (arrow), and the external surfaces are studded with granules (ribosomes). (×28,000.)

In addition to the situations just described it has also been observed that there is probably a continuity between the plasma membrane and the endoplasmic reticulum and also indirectly with the Golgi apparatus and other organelles.

Endoplasmic reticulum (ergastoplasm)

The cytoplasm of many cells, such as nerve cells, salivary gland cells, and the acinar cells of the pancreas, exhibits diffuse or discrete masses of material that stains with the same basic dye as does the chromatin material of the nucleus. This material, formerly known as chromophil substance, contains ribonucleoprotein and changes markedly during cellular activity.

With the electron microscope, regions of the cell exhibiting chromophil substance have been shown to consist of accumulations of osmiophilic granules approximately 150 Å in diameter. These granules, known as ribosomes, are made up of ribonucleoprotein and are believed to be the site of protein synthesis (Fig. 1-5).

The endoplasmic reticulum consists of a complex of cisternae and tubules, which often extend throughout the cytoplasm. It is enclosed by a membrane approximately 75 Å thick. Two varieties of reticulum have been identified: (1) agranular (smooth), in which the cisternae and vesicles do not exhibit osmiophilic granules on the surface of the membranes, and (2) granular (rough), in which the surface of the membranes are studded with granules (ribosomes). The lumen of the reticulum may contain material that has a greater density than the surrounding cytoplasm, and it is apparently in this region that synthesis of some cell products occurs.

Golgi apparatus

The Golgi apparatus (complex) consists of an irregular network that may be fairly discrete and localized in one part of the cell or diffuse and localized in several areas within the cytoplasm.

Electron microscopy shows that the Golgi apparatus consists of a series of parallel arrays of smooth-surfaced membranes. The contoured membranes bind flattened sacs piled one upon another (Fig. 1-6). In some instances the sacs appear dilated and are then known as Golgi vacuoles. The Golgi apparatus has been associated with secretory activities for some time. Recent studies have confirmed this concept, although many details regarding this mechanism await further clarification.

Centrosome (cytocentrum)

With the light microscope one may observe a small dark body, usually located near the nucleus, called the *centrosome*. The centrosome contains two or more small granules known as centrioles. In many instances the centrosphere (centrosome) is surrounded by a group of delicate, radially arranged fibrils called the *aster*. During the nuclear phase of cell division the centrioles separate and migrate to opposite sides sides of the nucleus. With the aid of the electron microscope the centriole appears to be a short, hollow cylinder having a dense wall in which are embedded nine longitudinally arranged tubular

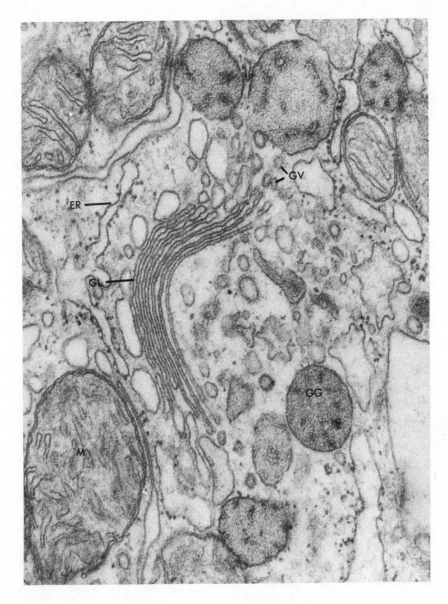

Fig. 1-6
Electron micrograph of part of calciferous gland of *Lumbricus terrestris,* showing Golgi apparatus. Note proximity of rough endoplasmic reticulum, **ER,** to the stacks of Golgi lamellae, **GL,** which transmit and modify protein derived from the **ER.** The material is then conveyed to Golgi vesicles, **GV,** which undergo further changes in the cytoplasm as represented by the Golgi granules, **GG,** which are eventually extruded at the free surface of the cell. **M,** Mitochondria. (×77,000.)

elements. In transverse section the centriole appears as a dense ring. It is usually located close to the Golgi apparatus.

Mitochondria

Mitochondria are present in all living cells and require special techniques for visualization at the level of the light microscope. They vary in number from a few to several hundred per cell. They appear as spheres and also as rods and filaments. When observed with the electron microscope, they all have basically a similar structure. They are bounded by a double-unit membrane. The outer membrane contains pores,

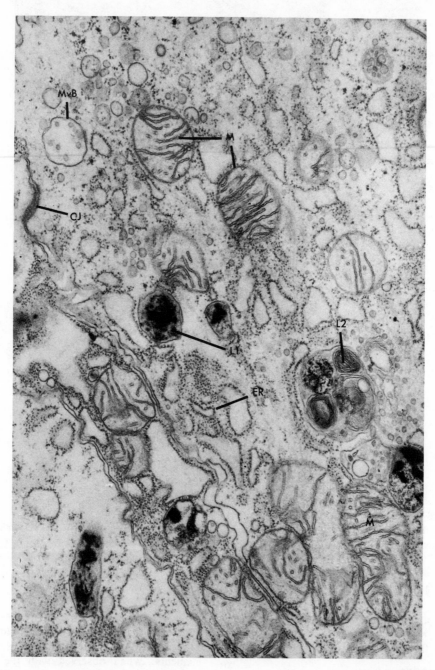

Fig. 1-7

Electron micrograph showing several organelles in the mantle epithelium. **CJ,** Cell junction; **ER,** endoplasmic reticulum; **L1, L2,** phagocytic vesicles (lysosomes); **M,** mitochondrion; **MvB,** multivesicular body. (×29,000.)

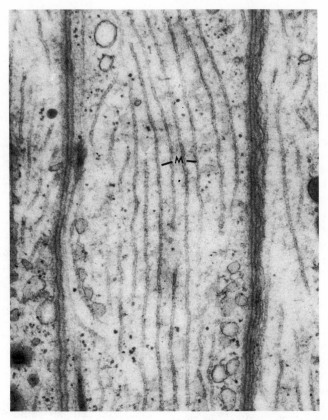

Fig. 1-8

Electron micrograph of longitudinal section of several microtubules, **M,** from marginal gland of Littorina. (×46,000.)

and the inner membrane is thrown into infoldings, usually in a transverse direction (Fig. 1-7). These infoldings are known as *cristae.* Minute granules, the elementary particles believed to be the source of several enzymes, are attached to the inner membrane. The core of the mitochondrion is filled with an amorphous fluid known as the *matrix.* A variable number of particles containing calcium and magnesium has been observed in the matrix. The mitochondria contain enzymes concerned with oxidative phosphorylation as well as electron and ion transport mechanisms. They are also involved in cellular respiration and in the storage and transfer of energy.

Fibrils and filaments

Fibrils occur in many cells. They are especially prominent in nerve (neurofibrils) and muscle cells (myofibrils). In epithelial cells of the skin they are known as *tonofibrils.* Structures formerly described as fibers at the optical

level have been shown to consist of subunits of much smaller dimension that can only be observed with the aid of the electron microscope. For example, the muscle fiber consists of numerous fibrillae, which are further subdivided into filaments. This is also true for collagen fibers.

Microtubules

In addition to the microfilaments mentioned cytoplasm frequently exhibits straight *microtubules,* having a diameter of approximately 200 Å (Fig. 1-8). The wall of the microtubule is composed of several filamentous subunits. Microtubules are numerous during mitosis and on other occasions when the cell alters considerably in size or shape. The exact function of these structures is not known for certain. It has been suggested that they may function as cytoskeletal elements or that they may be contractile and function in changes in cell shape or movement.

11

Nucleus

The nucleus of the cell at the interphase exhibits several morphological characteristics, which can be observed with the optical microscope. The nucleus usually appears as a spherical or ovoid body bounded by a nuclear membrane. The nucleus contains a fluid (nucleoplasm) in which is found one or more dark-staining, eccentrically placed spheres (nucleolus) and, in addition, a delicate, lacy network upon which dark-staining *chromatin granules* or flakes appear to be lodged (Fig. 1-9). Although the nucleoplasm is rarely stained, both the nucleolus and chromatin granules are strongly basophilic and stain a deep purple or blue with hematoxylin. When stained with toluidine blue, the two may be distinguished. The chromatin stains blue (orthochromasia), whereas the nucleolus, containing RNA, stains purple (metachromasia). In some cells, such as white blood cells and megakaryocytes, the nuclei appear to be lobed and connected by fine strands. In other cells, such as liver cells, osteoclasts, and skeletal muscle fibers, two, three, or more nuclei may be present—a condition sometimes referred to as a *syncytium*. In the red blood cell the nucleus is extruded, rendering these cells incapable of cell division.

The nuclear envelope consists of a double-layered structure interrupted at frequent intervals by openings or pores (Fig. 1-9). The membranes are separated by an interval known as the perinuclear space. The outer membrane is continuous at several sites with the cisternae of the endoplasmic reticulum and, like the latter, often bears ribonucleoprotein granules on the cytoplasmic surface. It is believed that a transference of large molecules such as RNA occurs in the region of the pores.

Nuclear sap (karyoplasm), which appears structureless at the optical level, has been shown at the electron microscope level to contain dispersed particles and delicate filaments. These dispersed materials are believed to condense at mitosis to form the chromosomes.

Chromatin particles previously mentioned represent portions of the chromosomes that were not dispersed during reconstruction following mitosis. There is a marked variation in the amount of chromatin present in the cells of various species.

Nucleolus

Each nucleus may contain one or more nucleoli, since they sometimes fuse and at times

new nucleoli arise. They consist in part of acidic and basic proteins, RNA, and at times DNA. They are especially large in neurons. It has been shown that there is a correlation between nucleoli size, number, cell growth, and protein synthesis. In actively growing or dividing cells and those actively synthesizing protein, the nucleoli are large and multiple, which is probably correlated with the fact that they are the site of RNA production. At the optical level one may observe in favorable preparations that the nucleolus is made up of two components: a structureless *pars amorpha* and a threadlike portion, the *nucleolonema*.

Nucleolonema

At the electron microscope level the nucleolonema has been shown to consist of a mass of granular material that is arranged in irregular strands embedded in an amorphous material (Fig. 1-9). The structure of the nucleolonema is further subdivided into a fibrillar component and a granular component. The latter is believed to consist of ribosomes.

Inclusions

Inclusions are granules that are present in the cytoplasm and vary in number during different physiological states of the cell. They consist of lipids, carbohydrates, proteins, and occasionally crystalline material. In routine histological preparations these structures are usually not well demonstrated. Lipids can be demonstrated after osmium fixation as dark brown or black granules or masses of material. Carbohydrate in the form of glycogen is readily demonstrated at the light level by the use of the periodic acid–Schiff reaction. When observed with the aid of the electron microscope, glycogen appears as particulate material—either as single granules or in the form of rosettes (Fig. 1-10).

Secretion granules

Secretion granules occur in a variety of cells, especially in epithelium. The appearance of these granules is cyclical in nature, depending upon the activity of the cell. In many instances the granules contain enzymes or precursors of enzymes and are periodically discharged at the free surface of the cell.

Pigment granules

Pigment granules occur in diverse tissues and are prominent in the skin and eye. They are either endogenous in nature, for example, hemo-

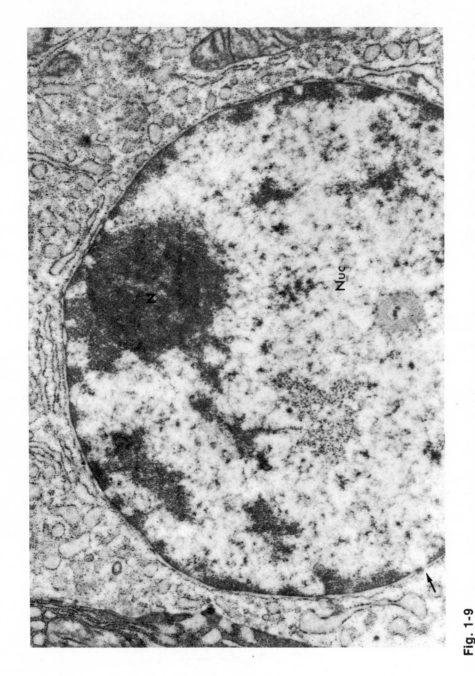

Fig. 1-9

Electron micrograph of a nucleus of a pancreatic acinar cell. The prominent nucleolus, **N**, is made up of granules arranged in irregular strands (nucleolonema). The nuclear envelope is made up of two membranes bonding a narrow perinuclear cisterna. At frequent intervals the nuclear membrane appears to be interrupted (arrow) by pores. Chromatin granules are scattered throughout the nucleus, **Nuc.** (×18,000.)

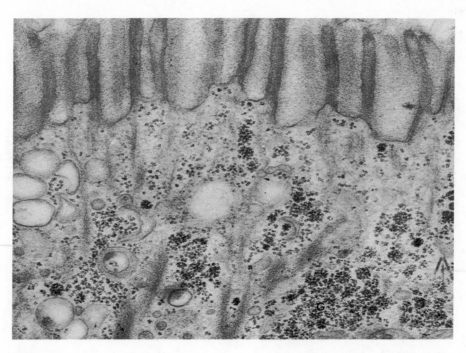

Fig. 1-10
Electron micrograph of part of epithelial cell of mollusc mantle, showing clusters of dark granules, **G**, glycogen, arranged in form of rosettes. (×45,000.)

Table 1. Staining characteristics of cell components

	Cell constituent	Chemical constituent	Characteristics
Nucleus	Chromatin	DNA	Purple, blue, or black with hematoxylin—basophilia
			Blue with toluidine blue—orthochromasia
			Blue-green with methyl green—pyronin
	Nucleolus	RNA	Purple, blue, or black with hematoxylin—basophilia
			Purple with toluidine blue—metachromasia
			Red with methyl green—pyronin
		Ribose	Red-purple with Feulgen reaction
Cytoplasm:	Ground substance	Protein	Pink-red with eosin—acidophilia, eosinophilia
	Mitochondria	Complex	Blue with Janus green B supravital; black with iron hematoxylin; red with acid fuchsin
Organoids	Centrioles	Protein	Rarely seen in hematoxylin and eosin; black with iron hematoxylin
	Chromophil substance	RNA	Same as nucleolus
	Fibrils	Protein	Special methods, argyrophil in nerve cells
Inclusions	Lipids	Fats	Blackened by osmic acid—osmiophilia
			Negative image in hematoxylin and eosin removed by solvents
	Zymogen	Protein	Red with eosin—acidophilia
	Mucigen glycogen	Carbohydrate	Unstained in routine hematoxylin and eosin negative image; red to purple with PAS

siderin, an iron-containing pigment, or melanin, a dark pigment responsible for skin color, or are exogenous pigments. those formed outside the organism.

Lysosomes

Lysosomes occur in a wide variety of cells and appear as scattered granules at the light level. When observed with the electron microscope, they appear as granules of varying size, being characterized by the presence of a membrane (Fig. 1-7). Lysosomes are pleomorphic; that is, they occur in diverse forms inasmuch as the appearance of the material enclosed by the membrane is concerned. They may arise by different methods, for example, as the result of the coalescence of pinocytotic vesicles, by the fusion of Golgi vacuoles, and possibly by other means. Their content may consist of a dense lipid or osmiophilic substance, myelin bodies, parts of organelles, and in some instances precursors of hormones. They contain hydrolytic enzymes such as acid phosphatase and aryl sulfatases and are concerned with intracellular digestion.

Table 1 summarizes the staining reactions of cell constituents most frequently mentioned in modern texts.

2
EPITHELIA

Epithelial tissues have two types of arrangement and two functions. First, they are arranged in sheets, one or more layers in thickness, covering the surface or lining the cavities of the body to form a protective sheath or limiting membrane. Second, they are grouped in solid cords, tubules, or follicles, which have developed as outgrowths from an epithelial sheet and are specialized for secretion, absorption, or excretion. The separation of function is not complete, however, since cells are present in many lining epithelia that have a secretory function.

EPITHELIAL CELLS AND INTERCELLULAR SUBSTANCE

Epithelial tissues are composed of cells of somewhat regular form without extensive protoplasmic processes. These cells are closely applied to each other, and a small amount of *intercellular substance* cements them together. In some cells it has been shown that the cementing substance consists in part of a mucopolysaccharide and is also rich in calcium, which is known to be necessary for cell adhesion. Near the free surface of certain epithelia the intercellular substance viewed under the optical microscope appears thicker and forms a *terminal bar* network. It has been shown by electron microscopy that these structures are areas of specialization of opposing cell membranes and, furthermore, that they encircle the entire cell.

Adjacent cells may on occasion appear to contact each other by *intercellular bridges.* However, this is the exception rather than the rule. These bridges can be readily observed in the stratum spinosum of the skin. They are protoplasmic extensions that were formerly believed to pass from a cell to an adjacent one. Electron microscopy has shown that the extensions contain tonofibrils. They do not extend into adjacent cells but terminate in specialized parts of cell membranes known as desmosomes (Fig. 2-1).

The specialization of cell membranes, known as desmosomes, occurs in most epithelial cells. They are made up of two plaques that consist of thickened parallel cell membranes separated by an intercellular space approximately 200 Å wide (Fig. 2-2). Attached to the cytoplasmic surfaces of the thickened membranes or plaques are numerous delicate tonofilaments. *Hemidesmosomes* occur in regions such as the basal layer of stratified epithelium of the skin adjacent to the basement membrane. As their name implies they consist of one half a desmosome.

The epithelia, which are arranged as coverings and linings, rest upon a *basement membrane,* or lamina. This was formerly believed to be a modification of the underlying connective tissues. At present there is evidence that it is derived from a secretion of the adjacent epithelial cells. At the optical level the basement membrane may appear to be hyaline and structureless or composed of a band of tightly or loosely packed (reticular) fibers. The hyaline material stains with the PAS method, whereas the fibers require special silver techniques for visualization. The basement membrane is often so fine that it is imperceptible in routine preparations. Some epithelia exhibit a well-marked membrane (pseudostratified of the trachea). Epithelial tissues are avascular, and blood capillaries are found only below the basement membrane.

Electron microscopy has shown that the basal lamina is separated from the basal epithelial cells by a light zone about 400 Å in width. The lamina exhibits a texture because of the presence of fine filaments embedded in the amorphous mucopolysaccharide (Fig. 2-3).

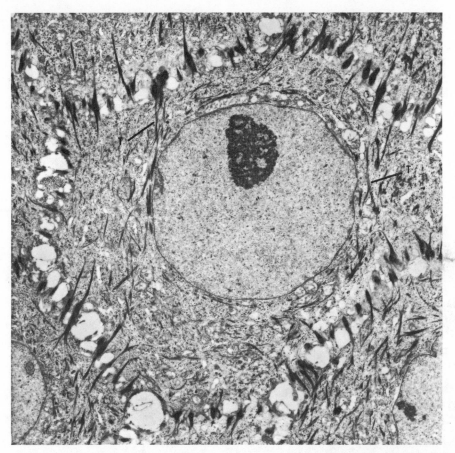

Fig. 2-1

Electron micrograph of cell from stratum germinativum of the gingiva. These cells exhibit many tonofibrils, **T** (the intercellular bridges of light microscopy). The fibrils terminate in desmosomes on the cell surface and do not, as was formerly supposed, extend to adjacent cells. (×6,000.)

The basal lamina is concerned with cell permeability and certain immunological reactions.

Epithelial cells lining moistened membranes or tubules usually exhibit free, smooth surfaces, whereas others exhibit protoplasmic projections known as *cilia*. Cilia of the motile variety are prominent structures in well-preserved material. They appear as slender elongated processes exhibiting an axial filament and a refractile basal body. The electron microscope has shown that cilia contain nine longitudinal filaments on the periphery and two centrally placed filaments. In transverse section the outer filaments appear double. The basal bodies appear similar to a centriole. They are hollow and contain nine peripherally located filaments (Figs. 2-4 and 2-5). Motile cilia are associated with the respiratory passages and the female reproductive tract. Stereocilia are elongate and nonmotile. Formerly described as cilia, they are now known to be attenuated microvilli. They occur in portions of the male reproductive tract.

When viewed with the electron microscope, striated borders are shown to be composed of many extremely thin, short, uniform, and closely packed protoplasmic projections known as microvilli. They are found in locations where absorption and secretion are the primary activities of the cell. In the small intestine the striated border is covered by a thin layer of mucoprotein secretion, and in poorly stained or preserved material an ill-defined layer is observable on the surface of the cell. This layer is sometimes referred to as a cuticle, or cuticular border.

Cell surfaces beset with protoplasmic pro-

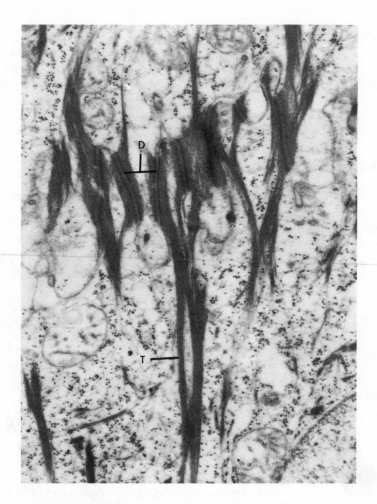

Fig. 2-2
Electron micrograph showing termination of tonofibrils, **T**, in desmosomes, **D**. The opposing plasma membranes of the desmosomes appear thickened, and a fibrillar material lies between the membranes. (×24,000.)

jections of an irregular arrangement are said to have a *brush border.* The projections known as brush borders are somewhat longer than those occurring as striated borders and appear at the electron microscope level as fingerlike projections on the distal surface of the cell. They, too, are known as *microvilli* (Fig. 1-3). They consist of a solid core enclosed by extensions of the plasma membrane. The heights of microvilli vary in diverse cells. They are numerous and relatively tall in the digestive tract. In some cells a fibrillar condensation of the apical part of the cytoplasm extends into the core of the microvillus, which is also continuous with fibrillar material in the region of the terminal bars. This fibrillar material is often referred to as the terminal web.

SIMPLE EPITHELIA
Squamous

The cells of simple squamous epithelium are flattened. Viewed from the surface they appear as fairly large cells with clear cytoplasm and a round or oval nucleus. Cell boundaries are not visible in ordinary preparations but may be demonstrated by the use of silver nitrate. In such preparations the outlines appear to be somewhat wavy and sometimes smooth (Fig. 2-6). In sections the cytoplasm is barely visible, but there is an enlargement of the cell at the center where the nucleus is situated. The boundaries between adjacent cells are not seen. This type of epithelium lines the blood vessels and, in fact, forms the entire wall of capillaries, giving ample opportunity for the diffusion of gases in

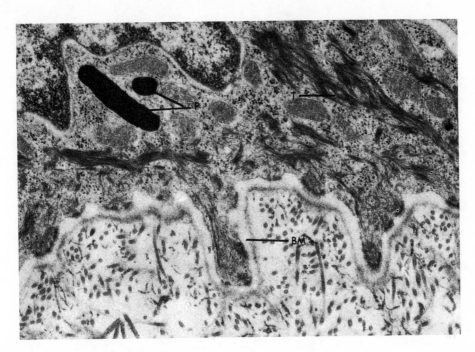

Fig. 2-3
Electron micrograph of the basal region of the epithelium of the monkey lip, showing the basal lamina, or membrane, **BM,** pigment granules, **P,** and tonofibrils, **T.** (×34,000.)

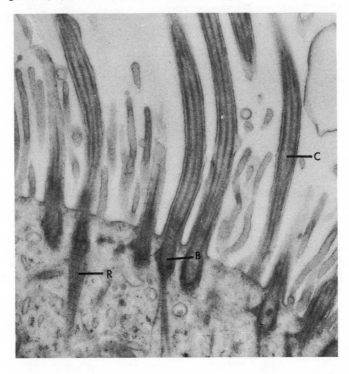

Fig. 2-4
Electron micrograph of longitudinal section of cilia, **C,** of epithelial lining of cat bronchiole; **R,** rootlet. The internal longitudinal filaments form a junction with the basal bodies, **B.** (×25,000.)

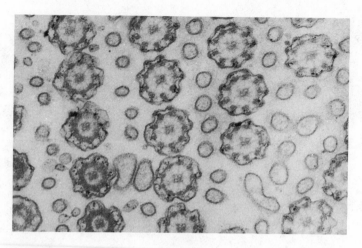

Fig. 2-5
Transverse section of cilia. (×45,000.)

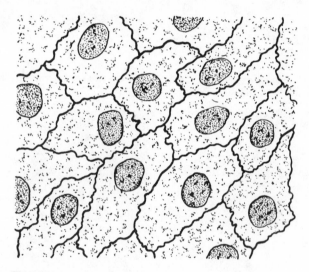

Fig. 2-6
Surface view of mesothelium of mesentery treated
with silver nitrate. (Redrawn from Bailey.)

these vessels. It is also present in other situations where diffusion rather than strength is required of a membrane. This is the case in Bowman's capsule of the kidney, which is used as an illustration of simple squamous epithelium (Fig. 2-7).

Table 2. Epithelia

A. Simple epithelia	B. Stratified epithelia
1. Squamous	1. Columnar
2. Cuboidal	2. Transitional
3. Columnar	3. Squamous
4. Pseudostratified	

The appearance of the tissue in the walls of blood vessels is shown in Figs. 8-3 to 8-5. When simple squamous epithelium lines the blood vessels, it is called endothelium; the same kind of tissue lining the body cavities is called mesothelium. These names refer entirely to the situation and embryological derivations of the tissues and are not morphologically descriptive terms. Mesenchymal epithelium, the lining of joint cavities, is not actually epithelial tissue at all, although it bears certain resemblances to simple squamous epithelium.

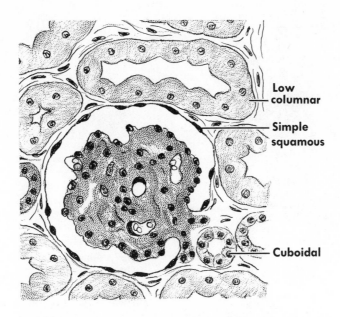

Low columnar

Simple squamous

Cuboidal

Fig. 2-7
Portion of kidney, showing types of epithelium.

Cuboidal

The cells of cuboidal epithelium are smaller in surface view than those of the simple squamous type and have more regular outlines. The shape, in surface view, is roughly hexagonal, and the cell boundaries are often clearly visible. In vertical section the cells are square with a round nucleus in the center of each. The square shape is modified to that of a truncated prism when the cells are grouped around a small opening or lumen. The cytoplasm may be either clear or granular; in the latter case the cell boundaries are indistinct. This type of epithelium lines small tubules such as are illustrated in Fig. 2-7. It also elaborates secretions (thyroid) or acts as a storage tissue (liver), although these functions are more commonly performed by columnar cells.

Columnar

The surface view of columnar epithelium is like that of the cuboidal epithelium. In sections, however, the cells are seen to be taller than they are broad; that is, they have the form of rectangles rather than squares. The nucleus is at the base of the cell. This type of epithelium is modified in many ways. The surface may be covered by a structureless protective cuticula, or it may have fine hairs or cilia projecting from it. The intercellular substance may form a net-work of fine bars near the surface ("terminal bars"). The cytoplasm may be clear or may contain granules or drops of secretion. As is the case in cuboidal epithelium the rectangular shape of columnar cells is changed to pyramidal when they are grouped around a small lumen.

The difference between cuboidal and columnar cells is not sharply differentiated; it depends on the height of the cells as seen in vertical section. An organ may be said by one author to be lined with cuboidal epithelium, while another writer will use the term *low columnar* in describing the tissue. An example of low columnar epithelium is shown in the illustration of the kidney (Fig. 2-7). Tall columnar epithelium is illustrated in Fig. 2-8, *A,* drawn from a section of the small intestine.

In studying a columnar epithelium it is important to select a region in which the section passes through the tissue in a plane perpendicular to its surface. When a slanting or tangential section is observed, the appearance is that of two or more layers of cells, and the tissue may be erroneously classified as stratified or pseudostratified epithelium (Fig. 2-8, *B*).

Columnar cells are the type that most frequently occur in secreting organs. They will be found not only in the lining of the greater part of the digestive tract but also in many glands,

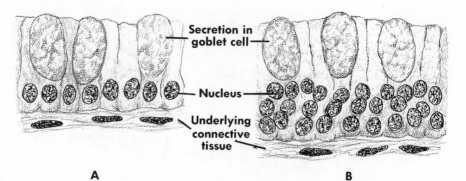

Secretion in
goblet cell

Nucleus

Underlying
connective
tissue

A

B

Fig. 2-8
Tall columnar epithelium from intestine. **A,** Vertical section. **B,** Tangential section.

where their function of forming limiting membranes is lost, and they serve as secreting elements only.

Pseudostratified

Pseudostratified epithelium consists essentially of columnar cells that are crowded very closely together. Because of this the rectangular form is distorted, and not all of the cells reach the free surface of the epithelium. Those that do reach the surface have an upper part like a columnar cell and a much constricted base. Others have a wide base and an irregular spindle shape, and still others are short and rounded. The nucleus of each cell lies at its widest portion, which gives the tissue the appearance of a stratified epithelium with nuclei at several levels. Only in the best preparations can it be demonstrated that while approximately only one cell in three touches the free surface, all have a portion touching the basement membrane. In all preparations there seems, at first glance, to be little difference between a vertical section of pseudostratified epithelium and the tangential section of simple columnar epithelium just described. The nuclei of the two kinds of tissue offer the best means of distinguishing between the two. In pseudostratified epithelium these are of several sorts, those at the base of the tissue being small and dark and those nearer the surface being larger and paler. In the tangential section of columnar epithelium, on the other hand, only one type of nucleus is present. The cytoplasm of the cells of pseudostratified epithelium is sometimes clear, sometimes granular. It may contain drops of secretion, and the surface cells are ciliated. The nuclei are round or oval according to the shape of the cells in which they lie. The usual appearance of this type of

epithelium is illustrated in Fig. 2-9. It is functionally adapted to serve as a fairly resistant limiting membrane. The secreting cells often found in it have the purpose of moistening the surface covered by the epithelium.

STRATIFIED EPITHELIA

In all the members of stratified epithelia a complete layer of small cuboidal or columnar cells lies next to the basement membrane. Above this, except in the case of a two-layered epithelium, there are one or more layers of polygonal cells. At the free surface lies a layer of cells that have a different shape in each subdivision of the group. It is, then, upon the shape of the cells at the *free surface* of a stratified epithelium that its classification in one of the three subdivisions is based.

Stratified columnar epithelium

Stratified columnar epithelium differs from the pseudostratified type in having a continuous layer of small, rounded cells next to the basement membrane. The columnar cells at the surface of the epithelium are thus entirely cut off from the basement membrane, and the epithelium is truly stratified. This type is of rare occurrence (male urethra).

Transitional epithelium

Transitional epithelium consists of several layers of cells. The basal cells are like those of stratified columnar epithelium. Above them are a varying number of layers of polygonal cells, of which those immediately below the surface layer tend to have an elongated pearlike form. The layer at the free surface is composed of large, somewhat flattened cells, generally described as dome shaped. One of these cells

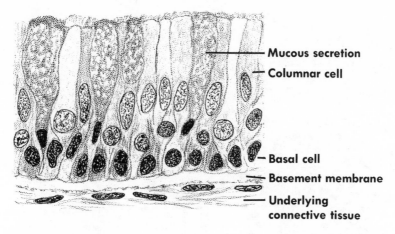

Fig. 2-9
Pseudostratified epithelium from trachea.

- Mucous secretion
- Columnar cell
- Basal cell
- Basement membrane
- Underlying connective tissue

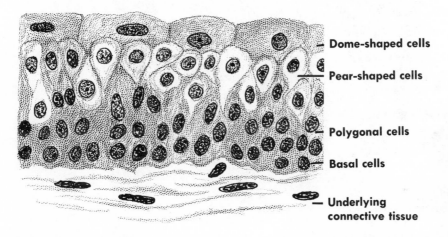

Fig. 2-10
Transitional epithelium from urinary bladder.

- Dome-shaped cells
- Pear-shaped cells
- Polygonal cells
- Basal cells
- Underlying connective tissue

often covers two or three of the underlying pear-shaped cells. The cells of this epithelium possess to an unusual degree the ability to change their position, sliding over each other so that when the organ they line is distended the epithelium is reduced to three or four layers. When it is empty, the cells heap up, forming several layers between the basal and surface cells. This is a nonsecreting epithelium, limited in its distribution to the urinary tract. It is illustrated in Fig. 2-10.

Stratified squamous epithelium

In stratified squamous epithelium the thickness and number of cells vary in different parts of the body; the shape and arrangement of component cells, however, follow the same general plan. In this epithelium the basal cells are covered by several layers of polygonal cells. Near the base the polygonal cells are quite small, but they gradually increase in size toward the middle of the tissue (hypertrophy); beyond this point they begin to flatten out and become smaller. As they approach the surface they may become flattened, shriveled (atrophy), and scalelike with pyknotic nuclei, which is the situation existing in the mucous membranes of the mouth and esophagus (Fig. 2-11). In more exposed, dry epithelia, such as the skin, the cells may incorporate a tough resilient material (keratin).

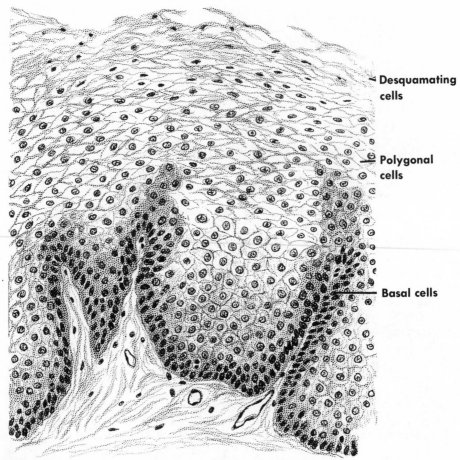

Desquamating cells

Polygonal cells

Basal cells

Fig. 2-11
Stratified squamous epithelium from esophagus.

When this condition exists, the epithelium is said to be *cornified* or *keratinized.* This tissue is particularly well adapted to perform its protective function because of (1) its great thickness and keratinization, (2) its ability to slough off surface cells under the impetus of abrasion, and (3) the replacement of these cells from below. Whereas surface cells are typically flattened, as on the surface of the cornea of the eye, or scalelike, as just described, they differ from simple squamous cells in that the flattened nuclei do not generally produce an enlargement of the cell. The addition of hair also increases the protective function of this epithelium.

The cells that make up the basal and polyhedral layers of this tissue, the so-called *stratum germinativum,* are characteristically basophilic, suggesting their great metabolic activity. In addition, shrinkage of this region produced during preservation (fixation) reveals prominent

intercellular bridges containing tonofibrils, a characteristic that has earned for them the name "prickle cells." Since none of the epithelia described are penetrated by blood vessels, their nutrition apparently depends on transmission through interstitial cellular fluids. This would create a serious nutritional problem for epithelia as thick as stratified squamous epithelia. At any rate it has been suggested that the death of surface cells and possibly keratinization may be the result of lack of nutrients. The thicker stratified squamous epithelia have fingerlike projections of connective tissue, known as *papillae,* penetrating quite deeply into the stratum germinativum, thereby increasing the surface area available for the diffusion of nutrients. In summary, then, we have surface cells that may be flattened or scalelike, keratinized or nonkeratinized. The epithelia appear papillate or nonpapillate.

24

3
CONNECTIVE AND SUPPORTING TISSUES

In the connective and supporting tissues the arrangement of cells and intercellular substance is quite different from that seen in the epithelia. Instead of being closely applied to each other in the form of a sheet or a cord, the cells lie more or less scattered, sometimes not in contact, sometimes touching only at the ends of long protoplasmic processes. The intercellular substance is much more prominent than among the epithelia and becomes the most important part of the majority of the tissues in the group.

The type of cell most frequently found in these tissues is of an irregular branching form, sometimes called stellate. Its nucleus is vesicular and its cytoplasm is somewhat granular and prolonged in the form of processes. Cells of this type make up the mesenchyme, the embryonic tissue from which all the members of the group are derived. The original shape of the cell is retained in some of the connecting and supporting tissues after they have been fully differentiated; in others it is modified. The intercellular components of the connective tissues consist of (1) fibers, (2) ground substance, and (3) tissue fluid.

FIBERS

The fibers are of three kinds, distinguishable by their appearance and chemical reactions: collagenous or white, reticular, and elastic.

White or collagenous fibers

White fibers are the most common. They possess little elasticity, are dissolved by weak acids, and yield gelatin when boiled. Collagenous fibers consist of bundles of fine fibrils, known as fibrillae, which lie parallel to each other and give the fiber its longitudinally striated appearance. The fibrillae are held together by a cementing substance. The fibrillae do not branch. The bundles or fibers, however, branch and anastomose and appear in section sometimes straight, but usually wavy. They stain fairly readily with eosin, giving a pink color to tissues containing many of them.

Studies made with the electron microscope have shown that the diameter of the collagen fibers varies considerably, averaging about 1,000 Å. The fibrils reveal characteristic periodic cross bandings with an interval of 640 Å in the mature fibrils. Information derived from electron microscope and x-ray diffraction studies have shown that the unit molecule of collagen is made up of long polypeptide chains and is known as tropocollagen. It measures approximately 2,600 to 3,000 Å in length and about 15 Å in width. These molecules arranged side by side in a staggered fashion make up collagen, exhibiting an average periodicity of 640 Å.

Reticular fibers

Reticular fibers are similar to white fibers, in some respects, in that they exhibit the same 640 Å periodicity present in collagenous fibers. They are finer in caliber, do not stain appreciably with eosin, but have an affinity for silver. Accordingly, they are not readily distinguished in sections prepared in the ordinary way. On boiling they yield reticulin, which differs slightly from gelatin obtained from white fibers. Reticular fibers also resist peptic digestion longer than do the white fibers.

Elastic fibers

Elastic fibers occur singly or in the form of sheets. In ordinary preparations they are hardly

distinguishable from the white fibers. If the sections are stained with resorcin, however, the elastic fibers will be sharply differentiated, as this dye colors them deeply but leaves the white fibers pale. In such slides the elastic fibers appear as stout, branching structures, heavier than the individual white fibrils or reticular fibers. On boiling they yield elastin, and they show a greater resistance to acids than do the white fibers. As their name implies, their most important physical characteristic is their elasticity, but this is not apparent in histological preparations.

GROUND SUBSTANCE

The ground substance of connective tissue is a homogeneous semifluid material that coexists with the tissue fluid and forms the fluid environment of the cells and fibers. The tissue fluid–ground substance complex is discernible, as a rule, only in especially well-preserved tissues. In the latter condition the ground substance stains metachromatically with toluidine blue. It has been shown to contain several polysaccharides, including hyaluronic acid. The enzyme hyaluronidase hydrolyzes hyaluronic acid, which in turn causes a reduction in viscosity and a consequent increase in the permeability of the tissues. The process by which intercellular structures are formed was, for a long time, controversial. Electron microscopy has now shown in a fairly conclusive manner that the fibers are elaborated by modified portions of the endoplasmic reticulum, which in turn is a prominent cell constituent.

From the foregoing description of the elements composing the tissues of this group it is evident that they have, in varying degree, the function of binding together the parts of the body and furnishing it with a supporting framework. Less obvious are other functions performed by the connective tissues. The fluid intercellular substance of connective tissue plays a part in the nutrition of the body, and the cells provide new phagocytes. Connective tissue of the loose variety is active in limiting the process of local infections and in the healing of tissue and organs. For the present we shall consider the connective tissues in relation to their connective and supporting qualities. From that point of view one may arrange them in order of their degree of differentiation and their solidity, as shown in Table 3; it must be pointed out that any classification is difficult and cannot be ad-

Table 3. Connective and supporting tissues

A. Connective tissues	B. Supporting tissues
1. Mucous connective tissue	1. Cartilage
2. Reticular tissue	a. Fibrous
3. Fibrous tissue	b. Hyaline
a. Areolar	c. Elastic
b. Dense fibrous tissue	2. Bone
c. Tendon	
d. Elastic tissue	
4. Adipose tissue	
5. Serous membranes	
6. Reticuloendothelial system	

hered to rigidly, since the different varieties have transitional forms.

CONNECTIVE TISSUES
Mucous connective tissue

Mucous connective tissue, which must not be confused with mucus-secreting epithelium, retains much of the appearance of mesenchyme, the primitive tissue from which it is derived. The cells are spindle shaped or branching. The intercellular fluid of mesenchyme is replaced by a mucoid jellylike mass from which the tissue derives its name. Fibers of the white or collagenous variety are present, lying in close proximity to the cells (border fibrils, or fibroglia). In microscopic preparations the jelly stains faintly, the fibers more deeply. In the adult body, mucous connective tissue is present only in the vitreous humor of the eye. It is usually studied in sections of the umbilical cord and is of interest chiefly because it illustrates a relation between fibers and cells that is less evident in the more highly differentiated tissues.

Reticular tissue

Reticular tissue also has an appearance in ordinary preparations which is somewhat similar to that of mesenchyme. The cells composing it are sometimes called primitive reticular cells. They are branching cells, the processes of which are generally in contact with each other. The intercellular substance consists of a nonstainable fluid and fine reticular fibers. The latter take the same color as the cell processes when the preparation is stained with eosin, and this fact makes it difficult to distinguish them. By careful examination, however, one may see, among the

slightly granular cytoplasmic processes, other fine hyaline strands that are intercellular fibers. With special stains (silver nitrate) the fibers may be more clearly demonstrated. They then appear as short fine fibers, for the most part closely associated with the cells (Fig. 3-3).

Reticular tissue such as has just been described is illustrated in Figs. 3-2 to 3-4. It forms the basis of the lymphoid organs, such as the lymph nodes, where it is combined with lymphocytes and other blood cells. The latter are present in such numbers as to obscure the reticular network in parts of the preparation, and care must be taken to avoid such regions in finding a place to study the fundamental tissue.

A more attenuated form of reticular tissue is found immediately subjacent to the epithelium of many organs (for example, the digestive tract). Here, the cells are more widely separated, and the appearance presented is like that of fine areolar tissue. Stains specified for the reticular fibers must be used in such cases to distinguish between the two kinds of tissue.

The primitive reticular cells apparently retain throughout life the ability to form phagocytic cells and certain types of leukocytes; that is to say, they combine the function of maintaining a connective tissue with that of phagocytosis. Preparations of reticular tissue contain, therefore, other cells in addition to the primitive reticular cells already mentioned. These are the macrophages and lymphoblasts, which are to be studied in connection with the development of blood. They do not contribute to the connective quality of the tissue that we are considering in this chapter.

Fibrous tissues

Fibrous tissues are all composed of cells, intercellular fluid, and fibers. They differ among themselves in the proportions and arrangement of the elements involved. In areolar tissue the white fibers predominate, but elastic fibers are also present. The white fibers are in bundles of varying thickness, irregularly disposed to form a network. In sections they are cut in all possible directions, and since they twist and interlace, one cannot trace any one bundle for a great part of its extent. The elastic fibers are also irregularly placed, and the whole presents a confused mass of fibers lying in a nonstainable fluid with cells in the spaces of the network. Areolar tissue from the submucosa of the digestive tract is shown in Fig. 3-1.

In some of the denser forms of fibrous tissue, also, the same irregular arrangement of fibers is to be observed, but more fibers are present than in areolar tissue, and the interfibrillar spaces are correspondingly reduced (Fig. 3-7). In the capsules of some organs, on the other hand, the fibers are oriented in a direction parallel to the surface of the organ that they invest (Fig. 3-2). Another form of dense fibrous tissue is tendon, in which the fibers are grouped in very thick parallel bundles. These bundles are so closely crowded together that the cells between them are flattened to a platelike shape. Tendon is composed almost entirely of white fibers (Fig. 3-9). Elastic tissue occurs also in dense arrangement. In the walls of the arteries the elastic fibers have developed and fused to such an extent that they form an incomplete (fenestrated) membrane, in the spaces of which are cells and a few white fibers.

It is clear that in these tissues the ability to bind together organs and parts of organs has reached a high degree of development through the elaboration of intercellular fibers. Cells called fibroblasts, which form or maintain the fibers, are present in all forms of fibrous tissue. There are, in addition, cells that have no part in carrying out the connective function of the tissue. They are fairly constant elements in the tissue, and their morphology will be described in this chapter, since they are to be distinguished from the fibroblasts; but their significance, like that of the cells of reticular tissue, will be discussed later.

Fibroblasts are present in all types of fibrillar tissue, from the finest areolar tissue to the tendons and elastic membranes. In loose areolar tissue, when seen in surface view, they appear as rather large branching cells with pale oval nuclei. The cytoplasm is so lightly stained as to be often barely perceptible, so that one may distinguish the nucleus alone. Often the cells lie in such a position that they are seen from the side; in that case they are fusiform and somewhat easier to see. In fully formed areolar tissue there are no fibroglia, or border fibrils, connected with the fibroblasts. The cells sometimes lie very close to the fibers, especially in the denser kinds of tissue, but careful examination makes it evident that cells and fibers are actually separate. The fibroblasts are sometimes called the fixed cells of connective tissue in contrast to the remaining ones, which are called wandering cells. Fibroblasts are the most common cells

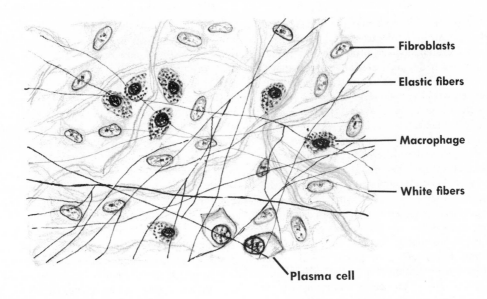

Fig. 3-1
Areolar tissue spread preparation.

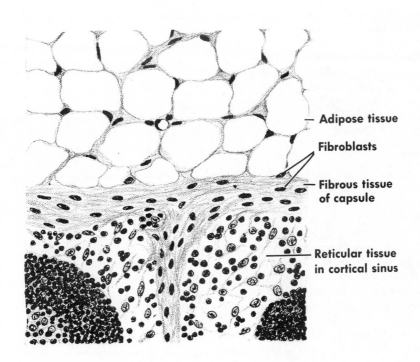

Fig. 3-2
Peripheral portion of a section of lymph node, showing reticular tissue in cortical sinus, fibrous tissue of capsule, and adipose tissue surrounding organ. Fibroblasts may be seen in capsule and adipose tissue.

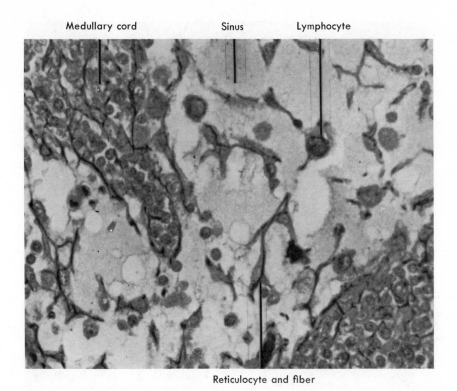

Medullary cord   Sinus   Lymphocyte

Reticulocyte and fiber

Fig. 3-3
Section of lymph node showing distribution of reticulocytes and reticular fibers in sinus. (Bielschowsky method; ×640.)

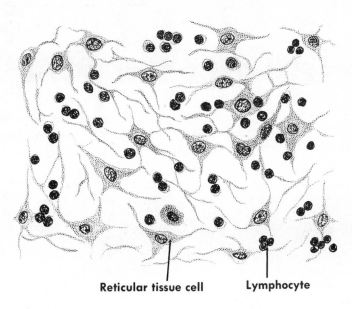

Reticular tissue cell   **Lymphocyte**

Fig. 3-4
Reticular tissue of lymph node stained with hematoxylin and eosin.

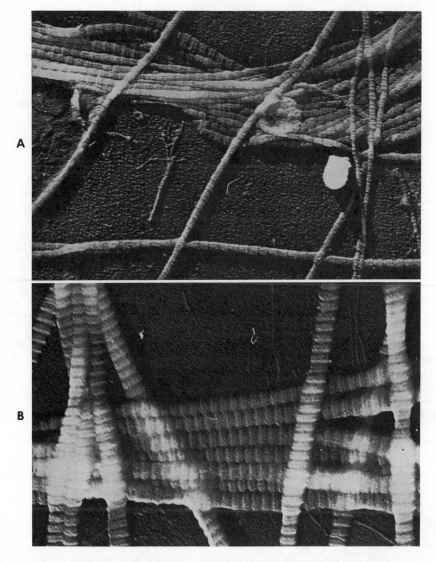

Fig. 3-5

Electron micrograph of connective tissue of skin. **A,** Reticular fibers (2 days). **B,** Collagenous fibers (90 days). Reticular fibers are smaller in diameter than collagenous fibers but apparently have the same periodicity. (×45,000.) (Courtesy Dr. Jerome Gross, Boston, Mass.)

of areolar tissue and usually the only kind to be found in the dense fibrillar tissues (Figs. 3-7 and 3-9).

The wandering cells, as we have said, belong to the phagocytic and blood-forming group. Several kinds may be distinguished. Clasmatocytes or histiocytes are smaller than fibroblasts and of less frequent occurrence. They have darker nuclei, and their cytoplasm is full of coarse granules and vacuoles that require special stains for adequate demonstration. The outline of the clasmatocyte is irregular. These cells are active in inflammatory conditions and are part of the reticuloendothelial system. They have also been called macrophages, pyrrole cells, and resting wandering cells.

Plasma cells are comparatively rare in most connective tissue (Fig. 3-1). They may be found in considerable numbers in the tunica propria of the digestive tract and in the loose connective tissue surrounding the secretive portions of the lactating mammary gland. They are smaller than

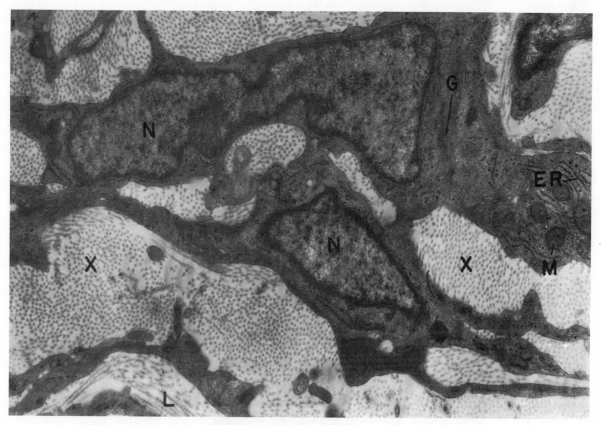

Fig. 3-6

Electron micrograph of collagenous connective tissue in mouse. (×27,000; reduced 2/3.) **ER,** Rough endoplasmic reticulum; **L,** longitudinal section of collagen fibrillae; **M,** mitochondria; **N,** nucleus of fibroblast; **G,** Golgi complex; **X,** cross section of collagen fibrillae. (Courtesy Dr. F. Gonzales, Chicago, Ill.)

clasmatocytes and differ from them and from fibroblasts in having a definitely rounded or oval shape without cytoplasmic processes. The cytoplasm is basic and nongranular. The nucleus is small and eccentrically placed. The chromatin of the nucleus is gathered in large granules along the nuclear membrane (so-called "cartwheel" nucleus).

Some connective tissue contains, also, cells that are full of large, deeply staining granules like those of basophilic and eosinophilic leukocytes. As the names indicate the granules have an affinity, in one case, for basic dyes such as azure and, in the other case, for acid stains like eosin. The basophilic cells of connective tissue are called mast cells. They are large, round cells with pale nuclei and abundant basophilic granules. They are said to be most numerous in the vicinity of blood vessels. The eosinophilic cells

found in connective tissue are thought by some authors to be leukocytes that have escaped from the blood vessels. Other workers regard tissue eosinophils and basophils as the same kind of cell in different stages of development. Both types require special stains for adequate demonstration, and neither is likely to be identified in a section of connective tissue stained with hematoxylin and eosin.

Blood cells. Fully formed leukocytes and other blood cells are often found in areolar tissue. These are corpuscles that have wandered into the tissue from blood and lymph vessels and do not, properly speaking, belong to it.

Adipose tissue

Adipose tissue is commonly included in the groups of connective and supporting tissues, although it differs from the other members of

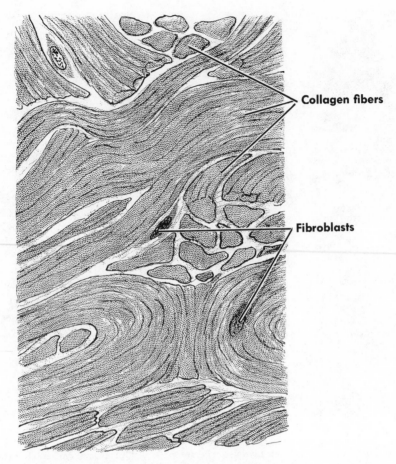

Collagen fibers

Fibroblasts

Fig. 3-7
Dense fibrous tissue, irregularly arranged, from section of scalp.

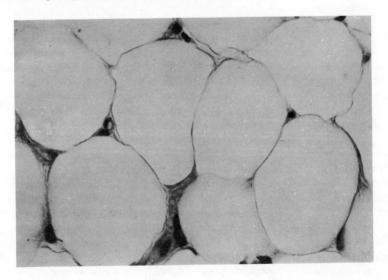

Fig. 3-8
Adipose tissue, showing fibroblast nuclei between fat cells. (Hematoxylin and eosin stain.)

32

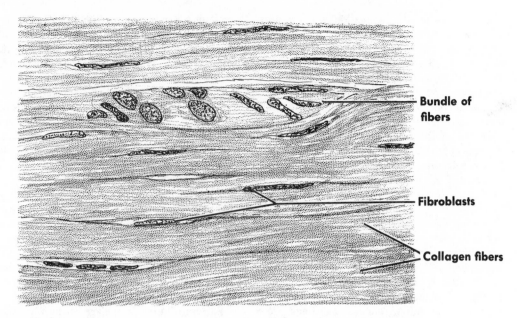

Fig. 3-9
Tendon cut longitudinally. A bundle of fibers appears in surface view with fibroblasts diagonally placed.

the group in several respects. The cells composing it do not form intercellular fibers or matrix but are specialized for the storing of fat. They thus form a reserve of foodstuffs as well as supporting pads of tissue. The cells are mesenchymal in origin, like those of connective tissue. They lose their protoplasmic processes early in the course of their transformation and become round, with abundant cytoplasm and central nuclei. The fat is deposited in the cytoplasm in minute droplets that gradually increase and unite in one large drop that pushes the nucleus to one side of the cell. As still more fat accumulates the nucleus becomes flattened, and the cytoplasm is reduced to a mere film enclosing the fat globule. In tissues that have been treated with ordinary fixatives followed by alcohol the fat is dissolved out, leaving the cytoplasm of the cells in the form of large irregular rings, each having a dark flat nucleus at one side. In preparations made with osmic acid the fat resists the action of the alcohol and appears as a deeply stained mass occupying the center of each cell. There is no intercellular substance elaborated by adipose tissue cells. They lie embedded in reticular or areolar tissue, the fibers among them being the product of reticular cells or fibroblasts. Adipose tissue is illustrated in Figs. 3-2 and 4-4.

Serous membranes

Serous membranes, the pleura, peritoneum, and pericardium, consist of a thin layer of loosely arranged connective tissues covered by a layer of relatively flat mesothelial cells. The membrane is made up of loosely arranged collagenous fibers, scattered elastic fibers, fibroblasts, macrophages, mast cells, adipose cells, and a varying number of other cells all suspended in a fluid, the serous exudate. The amount of fluid exudate and the variety and number of cells suspended in it increase greatly in adverse physiological or pathological conditions.

Reticuloendothelial system

The reticuloendothelial system, sometimes referred to as the system of macrophages, has as its most significant function the ingestion and removal of particulate matter. These cells are found in the loose connective tissue, in lymphatic and myeloid tissues, in the sinusoids of the liver, spleen, adrenal, and hypophysis, and also as "dust" cells in the lung and some perivascular cells.

The cells that occur in the sites mentioned here differ morphologically but react in a similar fashion when subjected to certain adverse conditions. When, for example, a weak solution of a dye such as trypan blue is injected into an animal, subsequent examination will show an appreciable accumulation of this dye in all the cells in the system to a degree not observed in any other cells. While this experimental confirmation shows the similarity in function of this group of cells, it has been shown that macrophages in specific tissues or organs phagocytize materials of a rather selective nature. The macrophages in the spleen and liver phagocytize degenerating red blood cells, retaining the iron for reutilization. In the lungs, dust and other particles of this nature are removed by the cells. Particulate matter of several kinds is removed by macrophages in the lymph nodes. The kinds of matter ingested by the macrophages may be relatively inert or noxious in character. Another function attributed to these cells is the production of antibodies. The function of macrophages is accordingly concerned with the defense mechanism of the body. The cells of this system arise from primitive reticular cells and from preexisting macrophages, lymphocytes, and monocytes.

SUPPORTING TISSUES
Cartilage

In the connective tissues just described the elements present are cells, fibers, and a fluid matrix, or ground substance. In the supporting tissues the fluid matrix is replaced by a solid substance that gives added firmness to the tissue. In cartilage this matrix is organic in nature and yields chondrin when boiled. It contains no mineral salts and lacks the hardness of bone, but it holds fibers and cells together in a solid plate of a definite shape. Cartilage forms the skeleton of the embryo and is exemplified in the adult by the tracheal rings. Through the matrix, fibers interlace much as they do in the fluid matrix of areolar tissue. The cells lie in minute spaces in the matrix, called the lacunae. These vary in shape, according to their position in the plate of cartilage. The cells, originally stellate like other mesenchyme cells, have lost their protoplasmic processes and have assumed the shape of the lacunae in which they lie. Unlike connective tissue, cartilage contains no blood vessels, so that nourishment must reach the cells by seepage through the matrix.

Cartilage develops from mesenchyme, as do the other tissues of this group. Mesenchyme cells first elaborate the fibers and later lay down the solid matrix upon them. Each cell forms a circumferential layer of matrix, thus enclosing itself in a lacuna. As growth and development proceed the amount of matrix between cells increases, pushing them farther apart, so that ultimately the condition is reached in which the cells lie in lacunae scattered through a relatively large amount of intercellular substance. For a time, at least, after the embryonic period, growth may be effected interstitially by the division of cartilage cells and the laying down of matrix around each daughter cell. Later, however, the increasing solidity of the matrix renders this type of growth more difficult, and increase in the size of the cartilage plate is brought about by the addition of new layers at the periphery by the cells of the perichondrium (appositional growth). In adult cartilage one may find two or four lacunae close together, separated by very thin walls of matrix. These and the lacunae that contain two cells indicate that interstitial growth is proceeding with difficulty.

Fibrocartilage. Cartilage occurs in three forms—fibrous, hyaline, and elastic—distinguished by the character of their fibers and the relative proportions of fibers and matrix. Of the three types, fibrocartilage most nearly resembles connective tissue (Fig. 3-10). In the intervertebral discs it blends on one side with connective tissue and on the other with hyaline cartilage, and as we shall see, it is intermediate between the two kinds of tissue, in qualities as well as in position. It consists of a network of coarse white fibers, which take the usual red color when stained with eosin. These fibers are embedded in a solid matrix that fills the interstices between them. The extent of the matrix varies somewhat in different specimens. In some cases it replaces the fluid matrix only partially and appears merely as fine purplish lines between the red fibers and as thin capsules surrounding the cells. In others its amount is greater, and it forms darker lines among the fibers and definite branching islands containing lacunae. In the former condition it is not easily distinguished from dense connective tissue; but one characteristic feature is always to be seen, namely, the round or oval lacunae that contain the cells. In connective tissue the cells are flattened by the pressure of the surrounding fibers; in cartilage they are protected by the capsules of matrix in which they lie.

Hyaline cartilage. The collagenous fibers of hyaline cartilage are not gathered in bundles but are dispersed throughout the tissue in a fine, close network, completely filled in by the

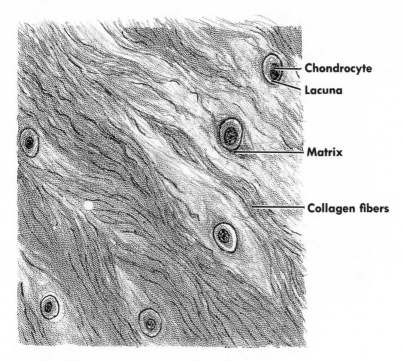

Fig. 3-10
Fibrocartilage.

substance of the matrix. The union is so close as to form a mass that, although pliable, is very firm. The fibers and matrix have, moreover, the same staining capacity and refractive index, so that in ordinary preparations they are not morphologically distinguishable. Hyaline cartilage is so called because the matrix appears clear ("glasslike"), and special techniques are required to demonstrate that the intercellular substance consists of fibers and matrix.

Hyaline cartilage occurs in the form of definite plates, in each of which the cells and matrix exhibit a definite plan of organization. If one studies a cartilage plate from the trachea, for instance, certain regions may be distinguished, and the plan will be found to be typical of all cartilage plates. At the periphery of the plate there is a fibrous layer, the perichondrium. This is, on the outside, similar to the surrounding areolar tissue with which it blends. It is well supplied with blood vessels. Toward the cartilage the perichondrium becomes more dense; that is, the fibers become heavier and more closely crowded, and the interfibrillar spaces containing the cells become smaller. The outer layer of the perichondrium is called the fibrous

layer, the inner the chondrogenetic layer. At the inner border of the chondrogenetic layer a condition is reached in which individual fibers are no longer distinguishable, their identity being obscured by the solid matrix in which they are embedded. Both fibers and matrix are pink in this region, in well-stained hematoxylin-eosin preparations. The cells are no longer free, as in the fluid matrix of the perichondrium, but are enclosed in spindle-shaped lacunae.

Toward the center of the plate, changes occur in cells and matrix. The ground substance (matrix), consisting chiefly of polysaccharide complexes, undergoes depolymerization. In this latter state it probably has an affinity for mineral salts. The color is pale except immediately around the lacunae, where it is often very dark. The shape of the lacunae also changes toward the middle of the plate, and they become round instead of flattened. Often they are found in pairs or groups of four, with the sides toward each other flattened. The cells occupying these central lacunae are spherical and in the living tissue fill the entire space. They are separated from the matrix by a fine capsule, which may rarely be distinguished. In fixed preparations

35

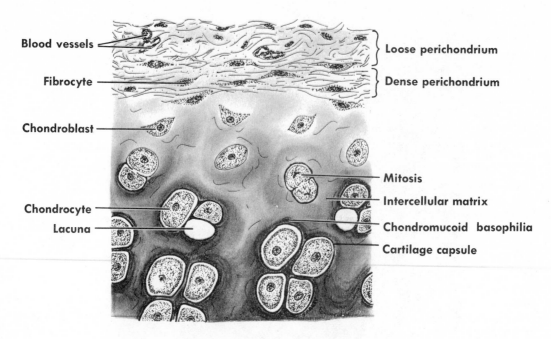

Fig. 3-11
Hyaline cartilage of trachea.

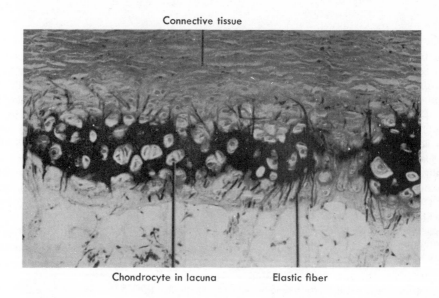

Fig. 3-12
Elastic cartilage. (Verhoeff's method; ×160.)

the cytoplasm is usually shrunken, and the only prominent feature is the nucleus. This is surrounded by an irregular cytoplasm. The shrinkage is due to the fact that fixatives penetrate slowly through the matrix and do not reach its center until after postmortem changes have taken place there and also to the fact that cartilage cells contain large amounts of glycogen and fat that are lost in processing. The appearance of hyaline cartilage in ordinary preparations is illustrated in Figs. 3-11 and 3-12.

Elastic cartilage. Elastic cartilage is like

hyaline in the arrangement of perichondrium, matrix, cells, and lacunae. The difference consists in the fact that elastic cartilage contains, in addition to the invisible collagenous fibers, a network of elastic fibers that may readily be demonstrated by the use of the appropriate stain. This type of cartilage occurs in the epiglottis and is present also in the external ear (Fig. 3-12).

Bone

The connective and supporting tissues hitherto described are found as components of various organs. Bone, on the other hand, forms a complete system of supporting structures, the skeleton. Like the other members of the group it consists of cells and intercellular substance. The latter is a solid matrix that, because of an extensive deposit of calcium carbonate, calcium phosphate, and other mineral salts, is not only solid but rigid. The matrix is laid down on a foundation of fibers that are, however, totally obscured by it. The proportion of organic matter is greatly reduced so that when it is destroyed by drying, the matrix appears little altered from the living condition. Sections of bone cannot be made in the ordinary way because of the hardness of the matrix. Two methods are used to prepare it for study; either it is softened by the use of acids, so that only its cells and collagenous groundwork remain, or pieces are dried and ground very thin.

Development of bone. The subject of the development and adult structure of bone is complicated by the presence of two types of ossification and two kinds of arrangement of the tissue in its fully formed state. It is advisable to consider the interrelations of these before describing any of them in detail. Differences in development arise from the fact that in the embryo some of the bones are laid down in undifferentiated mesenchyme, while in other parts of the body a temporary supporting system of cartilages precedes bone formation. The first type of ossification (intramembranous) is comparatively simple. In the second type (cartilage replacement) stages of cartilage erosion and of bone formation are intimately associated and form a more confusing picture. The essential process by which a bony matrix is formed is, however, the same in both cases. The difference between intramembranous and cartilage-replacement bone lies entirely in the tissue that precedes each in the place where it de-

Table 4. Development of bone

A. Formation of spicules of matrix
   1. Intramembranous
      Spicules laid down directly in mesenchyme
   2. Cartilage replacement
      Three steps:
      a. Bone formed around the outside of the cartilage (perichondrial)
      b. Erosion of the center of the cartilage
      c. Bone laid down on fragments of disintegrating cartilage (endochondrial)
B. Confluence of spicules to form spongy bone
C. Secondary erosion
D. Rebuilding
   1. In the form of new spongy bone
   2. In the form of compact bone

velops. The immediate result is also the same in both cases, namely, the formation of a mass of irregular trabeculae of bone, penetrated by blood vessels and connective tissue. Such bone is called spongy or cancellous bone.

In whatever manner it has been formed the newly developed spongy bone undergoes secondary changes. These consist of (1) erosion and (2) rebuilding. Differences in the manner and extent of rebuilding in different parts of the bone result in the development of two types of adult structure. In some regions the bone is eroded and rebuilt in its original form (spongy). In others rebuilding follows a new pattern and is more extensive, so that the tissue has the arrangement which is called compact bone. Compact and spongy bone are alike in their essential elements but differ in the arrangement and relative amounts of matrix, blood vessels, and marrow spaces.

In Table 4 the development of bone has been, for convenience, divided into four steps: spicule formation, confluence of spicules, erosion, and rebuilding. The division is arbitrary, and it should be remembered that different parts of the same bone may be in different stages of development at any one time, and the steps merge gradually into each other. Although all the processes involved are most active during fetal and early postnatal life, they continue slowly until old age is reached, and any one of them may be accelerated by metabolic or traumatic changes. In the following account of the development of bone we shall trace the histogenesis of intramem-

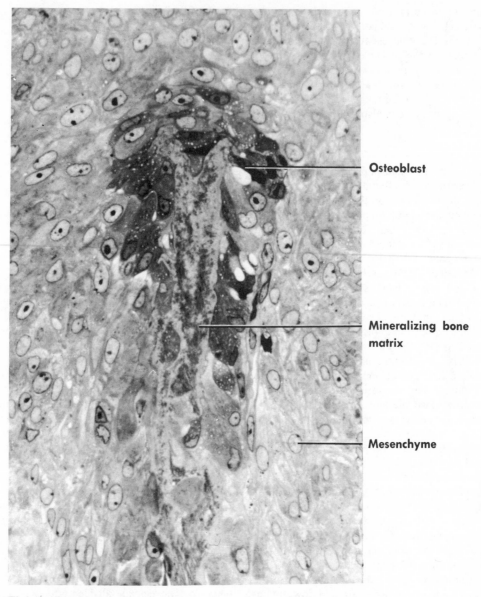

Fig. 3-13
Developing bone spicule. (×800.)

branous bone and cartilage-replacement bone, respectively, through the stages leading to the formation of adult bone.

Intramembranous bone. The regions in which formation of intramembranous bone occurs are determined by the proximity of the blood vessels. In an area where bone will develop, mesenchymal cells differentiate to form preosteoblasts. The cells are connected with one another by their processes and are

surrounded by delicate bundles of reticular fibers. The cells and fibers are loosely arranged in a semiviscid tissue fluid-ground substance (Fig. 3-13).

The initiation of bone formation consists of the production of an increased amount of ground substance between the cells, often trapping some cells within it. At the same time the cells increase in size and assume a polyhedral form, maintaining meanwhile the nu-

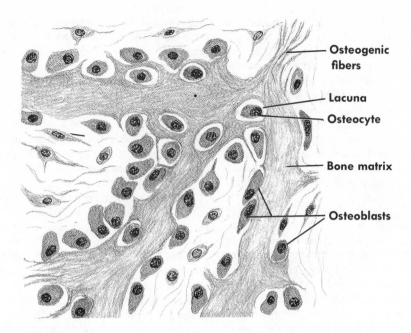

Fig. 3-14
Spicule of developing intramembranous bone from pig embryo, decalcified.

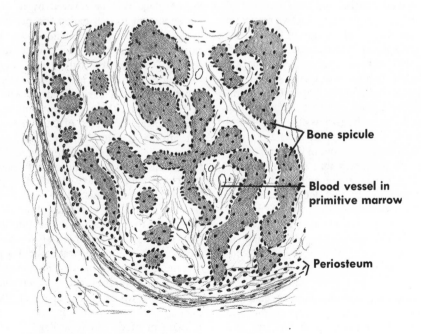

Fig. 3-15
Developing intramembranous bone of pig embryo under lower magnification than that shown in Fig. 3-14. Spicules are uniting to form spongy bone.

merous processes by which they are connected with adjacent cells. At this stage they are known as *osteoblasts,* and the bone in the nonmineralized state is referred to as *osteoid.* When certain conditions are attained in the elaboration of this complex of cells and matrix, the tissue undergoes mineralization of the matrix as crystalline hydroxyapatite. In addition, bone may contain other cations such as sodium, magnesium, carbonate, and citrate. The mineral or inorganic part of a bone may vary from 35% dry weight in young bones to 65% in adult bones.

The organic or interstitial component of bone contains numerous reticular fibers that are surrounded by an amorphous ground substance. In the embryonic state this substance contains mucoproteins and sulfated polysaccharides.

As development proceeds, new osteoblasts develop from the surrounding mesenchyme and lay down additional matrix on the peripheral side of the original layer of cells, thus enclosing them completely. An osteoblast, after it is surrounded by bone matrix, ceases to be active in the formation of new bones but remains in the tissue as a bone cell. The spicule thus formed contains all the essential elements of bone: fibers, a calcified matrix, and cells situated in lacunae. It differs from cartilage in two respects: first, in the chemical composition of the matrix; second, in the shape of the lacunae. In cartilage these are round or oval and entirely separate from each other. In bone each lacuna has a number of fine canals radiating from it and communicating with the canals of other lacunae. The shapes of the cells in the two tissues correspond to their lacunae. In cartilage the cells are round or oval without processes, but in bone the osteocytes have fine processes that extend into the canaliculi. The latter cannot be traced for any great distance in the ordinary decalcified section of developing bone, but their points of departure from the lacuna give the latter a somewhat jagged outline. The spicule itself is irregular in shape and is surrounded by a more or less complete layer of osteoblasts (Fig. 3-14).

As each spicule grows by the addition of new layers, or lamellae, of bone substance, it encroaches on the surrounding mesenchyme, and soon adjacent spicules come in contact and fuse with each other (Fig. 3-15). Thus, by union of originally separate masses a latticework of bony trabeculae is formed. It is characterized by the irregular shape and arrangement of its parts and of the enclosed spaces. The latter contain mesenchymal tissue that develops into bone marrow and is richly supplied with blood vessels (Fig. 3-15).

Cartilage-replacement bone. Bone in the condition just described (spongy bone) is ready for the processes of erosion and rebuilding, which may transform a part of it into compact bone. Before discussing these changes, however, we must consider the way in which spongy bone develops in situations where cartilage precedes it as a temporary supporting structure. In the long bones of the embryo a sort of model of the skeleton is laid down in cartilage. This must be replaced by bone in a gradual manner that will not leave the part unsupported at any time.

The first sign of the replacement of a cartilage by bone is the development of a cylinder of bone around its outside. This is the so-called perichondrial bone, laid down in a collarlike band about the middle of the cartilage, the ends of which are left free for growth (Fig. 3-23). In longitudinal sections of a developing bone of this type the perichondrial bone appears as a fairly dense strip of bone on each side of the cartilage. As soon as the perichondrial bone is well established, changes occur in the part of the cartilage that is covered by it. A mass of mesenchymal tissue, called the periosteal bud, invades the cartilage, breaking down the matrix as it grows. The periosteal bud contains blood vessels, osteoblasts, osteoclasts, and blood-forming elements. By its action on the cartilage matrix it forms a cavity in the central portion of the model, which is the primitive marrow cavity. Jagged spicules of cartilage matrix are left projecting into the cavity, and it is along these that the osteoblasts line up and begin the formation of bone that, because it lies within the outlines of the cartilage model, is called endochondrial bone (Figs. 3-16 and 3-17). The essential process of endochrondrial bone formation is like that occurring in membranous bone. Fibers are formed and matrix is deposited upon them, giving rise to separate spicules that later become confluent, resulting in a mass of bony trabeculae. The difference between the spicules of the two kinds of bone is that in endochondrial ossification each spicule is laid down around a fragment of calcified cartilage matrix, which may be seen at its center for some time after bone formation has begun, while in membranous bone spicules no such substrate is present.

While the processes just described are taking

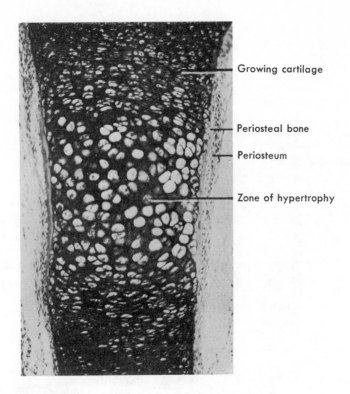

Growing cartilage

Periosteal bone

Periosteum

Zone of hypertrophy

Fig. 3-16
Central part of shaft of developing long bone.

place at the middle of the cartilage, the ends of the mass are growing rapidly, keeping pace with the growth of the embryo. If one examines a section of a cartilage that is being replaced by bone, he will see zones that represent different stages of development. At each distal end the cartilage is normal (hyaline). Toward the center, near the beginning of the region surrounded by perichondrial bone, is a zone of rapid growth, which is adding to the length of the model. This zone is characterized by the arrangement of the lacunae in rows lying in the long axis of the model. The lacunae in each row are flattened and separated from each other by thin plates of matrix, while the matrix between adjacent rows forms solid columns or bands. Still further toward the center, the lacunae are enlarged, and at the border of the marrow cavity they are confluent, and the matrix is reduced to jagged trabeculae. This is the place at which the erosive action of the invading marrow cells is apparent. The cartilage cells are said by some to be destroyed along with the matrix; other workers claim that they are transformed into osteoblasts.

Calcium salts are laid down in the remains of the cartilage matrix, in this part of the model, with the result that it stains more deeply with hematoxylin than does the normal matrix in other parts of the section. It is upon the bits of calcified cartilage, as we have already said, that the bone is laid down. In properly stained sections one may see spicules of dark purple cartilage matrix, coated with one or more layers of red bone, surrounded by osteoblasts.

The foregoing paragraphs describe the formation of the shaft, or diaphysis, of a long bone, in which there is at first one center of ossification. Later, however, new and independent centers develop in the ends of the cartilage model. These new centers, the epiphyses, spread radially. The growth zone of the cartilage, on which the increase in length of the bone as a whole depends, thus comes to lie between two centers of ossification that encroach on it from opposite directions (Fig. 3-19). The growth zone persists, however, during the early years of life, and so long as it remains the stature of the individual increases. Ultimately, at about the

41

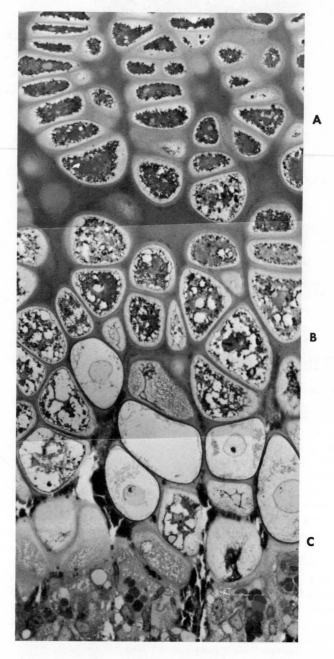

Fig. 3-17

Longitudinal section of epiphyseal portion of femur of 4-day-old rat. **A,** Zone of cartilage growth. **B,** Zone of cartilage hypertrophy. **C,** Invasion of marrow elements in areas of cartilage erosion.

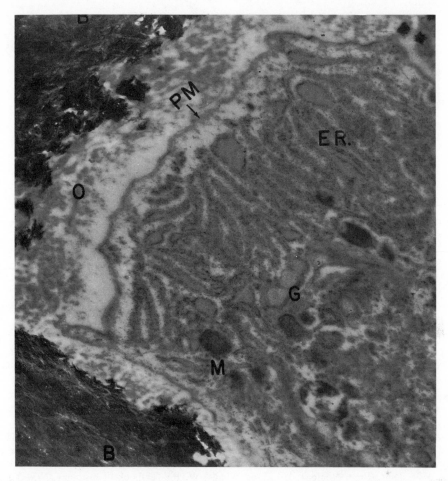

Fig. 3-18
Electron micrograph of osteoblast in rat. **B,** Bone; **ER,** endoplasmic reticulum; **G,** Golgi complex; **M,** mitochondria; **O,** osteoid; **PM,** plasma membrane. (×30,000.) (Courtesy Dr. F. Gonzales, Chicago, Ill.)

twentieth year of life, ossification outruns cartilage growth, and the epiphyses and diaphysis unite. After this has occurred growth of bone ceases, except for additions in thickness that may be made by osteoblasts in the surrounding tissue, or periosteum. The importance of this layer, as well as its structure, will be discussed in connection with the histology of adult bone.

The process of secondary erosion of bone actually begins soon after the first layer of spongy bone has been laid down and continues actively as long as the bones are growing. It starts at the point where bone formation began, namely, at the borders of the original marrow cavity. Thus, as ossification of the diaphysis of a long bone moves toward the ends of the carti-

lage model, it is followed by a secondary breaking down and resorption of part of the newly formed tissue. The result is an enlargement of the marrow cavity, which prevents the bone from becoming too heavy and solid.

The mechanism of erosion is carried out by osteoclasts. These are large cells in which the cytoplasm stains deeply, and in each of the cells there are several nuclei. The osteoclasts lie along the margin of the bone matrix, sometimes in definite spaces (Howship's lacunae) that they seem to have hollowed out.

Erosion of bone is not confined to the central portion of the bones, where, as we have said, its effect is a progressive enlargement of the marrow cavity. It occurs throughout the

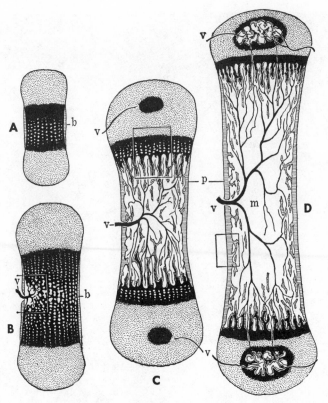

Fig. 3-19

Diagrams of ossification of long bone. **A,** Early cartilaginous stage. **B,** Stage of eruption of periosteal bone collar by osteogenic bud of vessels. **C,** Older stage with primary marrow cavity and early centers of calcification in epiphyseal cartilages. **D,** Condition shortly after birth with epiphyseal centers of ossification. Calcified cartilage in all diagrams is black; **b,** periosteal bone collar; **m,** marrow cavity; **p,** periosteal bone; **V,** blood vessels entering centers of ossification. (From Nonidez, J. F., and Windle, W. F.: Textbook of histology, New York, 1953, McGraw-Hill Book Co.)

mass of all bony tissue, but in all places except the marrow cavities it is followed by rebuilding. In the ends of the long bones and in the central portions of the flat bones the rebuilding keeps pace with erosion and follows the pattern of the original formation of the tissue, resulting in a renewal of spongy bone. In the peripheral parts of all bones, however, rebuilding is more rapid than erosion, and a compact layer of bone is established. This tissue is more regular in its arrangement than spongy bone. Its development may be described as follows: The marrow spaces, containing reticular tissue and blood-forming cells, are penetrated throughout by a rich vascular network. The vessels at the periphery of the bone follow a more or less regular pathway parallel to the surface. In long bones they run mainly in the long axis of the bone. In

places where compact bone is to be formed, erosion follows a definite plan, rounding out the marrow spaces so that they form cylindrical cavities around the blood vessels. After the marrow spaces have been thus reshaped they are lined by successive concentric layers of new bone. The process continues until the space is almost filled with lamellae of matrix and persists only as a central canal containing blood vessels and nerves. Such a grouping of layers of bone, with its central canal, is called a haversian system.

The remodelling of bone does not end when the primary haversian systems are laid down but continues into adult life. The primary systems are partially destroyed to make room for new ones in response to changes in mechanical requirements. The final result is a mass of bone

44

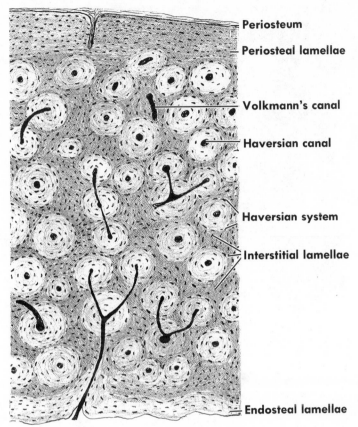

Periosteum

Periosteal lamellae

Volkmann's canal

Haversian canal

Haversian system

Interstitial lamellae

Endosteal lamellae

Fig. 3-20
Ground section of human compact bone, showing general plan of architecture.

composed of secondary and tertiary haversian systems embedded in the remains of earlier systems. The lamellae that form the background for the haversian systems, holding them together in a solid mass, are called interstitial lamellae. The surface of the bone is formed by circumferential lamellae that have been laid down by the osteoblasts of the periosteal tissue. This region contains no haversian systems, and the only blood vessels in it are those passing through to the marrow cavity. Endosteal lamellae of the same character line the shaft where it borders the marrow cavity (Fig. 3-20).

Adult bone. Since the development of bone has been so fully discussed, little remains to be said about its adult structure. Gross examination of a bone that has been sawed in two will show that it is composed of both spongy and compact tissue. In the long bones the spongy arrangement is confined to the epiphyses, and there is a cen-

tral marrow cavity entirely devoid of bone matrix. In flat bones the spongy tissue forms trabeculae crossing from one side to the other, so that there is no large marrow cavity but a number of small irregular marrow spaces. Either form of bone has an outer layer or cortex of compact tissue that is, in turn, covered by a tough fibrous coating called the periosteum.

Microscopically, sections of decalcified spongy bone present a picture much like that of developing intramembranous bone except for the greater extent of the trabeculae. Osteoblasts and osteoclasts are less common but may be found in portions of the tissue that are undergoing changes in arrangement. The matrix stains red with eosin and is lamellated; the cells are dark in color and disposed, one in each lucuna, between adjacent lamellae. With special techniques one may demonstrate the canaliculi and the fibers on which the matrix was deposited,

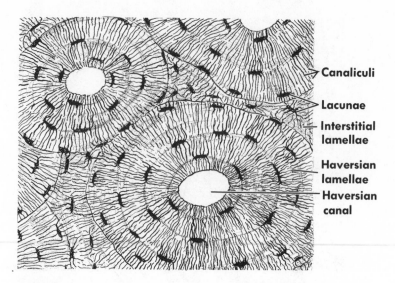

Fig. 3-21
Ground section of human compact bone, higher magnification than
that shown in Fig. 3-20.

Canaliculi

Lacunae

Interstitial
lamellae

Haversian
lamellae

Haversian
canal

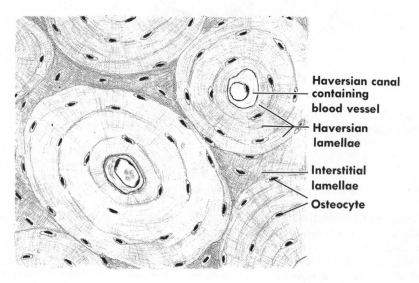

Fig. 3-22
Human compact bone decalcified, showing organic constituents.

Haversian canal
containing
blood vessel

Haversian
lamellae

Interstitial
lamellae

Osteocyte

but these are not ordinarily visible in hematoxylin-eosin preparations.

Ground sections of bone do not show the
cellular elements of the tissue, since these are
destroyed in the making of the preparation.
Such sections are useful in studying the architecture of compact bone. In transverse ground
sections the following features are to be noted
(Figs. 3-20 and 3-21): The haversian canals

appear as empty circular spaces, each of which
is surrounded by six to fifteen concentric lamellae of matrix. The lacunae and the canaliculi
radiating from them are readily visible. Between
haversian systems is the packing of interstitial
lamellae, and a piece taken from the periphery
of the bone will contain periosteal lamellae.
Canals running diagonally or at right angles to
those of the haversian systems are the canals of

Volkmann. They provide for transverse connections and anastomosis between the blood vessels and are distinguished from haversian canals because of their direction through the tissue and because they are not surrounded by concentric lamellae. The vascular pattern of bone is best seen in longitudinal ground sections, in which, however, the concentric arrangement of lamellae is not to be observed. The appearance of decalcified bone is shown in Fig. 3-22.

It will be seen from the description of bone that, despite its physical rigidity, it is a tissue that retains considerable ability to respond to environmental changes. The most obvious of these are traumatic changes such as fractures, which are repaired by the osteoblasts in the periosteum and at the border of the marrow cavity. Some disturbances of the ductless glands provide a stimulus to the osteoblasts of the periosteum that results in the laying down of additional cortical layers of bone (acromegaly). Also the skeleton serves as a storehouse for calcium, and the rates of erosion and rebuilding respond to variations of the mineral metabolism of the body. It is essential to life that a certain amount of calcium be present in the body fluids. When this amount is not supplied by the diet, it may be withdrawn from the bones, or conversely, excess calcium may be stored in them.

The skeletal system is under the influence of several hormones. One of these, the parathyroid, is responsible for the maintenance of normal levels of calcium in the blood. The activity of the parathyroids appears to depend upon calcium levels in the circulation. When blood calcium is low, secretion of the gland is stimulated. In hyperparathyroidism, bone is resorbed to an unusual degree and is replaced by fibrous tissue; this condition is known as *osteitis fibrosa,* or von Recklinghausen's disease. *Calcitonin* is a hormone that is derived from the thyroid gland. It has an action antagonistic to that of the parathyroid hormone in that it lowers blood calcium and inhibits bone resorption. In addition to the two hormones mentioned it has been shown that the growth hormone elaborated by the hypophysis is necessary for normal bone growth and that the gonadal hormones play a role in the rate of skeletal maturation.

It is obvious that normal bone growth and maturation are dependent on several nutritional factors. This is especially true of the adequate supply and availability of minerals such as calcium and phosphorus, which are the main inorganic components of bone. It has been shown that a dietary insufficiency of either calcium or phosphorus leads to a rarefaction and brittleness of bones. In situations where dietary calcium and phosphorus are adequate but vitamin D is deficient, interference with mineral absorption occurs and mineralization of the growing epiphysis is inhibited, giving rise to a condition known as *rickets.* When subjected to stress, bones in this state become deformed.

Adult rickets *(osteomalacia)* is a condition in which bone exhibits considerable amounts of osteoid tissue. The situation is caused by a long-term deficiency of dietary minerals and vitamin D. Deficiency in vitamin A results in an inhibition of the rate of growth of the skeleton by interfering with the ratio of osteoblasts and osteoclasts responsible for growth and resorption respectively. Retardation of growth and of healing of fractures is correlated with a deficiency of vitamin C resulting from insufficient production of the elements needed to form the bone matrix.

Periosteum. The periosteum is a connective tissue layer covering the bone except at the articular surfaces. It is divisible into two layers. The outer of these is a network of densely packed collagenous fibers with blood vessels. The inner layer provides the penetration fibers (of Sharpey), which are inserted into the bone and attach the periosteum to it. In the inner layer of the periosteum one may also find fine elastic fibers loosely arranged (Fig. 3-23). Osteoblasts occur here also whenever appositional growth of the bone is taking place. The endosteum is a thin layer of connective tissue lining the marrow cavity and the smaller cavities within the bone.

In addition to the more obvious function that the periosteum performs, such as anchorage for tendons and ligaments, it is also concerned with repair and regeneration of bone. While this is a somewhat disputed function, there seems to be little doubt that the osteogenic tissue which initiates bone repair is actually the inner component of the periosteum. The outer fibrous part of the periosteum is also important in bone repair inasmuch as it acts as a limiting membrane that restricts the extent to which new bone formation occurs.

Blood supply and nerves. The blood supply of bone comes by two routes. Near the middle of the shaft there is a medullary, or nutrient,

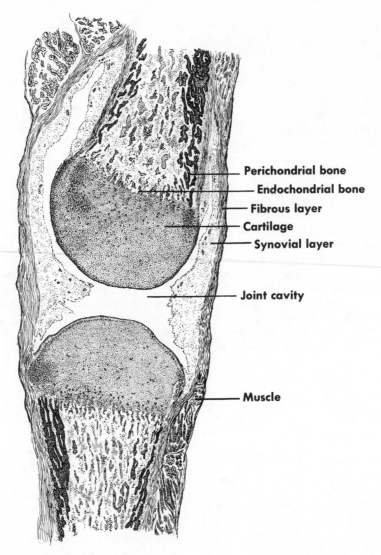

Perichondrial bone
Endochondrial bone
Fibrous layer
Cartilage
Synovial layer

Joint cavity

Muscle

Fig. 3-23
Joint from finger of newborn infant. The process of cartilage replacement is still going on, and one may distinguish between endochondrial and perichondrial bone.

canal that pierces the bone and leads to the marrow cavity. The nutrient artery passes through this canal, giving off branches to the haversian canals on the way. In the marrow cavity it divides into an ascending and a descending branch, both of which supply the marrow.

The other source of blood for the bone tissue is by way of the numerous arteries of the periosteum. These enter the substance of the bone through Volkmann's canals, which, in turn, lead to haversian canals.

Veins leave the bone through the nutrient

canal, and it is here also that the medullated and nonmedullated nerves enter. The latter accompany the blood vessels into the haversian canals.

Marrow. Although marrow is not, actually, a part of bone as a tissue, it is included in sections of decalcified bone and should be mentioned here. It is of two kinds, named red and yellow marrow, respectively, according to their color in the fresh state. Both kinds have a framework of reticular tissue. Red marrow is the chief site of the formation of certain types of blood cells, including the red corpuscles and contains

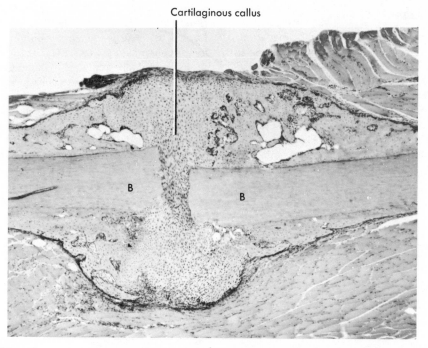

Cartilaginous callus

Fig. 3-24

Partial repair of bone fracture (rabbit rib). The space between the fractured ends of the bone, **B**, is filled in with fibrous tissue. On the periphery a cartilaginous callus, later replaced by bone, has developed. (× 40.)

a great number of blood vessels. The details of its structure will be considered in a later chapter. In yellow marrow the blood-forming elements have been replaced by adipose tissue, and the amount of reticular tissue is reduced. Red marrow is present in the cavities of all bones during fetal life and early childhood. It is gradually replaced by yellow marrow and is found in the adult only in the epiphyses of long bones and in the ribs, vertebrae, cranial bones, and sternum.

Joints. The bones are joined together to form the skeleton by a series of articulations, the structure of each varying with the degree of movability of the joint. Those articulations that are nearly or quite immovable are called synarthroses. In the skull, for instance, the bones are held together by ligaments composed of short fibers, of which some are elastic and others are continuations of the fibers of Sharpey. The vertebrae are less closely joined, allowing a limited amount of movement, and the spaces between them are occupied by intervertebral discs of fibrocartilage.

The movable joints, or diarthroses, are characterized by a space between the bones, which is the articular cleft. Each bone bordering on this space has at its end a cap of articular cartilage, which is the remainder of the embryonic cartilage model of the bone. This cartilage is of the hyaline type but has no perichondrial fibrous layer (Fig. 3-23).

The capsule that encloses the articular cartilages and the space between them is two layered. The outer part is the stratum fibrosum, composed of dense fibrous tissue, continuous with the outer layer of the periosteum of the bones. The stratum fibrosum is blended with the tendons and ligaments of the muscles attached at this point. The inner, or synovial, layer is of looser and more vascular connective tissue. In places where it borders on the articular cavity it is lined with the so-called mesenchymal epithelium. This consists of fibers and fibroblasts arranged around the border of the cavity and is not a free epithelium. The synovial layer sometimes forms projections into the joint cavity that may contain fibrocartilage.

BONE REPAIR

After bone fracture the following events occur in connection with the repair of the injured bone. First, there is a hemorrhage caused by the rupture of blood vessels, which is soon followed by the formation of a clot. Subsequently, fibroblasts and capillaries migrate into the area formed by the clot, which results in the formation of granulation tissue. The granulation tissue then becomes infiltrated with dense fibrous tissue, giving rise to a fibrous union *(procallus)*. The fibrous tissue soon is transformed to cartilage, which constitutes a temporary union or *callus* (Fig. 3-24). The cartilaginous callus is gradually replaced by bone because of the potential activity of the cells in the periosteum. Finally, excess bone present in the callus is partially or completely resorbed. The repair of bone as described here is dependent on an adequate blood supply, on the activity of the bone-forming cells in the periosteum, and also on adequate vitamin and mineral supplies.

4

MUSCLE

The fibers of muscle differ from those of connective tissue in structure and in function. In the connective tissues the fibers are intercellular and noncontractile and serve the purpose of binding or padding; in muscular tissue the cells are called fibers, and the property of contractility is highly developed. The function of muscle is to move parts of the body by its contraction. Only a small amount of intercellular substance is present in muscle, except as it is intermingled with connective tissue cells and fibers.

The morphological characteristics common to all types of muscle are as follows: The cells are elongated with well-defined nuclei. The cytoplasm (sarcoplasm) stains red with eosin and contains fibrils (myofibrils) that run parallel to the long axis of the cell. The fibers (cells) are surrounded by a limiting membrane, the sarcolemma. Three types of muscle are morphologically distinguishable: smooth muscle, skeletal muscle, and cardiac muscle. Of these the first and last are under the control of the autonomic nervous system and are called involuntary muscle. Skeletal muscle is innervated directly by the central nervous system and can, for the most part, be controlled by impulses from the higher centers of the brain. It is accordingly called voluntary muscle.

SMOOTH MUSCLE

Smooth muscle is derived from mesenchyme, the cells of which are not, originally, different in their appearance from those that give rise to the connective and supporting tissues. The muscle-forming cell, however, soon assumes a peculiar shape. It elongates into a spindle, elaborating at the same time a small amount of intercellular substance. At an early stage in the development of the connective tissue cell, fibers are visible along its border, to which the name *fibroglia* is given. In a similar way the developing smooth muscle cell is seen to have fibers along its border, here called myoglia. But whereas the border fibrils in connective tissue soon become separate from the cells, increasing to form the most conspicuous part of the tissue, those of smooth muscle remain in contact with the cell. They are said to persist throughout the life of the cell, connecting one fiber with another, although it is not certain that this is so. As the cells increase in size and become closely applied to each other, intercellular fibers become very difficult to demonstrate and will not be seen in ordinary slides.

Smooth muscle cells vary in length from 0.02 to 0.5 mm. and have a diameter at their thickest portion of about 4 to 7μ. (The average diameter of a red blood cell is 7μ.) From the middle they diminish gradually to a fine, rounded point at each end. The cells may best be seen in preparations made by shaking a bit of muscle in a weak acid solution. This dissolves the intercellular substance and makes it possible to study the forms of the isolated fiber. The myofibrils in the cells of smooth muscle are fine and not easily seen. The nucleus of the cell is elongated and centrally located at the thickest portion of the spindle. It lies in a small area of granular cytoplasm, and the myofibrils diverge to pass around this area. The sarcolemma is very fine. Branching fibers are very rare; they have been found in a few parts of the body but are to be regarded as exceptional.

Many of the features just described are imperceptible in longitudinal sections of smooth muscle (Fig. 4-1). The fibers normally occur in sheets, closely packed together, and it is seldom that an entire cell can be seen. In thick sections it is often difficult to make out the boundaries of adjacent fibers, since several of them are included, overlapping, in the depth of a section. One may see only the long nuclei and the cytoplasm faintly marked by the myofibrils. Longitudinal sections are best studied at the edge of a band or sheet, where the muscle shades off into the surrounding connective tissue and individual cells may be distinguished.

In transverse section the smooth muscle cells appear as discs of cytoplasm having various diameters. The largest of the discs are cut through the middle of the fibers and include the nucleus of the cell. The smaller sections pass through the ends of the fibers and therefore have no nuclei in them. The characteristics peculiar to smooth muscle in cross section are the small size and round shape of the individual fiber, the homogeneous appearance of the cytoplasm, and the central location of the nuclei in the cells (Fig. 4-1).

Smooth muscle occurs in bands or sheets surrounding glandular organs and forming a part of the wall of tubular organs. Such sheets are not surrounded by definite coverings but mingle with the areolar or reticular tissue around them. Isolated fibers of smooth muscle may also be found in the tunica propria of the digestive tract.

The smooth muscle fiber (Fig. 4-2) is enveloped by a plasma membrane studded with vesicles believed to be concerned with pinocytotic activity. External to the membrane is a homogeneous coat or layer similar to the basal lamina commonly observed in epithelial cells. External to the basal lamina, scattered reticular fibers occur. In certain regions of the cell surface, specializations occur that suggest by their appearance and relation to adjacent cells that they may be specialized desmosomes.

The myofilaments are delicate structures usually oriented in the direction of the long axis of the cell. Mitochondria occur in the region of the nuclear poles, beneath the cell membrane, and also between the myofibrils. The endoplasmic reticulum and the Golgi apparatus, also located at the nuclear poles, are poorly developed.

SKELETAL MUSCLE

Skeletal muscle, or striated voluntary muscle, presents a different appearance from smooth muscle. It develops from solid masses of mesoderm cells known as myoblasts. Some authors contend that striated fibers develop by an elon-

gation of the myoblast, which undergoes rapid mitotic nuclear division and in turn results in an elongated multinucleated cell. Other authors state that the elongated muscle cell or fiber is the result of the fusion of the growing myoblasts, giving rise to a syncytial arrangement. Another view is that both of these methods of development occur. The striated muscle fiber is longer and thicker than the smooth muscle fiber, maintains a uniform diameter throughout its length, and ends bluntly. Early in development the nuclei migrate from the center to the periphery of the cell, where they are to be found in adult muscle of this type.

The sarcolemma, which is barely perceptible in smooth muscle, can be observed with the light microscope. It is now apparent from electron microscope studies that the film investing the muscle fiber and visible with the optical microscope is not a single structure but consists internally of the plasmalemma of the muscle fiber and a coating of mucopolysaccharide and delicate reticular fibers. Sarcolemma is currently considered the plasmalemma of the muscle fiber.

The most striking morphological characteristic of striated muscle, to which it owes its name, is the transverse marking of the myofibrils (Figs. 4-3 and 4-4). These fibrils are thicker than those of smooth muscle and may be observed with the optical microscope. Each myofibril is composed of a succession of bands of different and alternating refractive indices. One set of these, the A band, appears dark and is doubly refractile or anisotropic. The alternating light, or I, band is isotropic. When the fibers are viewed with polarized light, the A bands appear light and the I bands appear dark. In specially stained preparations a dark transverse line bisecting the I band has been observed and is known as the Z line. The sarcomere, which is considered as the structural unit that is referable to the contractile cycle of muscle, is defined as the segment between the two successive Z lines. Accordingly, it includes one A band and part of the two bands adjacent to the A band.

At the electron microscope level the bands can be observed more clearly than at the optical levels (Fig. 4-5). The I band, as previously noted, is bisected by the dark Z band. Between the Z band and each margin of the I band a less distinct line occurs, marking the limits of the N band. The A band is bisected by a dark M

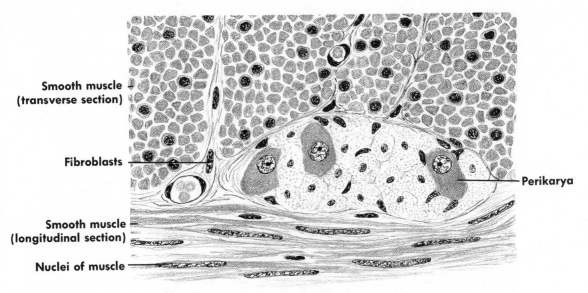

Fig. 4-1

Smooth muscle, from wall of intestine of monkey, showing longitudinal and transverse sections of fibers. Compare nuclei of muscle cells with those of fibroblasts, of connective tissue among muscle fibers. Note also perikarya, fibers, and supporting cells of Auerbach's nerve plexus.

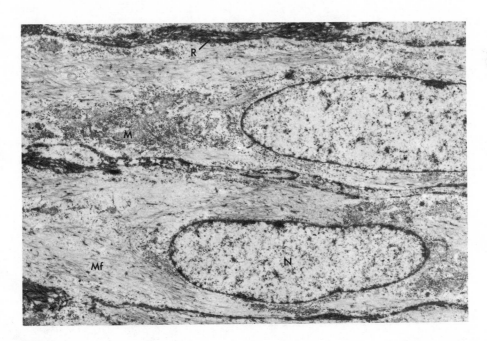

Fig. 4-2

Electron micrograph of parts of two smooth muscle cells from small intestine of mouse. **M,** Mitochondrion; **Mf,** myofibrillae; **N,** nucleus; **R,** reticular fibers. (×6,500.)

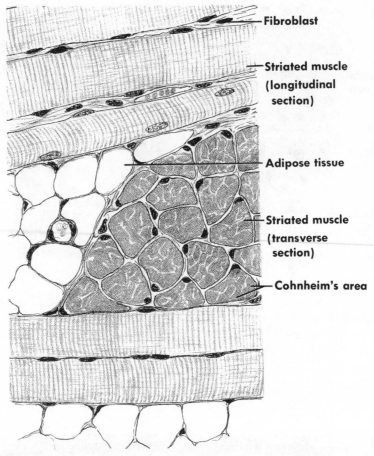

Fibroblast

Striated muscle (longitudinal section)

Adipose tissue

Striated muscle (transverse section)

Cohnheim's area

Fig. 4-3
Striated muscle from tongue of dog.

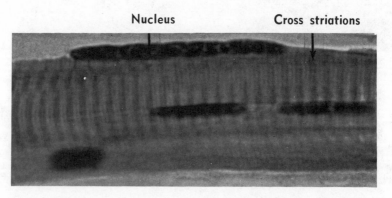

Nucleus   **Cross striations**

Fig. 4-4
Longitudinal section of human striated muscle. (×2,000.) (From Bevelander, G.: Essentials of histology, ed. 6, St. Louis, 1970, The C. V. Mosby Co.)

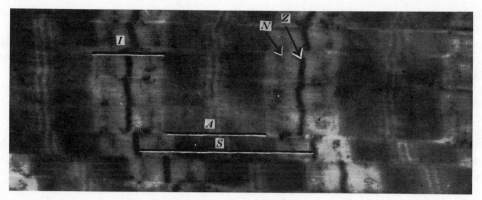

Fig. 4-5
Electron micrograph of striated muscle. (×45,000.) Longitudinal section of rest length of rabbit psoas. **I,** I band; **A,** A band; **N** and **Z,** discs, respectively; **S,** sarcomere. Note that myofibrils are further divided into myofilaments. (Courtesy Dr. D. Spiro, New York, N. Y.)

band. On both sides of the M band is a somewhat lighter and broader area marking the H band.

The myofibrils, the smallest contractile elements visible with the light microscope, are shown by the electron microscope to be divided into smaller units, the *myofilaments.* These are of two kinds and differ in their size and chemical compositions. The thicker filaments, containing *myosin,* are approximately 100 Å in diameter and 1.5μ long. These filaments are the chief constituent of the A band. The thinner filaments contain *actin,* measure 50 Å in diameter, extend approximately 1μ in either direction from the Z line, give rise to the I band, and continue for some distance into the A band. The length of the actin filaments observed in the A band is dependent upon the degree of contraction exhibited by the fiber. The arrangement and variation in the size of the filaments are responsible for the banding appearance observed in these structures. The I band contains thin filaments and appears light.

The central region of the A band contains only thick fibrils and is somewhat darker in appearance than is the I band. The portions of the A band adjacent to the I band contain both thick and thin fibers, which are densely packed and appear more dense or darker than other parts of the fibril.

With the electron microscope one may observe that the sarcoplasm or cytoplasm fills the spaces between the myofibrils and is most abundant in the region of the nucleus. Located within the sarcoplasm are mitochondria, which are large, abundant, and most numerous at the poles of the nucleus. They also occur between the myofibrils, where they are usually arranged with their long axis parallel to the long axis of the myofibrils. In addition, a small Golgi network is located at the pole of the nucleus, and lipid droplets and particles of glycogen are between the myofibrils.

The sarcoplasmic reticulum, which corresponds to the endoplasmic reticulum of other cells, is visible only with the electron microscope. It is a continuous system of fine, membrane-bound, interconnecting tubules forming a meshwork around each myofibril. The system exhibits a constantly repeating pattern. It is longitudinally arranged in reference to the A and I bands and exhibits three transversely arranged channels located near the A-I junction in mammalian muscle. This complex is known as a *triad.* The triad is believed to facilitate the transmission of excitatory impulses to the muscle fibers.

The appearance of ordinary sections of skeletal muscle is as follows: In longitudinal section the myofibrils are marked by alternating light and dark transverse bands. There are many nuclei in one fiber, lying at its periphery immediately beneath the sarcolemma. Occasionally, one sees a nucleus that seems to be in the center of a fiber. Careful focusing of the microscope will show, however, that in such a case one is looking down on the surface of a tangential section and that the nucleus is on the outside of the cell (Figs. 4-3 and 4-4). In transverse sections it is apparent that the fibers are larger than those of smooth muscle, having diameters that range from 17 to 87μ. Their shape is round or polygonal, and the peripheral position of the nucleus is noticeable. It is also possible to see the cut ends of the sarcostyles, which give the cytoplasm a finely stippled appearance. In transverse section one may see that the myofibrils are gathered in groups instead of being evenly distributed throughout the cytoplasm. Some writers use the term *sarcostyle* to describe such a group of myofibrils, but the name is usually applied to the myofibril itself. Large fibrils are sometimes called a muscle column of Kölliker. In a cross section of a muscle fiber one may sometimes see such a group of fibrils separated from adjacent groups by clear sarcoplasm. Such cross sections of muscle columns are called Cohnheim's areas.

Skeletal muscle, as the name implies, is attached to the bones, the attachment being made through the tendons. At the point where the muscle joins the tendon the nuclei are especially numerous, indicating that this is the region of the most rapid growth. The sarcostyles may be traced to the sarcolemma, which covers the end of the fiber, and tendon fibers may be seen in close contact with the outside of the membrane. It is believed by some writers that the tendon fibers actually pierce the sarcolemma and are continuous with the sarcostyles. Such a continuity cannot, however, be observed in ordinary slides, which give the impression that the muscle is attached to the tendon by its sarcolemma.

The fibers that compose a muscle are gathered together in fascicles, or bundles. Fine connective tissue surrounds the individual fibers; this is called the endomysium. The covering of a fascicle is the perimysium, and the sheath surrounding a group of such bundles is the epimysium.

Muscle of exactly the same morphological appearance as the skeletal muscle is found in various places where it is not attached to the bones. In such situations it has no surrounding connective tissue sheath but merges with the connective tissue about it. Such muscle is not truly skeletal, since it does not move parts of the skeleton. In the tongue, for instance, it is more accurately described by the name voluntary muscle. In other regions muscle of this type is not, strictly speaking, either skeletal or voluntary. The wall of the esophagus contains, in its upper portion, striated muscle that is not under the control of impulses from the higher centers of the nervous system or attached to bone. It is morphologically indistinguishable from skeletal muscle, however, and is therefore called by the same name.

CARDIAC MUSCLE

The third type of muscle is that of the heart. The functional peculiarity of cardiac muscle is its ability to contract rhythmically and continuously—entirely independent of the will. Morphologically, cardiac muscle may readily be distinguished from smooth and skeletal muscle, although it shares some of the characteristics of each.

The fibers branch freely and anastomose (Fig. 4-6). This arrangement is evident under the low power of the microscope. The nuclei of cardiac muscle are centrally located like those of smooth muscle. The myofibrils are transversely striated, in somewhat the same way as those of skeletal muscle, but the striations are not so marked. The sarcolemma is also less noticeable than that of skeletal muscle. In longitudinal sections the fibers are recognizable because of their branching. They are distinguished from sections of striated muscle by the central position of their nuclei. In some preparations of cardiac muscle one may see transverse markings on the fibers that are different from the striations of the sarcostyles. These are the intercalary discs. They are fairly heavy lines, sometimes running directly across the fiber or, more often, traversing it in a series of steps. Electron microscope studies have shown that the intercalated discs are composed of membranes marking the cell boundaries at the junction of the fibers. This observation demonstrates that the cells or fibers of cardiac muscle are not of the syncytial type as was formerly believed (Figs. 4-6 and 4-7).

In transverse as in longitudinal section the position of the nuclei differentiates cardiac from skeletal muscle (Fig. 4-6). In distinguishing it from cross sections of smooth muscle one must observe the extent and character of the cytoplasm. The fibers of cardiac muscle are thicker than those of smooth muscle, having diameters of from 9 to 20μ. It is possible to see in cross sections the cut ends of the sarcostyles, which give the cytoplasm a stippled appearance except in the region immediately around the nucleus.

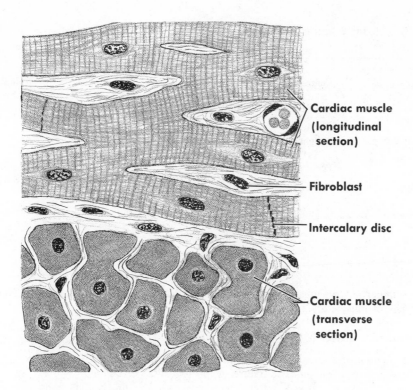

Fig. 4-6
Cardiac muscle of monkey.

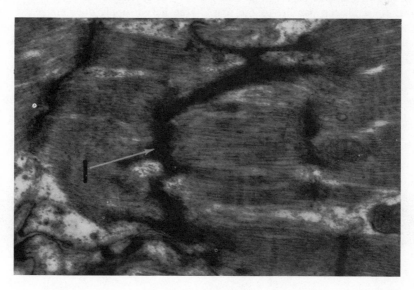

Fig. 4-7
Electron micrograph of cardiac muscle of snake, showing junction of fibers of intercalary disc (**I**). (Courtesy Dr. F. Gonzales, Chicago, Ill.)

Table 5. Diagnostic features of muscle

Type	Nucleus	Myofibrils	Sarcolemma	Shape and size
Smooth				
Longitudinal section	Central	Faint, no striations	Very thin	Spindle
Cross section	Central	Invisible	Very thin	Circular, 7μ
Skeletal				
Longitudinal section	Peripheral	Well-marked striations	Definite sheath	Uniform thickness
Cross section	Peripheral	Visible as dots, in groups	Definite sheath	Rounded poly-gons, 17 to 87μ
Cardiac				
Longitudinal section	Central	Lightly striated	Thin sheath	Branching
Cross section	Central	Visible as dots	Thin sheath	Round, 9 to 20μ

The most important diagnostic features of the three types of muscle are given in Table 5.

MUSCLE-TENDON JUNCTION

At the termination of a muscle, many of the fibers are attached to a tendon. The nature of the muscle-tendon attachment was not clarified until recently. With ordinary staining methods the impression obtained was that the muscle fiber and the tendon fibers were continuous and blended with one another. Recent studies have shown that this concept is not correct. It has been shown that fine argyrophilic fibers thicken near the end, run parallel to the axis of the muscle fiber, and then converge over its termination to form a strand that is continuous with the fiber bundles of the tendon. It has also been shown in electron microscope studies that the connective tissue fibrils are inserted into indentations of the sarcolemma of the muscle fibers.

CIRCULATION AND INNERVATION OF MUSCLE

All muscle has a plentiful supply of blood vessels and nerves. In striated muscle the network of capillaries is so extensive that each fiber lies in contact with at least one blood vessel. The innervation consists of myelinated fibers from the central nervous system, and each muscle fiber is in connection with a nerve fiber. In smooth muscle, which is composed of smaller fibers, the individual cell is not as well supplied. Capillaries ramify through the tissue but not to the extent of reaching every cell. Similarly, the nerve supply does not reach every smooth muscle fiber. It is believed that smooth muscle is a syncytium and that nerve impulses pass from one fiber to another.

The capillaries of cardiac muscle are supplied through the coronary artery. Its nerve supply is derived from the sympathetic and parasympathetic nervous systems.

5
NERVOUS TISSUE

The nervous system is divided into two parts: (1) the central nervous system (CNS), composed of the brain and spinal cord, and (2) the peripheral nervous system (PNS), consisting of all other nervous tissue, that is, ganglia and nerves. This system is composed of functional units known as *neurons* (nerve cells), which are arranged in chain formation extending throughout the body. Neurons are highly differentiated in that they are hyperirritable but have lost the ability to move and to reproduce and usually have limited powers to repair damage. It is this combination of irritability and arrangement that permits the nervous system to receive impulses, integrate them, and transmit them in such a way that coordinated activity occurs.

A neuron consists of a cell body, or *perikaryon;* one or more branching afferent processes known as *dendrites,* which transmit impulses toward the perikaryon; and one efferent process known as the *axon,* which conducts impulses away from the perikaryon. The dendrites and axons are collectively called processes, or *nerve fibers.* Branches occurring along the length of nerve fibers are called *collaterals,* those at the ends are called *terminal arborizations.* A *synapse* is a region in which the terminal arborizations of the axon of one neuron come in proximity to the dendrites or perikarya of succeeding neurons. Synapses are not regions of protoplasmic continuity, since minute but definite gaps between adjoining plasma membranes are demonstrable (Fig. 5-14).

PERIKARYON

The perikaryon is a cytoplasmic thickening that includes a nucleus (karyon). The nucleus is usually a large, lightly staining vesicular struc-

ture with a single prominent nucleolus and several fine chromatin granules (Fig. 5-1, *A*). The cytoplasm contains a conspicuous number of angular pieces of basophilic, metachromatic, RNA-containing *chromophil substance,* usually referred to as Nissl, or tigroid, bodies. With toluidine blue the Nissl substance stains a purplish color and gives the cytoplasm a mottled appearance (Fig. 5-1, *B*). Chromophil substance extends into the dendrites but is absent in a well-defined funnel-shaped area adjacent to the axon known as the *axon hillock* as well as in the axon itself. The amount of chromophil substance in the perikaryon varies considerably. By the use of special stains (for example, silver) minute *neurofibrils* (Fig. 5-1, *C*) may be demonstrated as a fine network embedded in the clear cytoplasm, or *neuroplasm.* The neurofibrils are found in perikarya as well as in both dendrites and axons. The fibrils are most readily visible in the axon hillock. With special techniques the Golgi apparatus and mitochondria may be demonstrated.

FINE STRUCTURE OF MOTOR NEURON

At the electron microscope level the structure of the neuron may be observed in greater detail than at the optical level. The nucleus is relatively large and has, as a rule, a single nucleolus and sparsely distributed chromatin material. The Golgi apparatus is usually prominent and may be present in the form of cisternae, vesicles, or both. The chromophil substance, or Nissl bodies, are prominent features of the cytoplasm and are widely distributed throughout the cell, except at the periphery of the cell body. They are composed of short parallel cisternae of the endoplasmic reticular system and densely

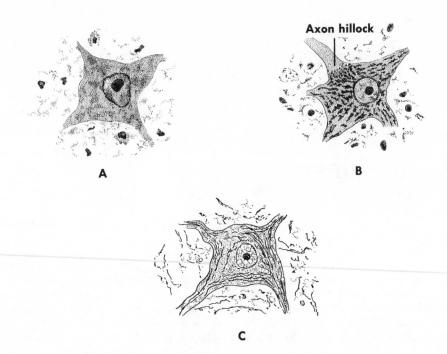

Fig. 5-1
Motor neurons stained in three different ways. **A,** Hematoxylin and eosin. **B,** Toluidine blue, showing Nissl substance. **C,** Silver nitrate, showing neurofibrillae.

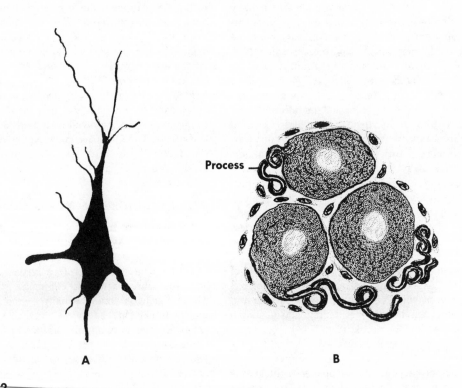

Fig. 5-2
A, Motor neuron, Golgi method, from spinal cord of cat. **B,** Sensory neuron, Golgi method.

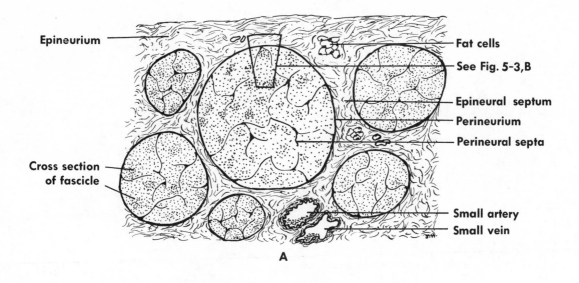

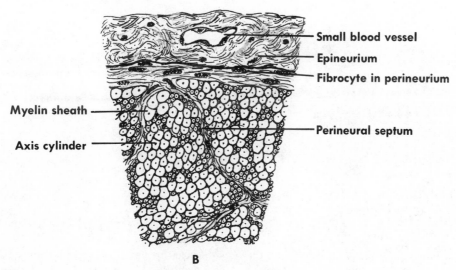

Epineurium

Cross section
of fascicle

Fat cells

See Fig. 5-3,B

Epineural septum

Perineurium

Perineural septa

Small artery

Small vein

A

Small blood vessel

Epineurium

Fibrocyte in perineurium

Myelin sheath

Axis cylinder

Perineural septum

B

Fig. 5-3

·A, Portion of transverse section of nerve trunk. **B,** Medium-power view of nerve fibers and surrounding connective tissue.

packed ribonucleoprotein granules. Neurofilaments appear as a fine meshwork extending throughout the cell. Aggregations of neurofilaments make up the neurofibrils. The mitochondria are usually rod shaped and are scattered among the several organelles present. In addition to the organelles mentioned there may be granules and vacuoles of a transitory nature. The function of these inclusions is not clear at present.

Perikarya are sometimes classified according to the number of processes they bear. The so-called *unipolar* perikarya found in the dorsal root ganglion of the spinal cord bear a single process, which soon branches into an axon and dendrite (Fig. 5-2). *Bipolar* perikarya bear one axon and one dendrite, as in the retina of the eye. *Multipolar* perikarya bear several dendrites and one axon, as in the ventral horn of the gray matter of the spinal cord (Fig. 5-1).

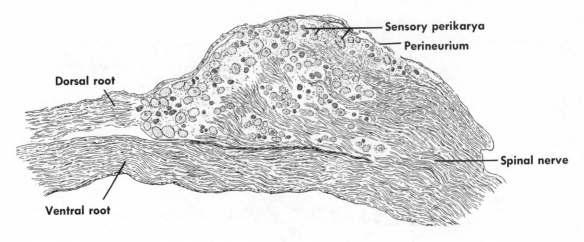

Fig. 5-4
Longitudinal section through spinal ganglion.

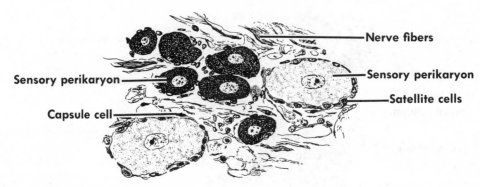

Fig. 5-5
Sensory cells from spinal ganglion.

Perikarya occur exclusively in *ganglia* of the PNS (Figs. 5-4 and 5-5) and in the gray matter of the CNS (Fig. 5-12).

NERVE FIBERS

Histologically, nerve fibers are of four types: (1) fibers without an observable sheath, (2) fibers with a prominent fatty myelin sheath only, (3) fibers with a cellular sheath enclosing a minute quantity of myelin, and (4) fibers with a cellular sheath enclosing a thick layer of myelin.

Both axons and dendrites may or may not bear these sheaths, and one cannot differentiate between these processes in routine histological preparations of nerves (PNS). By the use of Nissl body stains—for example, toluidine blue

—one can frequently distinguish between axons and dendrites in the gray matter of the CNS. Because of this difficulty in histological identification it is customary to describe all "fibers" as one would an axon.

The axonic protoplasm itself is called the *axis cylinder* and consists of argyrophilic *neurofibrils* embedded in neuroplasm or *axoplasm*. The axoplasm shrinks badly in routine preparations so that it frequently appears as a thin acidophil structure with hematoxylin and eosin stains. The term *axon* is frequently used interchangeably with axis cylinder. In the gray matter of the spinal cord, where visible sheaths are absent, the axis cylinder is usually referred to as a *naked axon*. The axis cylinder also appears exposed, that is, without a visible covering,

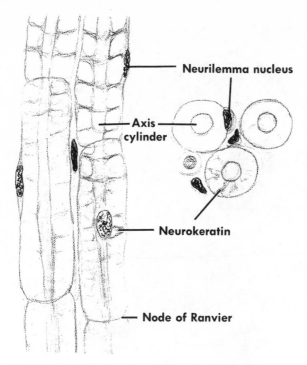

Fig. 5-6
Myelinated nerve fibers in longitudinal and transverse sections.

near the sites or within effectors (for example, muscles and glands). In gray matter freely branching dendrites may sometimes be distinguishable from the single axon. Naked fibers frequently give rise to collateral branches along their length and form the freely branching terminal arborizations.

In the white matter of the spinal cord the axis cylinder is surrounded by a *myelin sheath,* a phospholipid-containing component that appears black when treated with osmic acid (osmiophilia). The periodic acid–Schiff test reveals that simple sugars are a component of myelin. When the myelin is removed by fat solvents, such as absolute alcohol or xylene, certain stains indicate that myelin is penetrated by a protein-containing network of *neurokeratin.* In longitudinal sections of these nerve fibers one may observe interruptions in the myelin sheath. They are known as the *nodes of Ranvier* (Fig. 5-6). In fresh tissue preparations myelin sheaths appear as white glistening coverings. The presence of this substance gives the characteristic color to the white matter of the CNS.

In the autonomic division of the peripheral nervous system the so-called gray fibers contain only a small amount of myelin surrounding the axis cylinder. These are still referred to as "nonmyelinated" fibers. They are found in the vagus nerve, sciatic nerve, and the nerve plexi in the digestive tract and peritoneal cavity. These fibers are enclosed in a cellular covering known as *Schwann's sheath,* and the cells are called *Schwann's cells* (Figs. 5-7 and 5-8). In gray fibers the Schwann cells are flat and overlap each other so that the sheath appears discontinuous. In longitudinal sections the nuclei of these cells may be seen in irregular rows following the wavy contours of the axis cylinders. In hematoxylin and eosin preparations these nuclei may be confused with those of the surrounding connective tissue cells. The attenuated cytoplasm of Schwann's cells is visible only in special preparations and is also known as the *neurilemma.* In cross sections through certain nerves, several axis cylinders may lie in a small amount of myelin enclosed within one and (Fig. 5-8) the same Schwann cell. The latter are nevertheless considered nonmyelinated fibers.

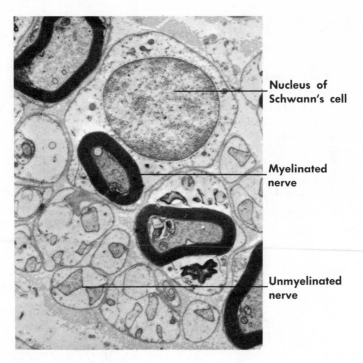

Nucleus of Schwann's cell

Myelinated nerve

Unmyelinated nerve

Fig. 5-7
Electron micrograph showing transverse section of nerves. (×4,000.)

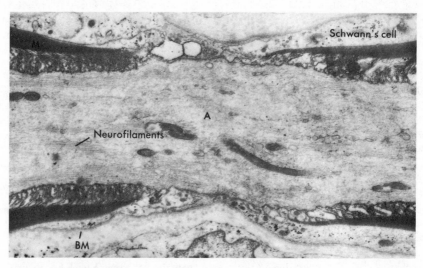

Schwann's cell

M

Neurofilaments

A

BM

Fig. 5-8
Electron micrograph of longitudinal section of a human myelinated nerve fiber in region of a node of Ranvier. **A,** Axis cylinder; **BM,** basement membrane of Schwann cell; **M,** myelin. Note that myelin is lacking in region of node. (×17,000.)

The fourth type of fiber consists of a single axis cylinder surrounded by a thick myelin sheath as well as a smooth, definitely delineated neurilemma (Schwann's sheath) (Fig. 5-6). This type of white fiber is found in the peripheral nervous system. As in all heavily myelinated fibers there are periodic interruptions in the myelin where the neurilemma dips to touch the axis cylinder at the *nodes of Ranvier.* These nodes are observed only in longitudinal sections or in teased preparations. In routine preparations the nodes appear as slender transverse striations. In silver preparations a black precipitate forms on the node and on the axis cylinder for a short distance on each side of it, so that the fibers are marked at intervals by small black crosses. In osmium preparations the blackened myelin region is seen to be interrupted at the site of the node. When the nucleus of the Schwann cell is visible, it may appear to lie in an indentation of the myelin. In fixed preparations of peripheral nerves the myelin of each segment is interrupted by oblique incisions, the Schmidt-Lanterman clefts.

FINE STRUCTURE OF MYELIN SHEATH

Electron microscopy has shown that the myelin sheath consists of a system of concentric lamellar membranes approximately 30 Å thick, varying in number from a few to fifty or more. The membrane is derived from the Schwann cell membrane, which wraps around the nerve fiber in concentric layers. It consists of lipids and alternating layers of neurokeraton (Fig. 5-9).

In the CNS the oligodendrocytes form myelin by wrapping their plasma membrane around the nerve fiber in a manner similar to that described for the peripheral nervous system.

In fibers bearing both myelin and neurilemma, collaterals arise only at nodes, whereas branches of the axis cylinder may arise anywhere along a naked axon. It should be emphasized that with rare exception the descriptive terminology set forth previously in reference to axons is equally applicable in describing dendrites.

In passing it should be noted that some fibers are but a few millimeters long, while others are greater than 1 meter in length. The sum total of protoplasm in the fibers of a neuron is many times greater than the amount of protoplasm in the perikaryon. White, or myelinated, fibers conduct impulses at a higher rate than do gray, or slightly myelinated, fibers. This would ac-

count for the fact that somatic reflexes (involving myelinated fibers and striated or skeletal muscles) are more rapid than visceral reflexes (involving slightly myelinated fibers and smooth muscle fibers). Fibers possessing a neurilemma can slowly regenerate if damaged, but the fibers of the CNS, lacking a neurilemma, do not regenerate.

NERVES

Nerves, or nerve trunks, are groups or bundles of fibers (axons, dendrites, and their collaterals) bound together by connective tissues and invested with blood capillaries. Nerves per se do not include perikarya. A single discrete bundle of nerve fibers and connective tissue is called a *fascicle* (Fig. 5-3). Some of the larger nerve trunks are composed of numerous fascicles, with an attendant increase in the amount of connective tissue and capillaries. The terminology used to designate the topography of the connective tissue associated with the nervous system is similar to that established for connective tissues found in skeletal muscles.

In nerve trunks comprised of several fascicles the entire structure is enclosed by a loosely arranged covering of collagenous and elastic fibers known as the *epineurium* (Fig. 5-3). In the large nerve trunks the epineurium is frequently prominent and contains many blood vessels. It also may give rise to extensions, known as epineural septa, occupying spaces between adjacent groups of fascicles. As the nerve trunk divides the epineurium is reduced until it can no longer be distinguished from fine areolar tissue.

A single fascicle is held together by a concentrically arranged layer of dense collagenous fibers called the *perineurium.* The perineurium varies from a thick prominent structure in large nerves to a very thin one in small nerves. Branches, or trabeculae, of the perineurium (perineural septa of some authors) penetrate the fascicle and give rise to the *endoneurium,* which in turn separates the individual nerve fibers. The endoneurium is composed of fine connective tissue sheaths that completely enclose and are intimately associated with the neurilemma of individual fibers. These sheaths are known as the *sheaths of Henle,* or *endoneural sheaths.*

Small nerve trunks occurring in connective tissue are distinguishable from the fibers of connective tissue by the following features (Fig. 5-10): In longitudinal section, nerves appear

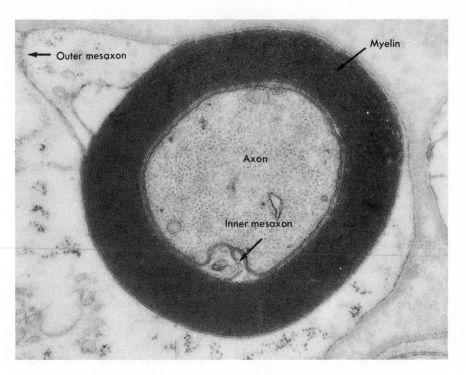

Fig. 5-9
Electron micrograph of transverse section of a myelinated nerve. (×38,000.)

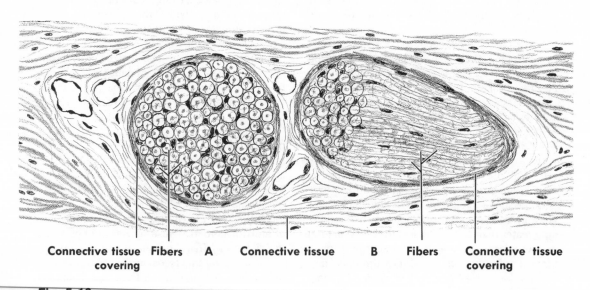

Connective tissue **Fibers** **A** **Connective tissue** **B** **Fibers** **Connective tissue**
covering **covering**

Fig. 5-10
Myelinated nerve fibers forming small trunks in areolar tissue. **A,** Cut transversely. **B,** Cut tangentially.

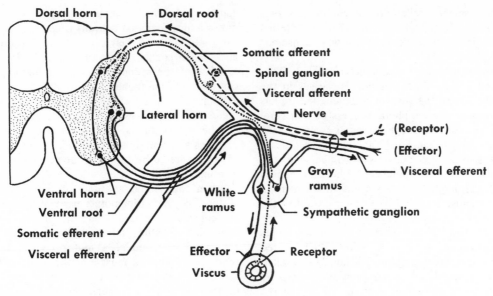

Fig. 5-11
Diagram showing relationship of somatic and visceral neurons to spinal cord, sympathetic ganglia, and viscera.

as groups of fine fibers arranged regularly and parallel. The myelin sheaths may be completely dissolved, and if this is true, each axis cylinder is then separated from its neighbor by a space bounded by the neurilemma sheath. The axis cylinder and neurokeratin are less eosinophilic (or more basophilic) than the surrounding connective tissue fibers. Sections through nerves containing a majority of nonmyelinated fibers are somewhat more difficult to distinguish and may even be confused with smooth muscle fibers by the novice. In nonmyelinated fibers the neurolemma sheaths are irregular and nearly in contact with the somewhat basophilic axis cylinders.

REFLEX MECHANISM

The simplest manner in which the central and peripheral divisions of the system act to respond to environmental change is shown diagrammatically in Fig. 5-11. An impulse arises in a sensory end organ by stimulation of the latter. From there it is carried by the peripheral fiber of the sensory neuron to its perikaryon, which is located in the spinal ganglion. It then travels by way of the central process of this cell to the spinal cord. The impulse then passes through the dendrite and perikaryon of an intercalated (association) neuron, which is located in the dorsal horn of the gray matter of the

spinal cord. The axon of the intercalated neuron is in synaptic relation with one of the dendrites of the third or motor neuron of the chain. This cell lies in the ventral horn of the gray matter. The impulse goes out by way of the axon of the motor neuron, passing through the ventral root of the spinal nerve and one of the peripheral nerves to an effector or organ that performs an action as a result of the impulse it receives.

The part of the peripheral nervous system that serves to distribute impulses to the viscera is known as the autonomic system. This subdivision of the nervous system is made on a functional rather than a morphological basis, but there is a difference between the number of neurons involved in the efferent pathways of the two divisions. Fibers of the cerebrospinal nerves pass directly from their central origins to the muscles they control. Those of the autonomic system on the other hand have two two neurons in the efferent arm. The perikaryon of the first is located within the central nervous system and gives rise to a preganglionic fiber. The second is located in a peripheral ganglion and gives rise to a postganglionic fiber that, in turn, reaches the effector. The fibers that constitute the craniosacral outflow are known as the parasympathetic system; those of the thoracolumbar region, the sympathetic system.

The pathway just described illustrates a

simple somatic reflex arc, or circuit. It serves to produce quick reaction to a change of eternal conditions without the intervention of conscious processes.

The course of a sympathetic reflex is illustrated in Fig. 5-11. An impulse arises in the epithelium of the gut, for instance, and travels by way of the peripheral process of a visceral afferent neuron through the ramus communicans to the spinal ganglion. The central process of this sensory cell conveys the impulse to the lateral horn of the spinal cord, where it synapses with the dendrites of a visceral motor neuron. The impulse leaves the spinal cord through the axon of the latter (preganglionic fiber), which goes by way of the ventral root and the ramus communicans to synapse with a cell located in a sympathetic ganglion. The impulse is picked up by a neuron in this ganglion and carried by its axon to the effector of the viscus. In the case we have illustrated this would be the smooth muscle of the gut. The axon of the ganglion cell is called the postganglionic fiber. Thus, in the autonomic system there are two neurons involved in the pathway from the central nervous system to the viscera.

The two circuits just described are simple ones, requiring few neurons for the transmission of a stimulus from the receptor to the effector. The vast majority of responses to external stimuli, however, include much longer and more complicated chains of neurons. The study of such responses forms a separate branch of anatomy—neurology. We can mention in this text only a few facts concerning these processes.

A single sensory neuron may connect with several association (intercalated) neurons, some of which carry the impulse to the brain. A single association neuron usually receives impulses from several sensory and association neurons. The chains of neurons in the central nervous system are interconnected to form a network in which single neurons are brought under the influence of impulses arising from several different sources. In the spinal cord and brain, impulses are received from various parts of the body and are integrated so that the outflow of impulses along the efferent neuron is adjusted to the needs of the body as a whole.

It is evident from the foregoing description that perikarya are not evenly distributed throughout the nervous system but are collected into groups. The largest collection of these groups is in the gray matter of the brain and

spinal cord, which contains the perikarya of motor and association neurons (Fig. 5-12). Sensory neurons have their perikarya in the spinal and cranial ganglia, while the visceral efferent neurons of the second order are gathered together in the autonomic ganglia. All these collections of nerve cells are connected among themselves by fibers, groups of which make up the nerve trunks. A nerve trunk consists of axons and dendrites of neurons, the perikarya of which are to be found in the ganglia, cord, or brain.

When the spatial relations of the nervous system and the various other parts of the body are considered, it is obvious that it would be impossible to study microscopically an entire neuron. For example, a motor neuron that sends impulses to a muscle of the foot has an axon that extends from the lumbar region of of the spinal cord through the entire length of the leg. Other neurons, although not so extensive, have processes of such length that they cannot be dissected out and studied in their true relation to the cells. It is most convenient to divide the subject into two parts and study separately the nerve trunks and the collections of perikarya, but in so doing we must bear in mind the true relation of these parts to each other.

NERVE ENDINGS
Motor endings

The motor endings are the terminal parts of the efferent nerves that are in contact with either muscles or glands. Striated muscles may exhibit two types of motor endings: (1) The motor plate, shown in Fig. 5-13, consists of a terminal ramification of the nerve fiber that ends in a mass of granular modified sarcoplasm; this structure appears in section to be an elevated area that measures from 40 to 60μ in diameter. (2) In some cases the motor terminations consist of a simpler bulblike arrangement of small loops that end within or outside the sarcolemma.

The efferent fibers that supply cardiac muscle, smooth muscle, and glands are part of the autonomic nervous system. These fibers are usually nonmyelinated and often terminate in nodular thickenings. In muscle these terminations end near the nucleus of the muscle fiber; in glands the fibers run to the base or sides of the gland cell where they end freely or penetrate the cell and end in an expanded terminal loop.

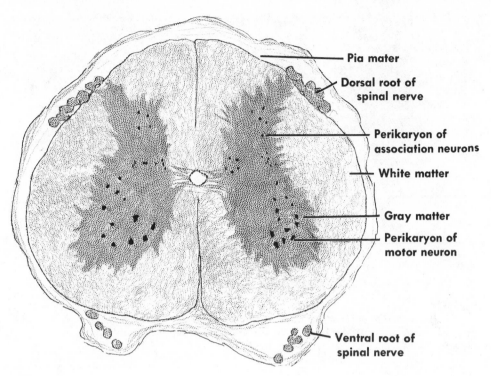

Pia mater

Dorsal root of
spinal nerve

Perikaryon of
association neurons

White matter

Gray matter

Perikaryon of
motor neuron

Ventral root of
spinal nerve

Fig. 5-12
Spinal cord of cat, low magnification.

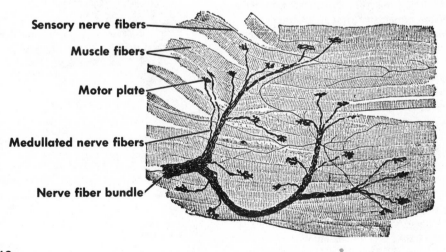

Sensory nerve fibers

Muscle fibers

Motor plate

Medullated nerve fibers

Nerve fiber bundle

Fig. 5-13
Motor nerve endings of intercostal muscle fibers of rabbit. (×150.) (From Bremer, J. L., and Weatherford, H. L.:
A text-book of histology, New York, 1948, McGraw-Hill Book Co.)

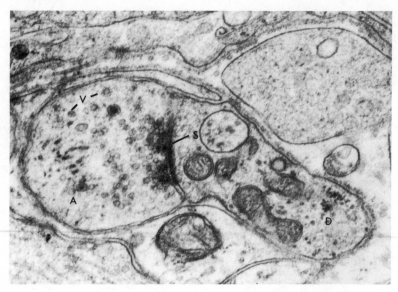

Fig. 5-14

Electron micrograph of an axon-dendritic synapse of sympathetic ganglion of guinea pig. **A,** Axon showing presynaptic vesicles, **V; D,** dendrite; **S,** synaptic cleft. (×32,000.) (Courtesy Mrs. Dorothy Sulkin, Winston-Salem, N. C.)

Sensory endings

Aside from those located in specialized organs such as the eye and ear the sensory endings consist of the following types.

Free endings. Free endings are the simplest type from the structural standpoint. They consist of terminal branches of delicate fibers that often show slight enlargements. These endings have been observed in stratified epithelia, tendon, and connective tissue.

Encapsulated endings. Encapsulated endings are characterized by the presence of a central nerve fiber or several branches embedded in tissue fluid that is enclosed within a connective tissue capsule. There are several varieties of encapsulated endings: (1) the tactile corpuscle of Meissner, (2) genital corpuscles, (3) bulbous and cylindrical corpuscles of Krause, and (4) the lamellar corpuscles (Fig. 5-15).

Muscle spindles. Muscles have sensory nerves that terminate about slender, poorly developed bundles of muscle fibers. The terminal parts of the nerve fibers are arranged spirally around these muscle cells. This complex of nerve and muscle is enclosed within a dense connective tissue sheath and is known as a muscle spindle. Structures analogous to the muscle spindles also occur in tendons.

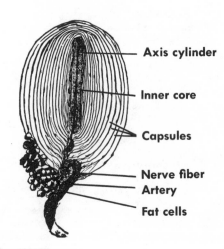

Fig. 5-15

Small lamellar corpuscle from mesentery of cat. (×50.) Nuclei of capsule cells appear as thickenings. Myelin of nerve fiber may be traced to inner core. (From Bremer, J. L., and Weatherford, H. L.: A textbook of histology, New York, 1948, McGraw-Hill Book Co.)

Axis cylinder

Inner core

Capsules

Nerve fiber
Artery
Fat cells

NEUROGLIA

In addition to cells that are specialized for the transmission of stimuli the nervous system contains a large number of supporting cells. The

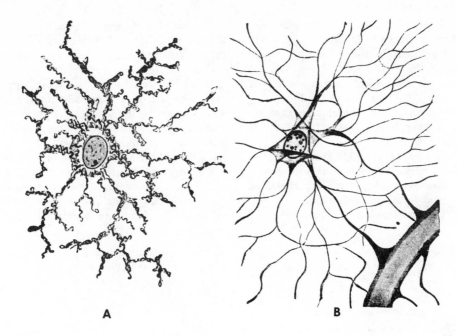

Fig. 5-16

Astrocytes. **A,** Protoplasmic. **B,** Fibrous. (After Hortega. From Bremer, J. L., and Weatherford, H. L.: A text-book of histology, New York, 1948, McGraw-Hill Book Co.)

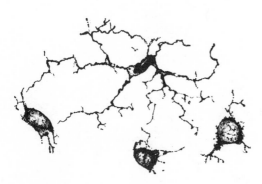

Fig. 5-17

Neuroglia cells from brain of rabbit. Microglia (above) and oligodendroglia. (Stained by Penfield's method.) (From Bremer, J. L., and Weatherford H. L.: A text-book of histology, New York, 1948, McGraw-Hill Book Co.)

interstitial tissue of the spinal cord and brain is called neuroglia, and the term is also sometimes extended to include the cells of the neurilemma and the inner cells of the capsules surrounding ganglion cells. In sections of the spinal cord that have been stained to demonstrate nerve cells and fibers one may see the nuclei of the neuroglia cells among the nervous elements. They are smaller than the nuclei of nerve cells and have no conspicuous nucleoli. The detailed study of this tissue involves the use of special methods and is not usually undertaken in an elementary course. The following facts may be mentioned concerning the cells. The most common type of the neuroglia cells is the astroglia. These are branching cells, some of which (fibrous) have along their borders and in contact with their cytoplasm fibrils that are similar to fibroglia and myoglia fibrils. Others (protoplasmic) lack these fibrils. In either kind of astroglia the cells have specialized processes that are in close contact with the walls of the blood vessels of the nervous system. These "sucker feet" have been thought to enable the cell to derive nourishment from the blood; it is also stated, however, that their function is to provide a special limiting membrane around the vessels (Fig. 5-16).

A second type of neuroglia cell is the oligodendroglia (or oligodendria). These cells have very fine processes and no neuroglia fibrils. Their nuclei are larger and paler than those of the astroglia cells. They are grouped around nerve cells in the brain and around fiber tracts in the spinal cord.

A third type is the microglia, the smallest of the neuroglia cells. They have deeply staining nuclei, are irregular in shape, and have no fibrils or sucker feet. They are said to be phagocytic (Fig. 5-17).

The ependyma, or layer that lines the central canal of the nervous system, forms the fourth group of neuroglia cells. These are elongated cells arranged in a layer like a columnar epithelium. They contain fibrils and are sometimes ciliated.

The neurilemma and satellite cells are sometimes considered as a fifth group of neuroglia cells. They are called, respectively, lemmocytes and amphicytes.

It is of interest to note that these supporting cells, although they are similar in appearance and function to the simpler mesenchymal derivatives such as reticular tissue, are for the most part ectodermal in origin. This is certainly true of the ependyma and of the astroglia, which form the greater part of the tissue. The microglia are probably mesodermal in origin; the oligodendroglia are said by some authors to be mesodermal but are ectodermal according to others.

6
BLOOD AND LYMPH

Blood and lymph are the fluid tissues of the body. Their function is the distribution of oxygen, nutritive substances, and the products of the endocrine glands to all parts of the body and the removal of waste substances and toxins. Both consist of a fluid matrix called the plasma and of cells of various types. The cells, or corpuscles, of blood are of two types: the red and the white. Together, they are about equal in bulk to the plasma. The red cells are much more numerous than the white; there are four to five million of them in a cubic millimeter of normal blood, in which there are but 8,000 or 10,000 of the white cells.

RED BLOOD CORPUSCLES (ERYTHROCYTES)

When a drop of freshly drawn blood is examined under the microscope, the red corpuscles are seen as biconcave discs, having a diameter of approximately 8μ. In the fresh state they appear greenish in color rather than red. The depression in the center of each corpuscle makes a light spot that might at first sight be mistaken for a nucleus. The adult red cells are, however, nonnucleated in mammalian blood. Often they stick together in rows, or rouleaux. As a drop of blood dries at its edges the red cells lose fluid and change their shapes. Some are cup shaped; others are very irregular in outline. In sections of organs and tissues stained with hematoxylin and eosin the red blood cells have a bright orange or red color. The disc shape is the most common in such preparations; but especially in small vessels, the cells are sometimes cup shaped, sometimes compressed into angular forms. The usual method of preparing blood for microscopic study is to spread a drop on a slide so that it forms a thin smear and then to stain it with a special stain. Wright's stain is commonly used. The red corpuscles, when so treated, lose volume without changing shape. Those at the center of the smear, when there have been no changes because of rapid drying, have the form of biconcave discs that average about 7.5μ in diameter. The cells are nongranular and colored pale brown or pink by the stain.

Since the red blood cells are nonnucleated, it is sometimes said that they should not be called cells. The name erythroplastic may be used, but erythrocyte is the most common term. The cytoplasm of the red corpuscles contains a substance called hemoglobin, which is very readily oxidized and reduced, and it is this substance that enables the erythrocytes to perform their function of carrying oxygen from the lungs to the tissues. Hemoglobin imparts a reddish tint to cells containing it if the latter are stained with Wright's stain. This fact is important in the recognition of early stages of development of red blood cells (see Bone marrow, Chapter 7).

WHITE BLOOD CORPUSCLES (LEUKOCYTES)

The leukocytes as a group respond differently from the red cells to the treatment involved in making a smear. Erythrocytes lose a slight amount of volume and are, therefore, smaller in the smear than in the fresh state. Leukocytes, on the contrary, are flattened by the treatment and acquire a greater diameter.

The colorless leukocytes are true cells and contain a nucleus and cell organelles. Some exhibit amoeboid movement, and for convenience, they may be divided into two main groups: the granular variety and the nongranular, or lymphoid, types. In sections stained with hematoxylin and eosin the leukocytes stand out among the erythrocytes because of their darkly stained nuclei. It is sometimes possible to iden-

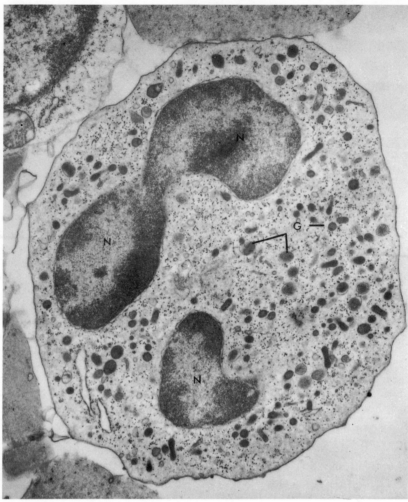

Fig. 6-1

Electron micrograph of neutrophilic leukocyte from the bone marrow of a cat. The granules are bounded by a membrane and vary in density. They contain hydrolytic enzymes. Ribosomes are scattered throughout the cytoplasm. **G,** Specific granules; **N,** lobes of nucleus. (×19,000.)

tify lymphocytes, granulocytes, and monocytes in such preparations, but for critical examination of white cells one must use preparations made with special stains.

Granular (polymorphonuclear) leukocytes

An outstanding feature of the granulocytes is the presence of granules in the cytoplasm. Each variety of granulocyte has a different kind of granule readily identified at both the optical and the electron microscope levels. A second characteristic feature of these cells is the nucleus, which is multilobed. Although several criteria may be used to distinguish and classify the granulocytes, the one most commonly used is

based on the morphological characteristics of the nucleus and the size, shape, and tinctorial properties of the granules. The granulocytes make up from 60 to 70% of the white cells. In a blood smear treated with Wright's stain the types of cells illustrated in Plate 1 may be distinguished.

Neutrophilic (heterophilic) leukocytes. The nucleus of neutrophilic leukocytes consists of from three to five irregular oval lobes connected by thin chromatin strands. In dry smear preparations an appendage appears on one of the lobes in approximately 3% of the cells. This chromatin appendage, known as a "drumstick" (not to be confused with irregu-

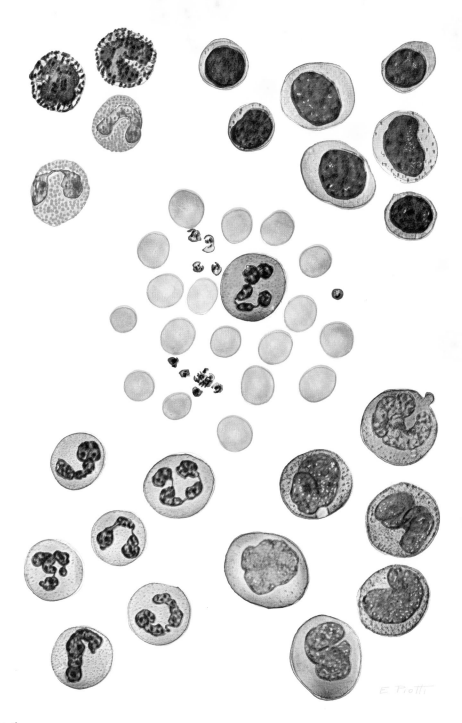

Plate 1

Cells from smear preparation of normal human blood. (Wright's stain.) In center: Adult red blood corpuscles, blood platelets, and a polymorphonuclear neutrophil. At left above: Two polymorphonuclear basophils and two polymorphonuclear eosinophils. At right above: Three large and four small lymphocytes, some with granules in protoplasm. At left below: Polymorphonuclear neutrophils; two of these cells, the uppermost and the lowermost of the group, are young, with merely crooked nuclei, sometimes known as band, stab, or nonfilamentous forms; mature cells have multilobed nuclei. At right below: Six monocytes, some containing more protoplasmic granules than others; in the younger cells nuclei tend to be rounded and in the adult cells they are horseshoe shaped, indented, or lobed. (From Bremer, J. L., and Weatherford, H. L.: A text-book of histology, New York, 1948, McGraw-Hill Book Co.)

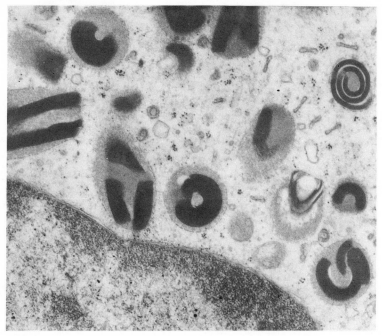

Fig. 6-2
Electron micrograph of part of eosinophilic leukocyte from bone marrow of a cat, showing detail of organic crystals in membrane-bound granules. (×33,000.)

larities on the margin of the nuclei), represents the chromatin material in which the female (XX) chromosomes are located. The cytoplasm (except for a clear homogeneous peripheral zone) is slightly acidophilic and contains numerous fine granules, which appear purple or lavender. These cells measure about 8μ in the fresh state and attain a size of 12μ in a dry smear preparation. At the electron microscope level the granules appear diverse in size and shape (Fig. 6-1).

Acidophilic (eosinophilic) leukocytes. The acidophilic leukocytes, which are approximately spherical, measure 9μ in diameter in the fresh condition and in dry smears may attain a diameter of nearly 12μ. They make up from 2 to 5% of the total leukocytes in the peripheral blood. In contrast with the nuclei of the neutrophils, the nuclei of the acidophils usually consist of two oval lobes connected by chromatin strands. Except for a centrally located area occupied by the cytocentrum the cytoplasm contains numerous coarse granules, which in man are spherical. When stained with acid dyes, the granules vary in appearance from pink to bright red. When observed with the electron microscope, the granules exhibit dense crystal-

line bodies that vary in appearance in different species (Fig. 6-2).

Basophilic leukocytes. The basophils are least numerous of the leukocytes and comprise less than 0.5% of the total count. They are approximately the same size as the neutrophils. The nucleus often appears S-shaped, is constricted in two or more regions, and stains less intensely than the other varieties. The granules are extremely coarse and with Wright's stain appear a dull blue. They also give the impression of being partially extruded from the cell surface and often partially obscure the nucleus. When viewed with the electron microscope, the granules appear membrane bound; the material enclosed by the membrane varies in appearance in diverse species. Scattered mitochondria and Golgi vesicles are usually present.

Nongranular leukocytes

Lymphocytes. In the human the lymphocytes make up from 20 to 25% of the total number of white cells of the blood. They are spherical and measure from 6 to 8μ in diameter, although some of them may be slightly larger. The most characteristic morphological feature of these cells is the presence of a large, dense

75

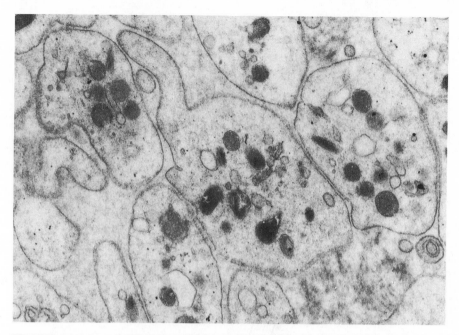

Fig. 6-3
Electron micrograph showing several blood platelets (thrombocytes). (×29,000.)

nucleus with a distinct indentation on one side, which is not, however, observed in dry smear preparations. Prominent nucleoli may be observed in well-prepared sections at both the optical and the electron microscope levels. The cytoplasm appears as a thin rim surrounding the nucleus. It is homogeneous and basophilic, which is referable to numerous ribosomes observed at the electron microscope level. Occasionally, purple *azurophilic* granules may be observed in the cytoplasm, but these are inconstant features.

The larger lymphocytes are relatively few in number, and their increase in size is due to the presence of a greater amount of cytoplasm. The cytoplasm usually contains a few scattered mitochondria and granules.

Monocytes. The monocytes resemble the lymphocytes, especially in forms that appear to be transitional. A typical monocyte measures from 9 to 12μ in diameter. In dry smear preparations, however, they may appear 20μ or larger. The mature monocyte exhibits considerably more cytoplasm than does the lymphocyte and often, though not invariably, has an eccentrically placed nucleus, which is oval or kidney shaped. It stains less intensely than those of the lymphocytes. Organelles such as mitochondria and a Golgi apparatus are usually

observed. The monocytes comprise from 3 to 8% of the leukocytes of the circulating blood.

Functions of leukocytes

The leukocytes in the bloodstream appear to be inactive, and their function is not well understood. Outside the bloodstream they exhibit amoeboid movement. Leukocytes constantly migrate from the vessels to the tissues. This is particularly noticeable at the site of local injury or infection, where the granulocytes migrate in response to chemotactic stimulation. Later, monocytes also accumulate in these areas. Among the granulocytes only the neutrophils exhibit phagocytosis. Many types of bacteria are ingested by this process. During this process the specific granules of the cell break down and disappear, meanwhile liberating hydrolytic enzymes, which are responsible for the destruction of bacteria. Various other enzymes are present in leukocytes, but their function is not known at present.

PLATELETS

In addition to the cells just described, blood contains groups of very minute cytoplasmic fragments that are called platelets, or thrombocytes, and are not generally included under the head of corpuscles. The individual platelet, about 2μ in diameter, is composed of a cytoplasm, which stains blue with Wright's stain. It has a dark granular center, the chromomere, and a light peripheral area, the hyalomere.

Thrombocytes, or platelets, are believed to liberate the enzyme *thromboplastin* involved in the clotting of blood (Fig. 6-3). Thromboplastin transforms prothrombin to thrombin, which, in turn, transforms fibrinogen to fibrin. Thromboplastin also has been identified in blood plasma.

PLASMA

Blood plasma is a homogeneous, slightly alkaline fluid. It contains 10 mg/100 ml. of calcium, also sodium chloride, bicarbonate, phosphate, globulins, and albumin. Plasma comprises about 55% of the blood; formed elements make up the other 45%. These proportions vary under diverse physiological and pathological conditions. One of the constituents of the plasma, *fibrinogen,* separates from the plasma during injury of the vessels to form delicate filaments of *fibrin,* which in turn form a network in which blood cells become enmeshed to form a blood clot. Plasma mediates the nutritive substances derived from food, the waste products of the various tissues, and secretions of the endocrine glands.

LYMPH

Lymph is of less interest to the student of histology than blood. It consists of a fluid plasma that is somewhat different chemically from blood plasma. In it are floating leukocytes, principally lymphocytes and large mononuclear leukocytes. In sections of lymph vessels one sees only a fine granular coagulum with occasional nucleated corpuscles.

7
BLOOD-FORMING ORGANS

BONE MARROW

In the adult body, blood cells are normally formed in two organs that are alike in having a framework of reticular tissue but different in the kinds of corpuscles that they produce. Bone marrow is the normal source of the red blood cells and the granulocytes and lymph nodules, of the lymphocytes.

It will be remembered that in the formation of a bone a space is left at the center by the resorption first of the cartilage and later of endosteal bone. This space is invaded by mesenchyme that develops into an organ having no part in the supportive function of the bone itself. This is the red bone marrow, which in the adult is the source of most blood corpuscles. The primitive mesenchyme of the embryo develops in this location into three main types of cells: first, a framework of reticular tissue; second, adipose tissue; and third, hematopoietic, or blood-forming, cells. In early life all three kinds of cells are present in the marrow of any bone. Later, the hematopoietic cells disappear from the marrow of some of the bones, leaving only reticular tissue and fat cells, which make up the yellow marrow. In other bones the marrow continues to form blood cells throughout life, and their presence makes the tissue red.

Marrow may be studied in smear preparations or in sections. For critical examination a blood stain must be used. In such a preparation one may recognize the cells shown in Plate 2.

Reticular tissue cells

In sections reticular tissue cells are somewhat obscured by the hematopoietic cells, but they may be distinguished in smears or thin section.

Adipose tissue cells

Adipose tissue cells are generally scattered in red marrow and appear under low-power magnification as holes in the marrow.

Hemocytoblasts (stem cell)

Hemocytoblasts are from 10 to 12μ in diameter and have a basophilic, nongranular cytoplasm. The form of the cell is pear shaped or polygonal, without cytoplasmic processes. The nucleus is large and pale and is situated at the widest part of the cell.

Promyelocytes, myelocytes, metamyelocytes

There are three intermediate stages between the hemocytoblast and the granular leukocyte. They are characterized in general by the development of cytoplasmic granules which are neutrophilic, eosinophilic, or basophilic, according to the kind of leukocyte destined to develop from each. It is possible, with sufficient care, to recognize three main types or stages of this group. The youngest (promyelocyte) is a spherical cell with a basophilic cytoplasm much like that of the hemocytoblast except that it contains a few granules. The nucleus of the promyelocyte is large and pale. The second stage (myelocyte) is the most common of the group and the most easily distinguished. The myelocytes divide rapidly, giving rise to successive generations of cells in which one may trace a gradual increase in the number of specific cytoplasmic granules and an accompanying loss of affinity for basic stains. Also, as divisions occur there is a slight loss in size and increase of density of the nucleus. The products of the last divisions of the myelocytes are the

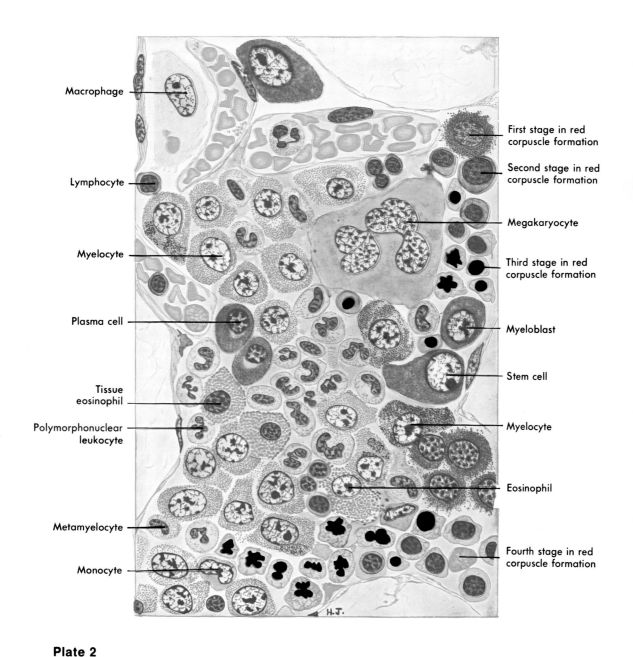

Macrophage

Lymphocyte

Myelocyte

Plasma cell

Tissue
eosinophil

Polymorphonuclear
leukocyte

Metamyelocyte

Monocyte

First stage in red
corpuscle formation

Second stage in red
corpuscle formation

Megakaryocyte

Third stage in red
corpuscle formation

Myeloblast

Stem cell

Myelocyte

Eosinophil

Fourth stage in red
corpuscle formation

H.J.

Plate 2

Normal vertebral bone marrow, male adult. (Zenker fixation, decalcified and stained with phloxine–methylene blue.) In one field representative cells have been brought together in the proper proportion and relation one to another in order to illustrate typical normal picture. Zeiss ap. obj. 90, oc. 10. (From Bremer, J. L., and Weatherford, H. L.: A text-book of histology, New York, 1948, McGraw-Hill Book Co.)

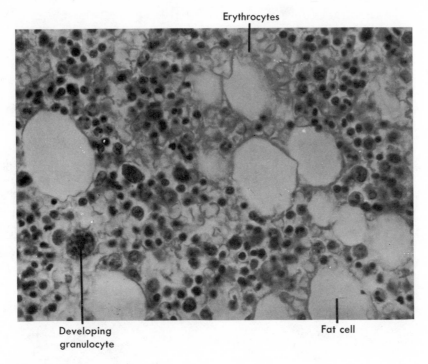

Erythrocytes

Developing
granulocyte

Fat cell

Fig. 7-1
Section of bone marrow in monkey. (Eosin-azure; × 640.)

metamyelocytes. These cells develop without further division into polymorphonuclear leukocytes. Metamyelocytes are, in fact, early stages of granulocytes, which are not sufficiently mature to enter the circulation under normal conditions.

Proerythroblasts, erythroblasts, normoblasts

The proerythroblast is the earliest recognizable stage in the development of the red blood cell. It differs from a promyelocyte in the following ways: It is slightly smaller and has a more chromatic nucleus; hemoglobin is beginning to develop in its cytoplasm; at this stage the cytoplasm is basic, like that of the hemocytoblast and the promyelocyte, but the presence of hemoglobin gives it a slightly purplish or grayish tinge. In the next stage, the erythroblast, a series of changes develops gradually as the cells divide. These changes are of two sorts: an increase in the amount of hemoglobin in the cytoplasm and a decrease in the size of the cell and its nucleus. The former change is expressed morphologically as a shift in color

from the grayish blue of the proerythroblast toward the pink that is characteristic of the erythrocyte. When the pink color is fully developed, the cells are called normoblasts. A normoblast is only slightly larger than an erythrocyte but differs from it in having a nucleus. Normoblasts undergo a number of divisions, during which their nuclei become progressively smaller and darker. Ultimately, the nucleus of the normoblast is reduced to a compact, deeply staining mass, and when this is extended from its surface, the cell is a fully developed red blood corpuscle.

DEVELOPMENT OF BLOOD CELLS IN THE EMBRYO

While the most important permanent source of blood cells is the red bone marrow, there are several other sites of blood formation that occur during embryonic development. The cells that differentiate into blood islands in the extra-embryonic mesoderm of the yolk sac give rise to hemocytoblasts. The liver and the spleen also have an important hematopoietic function during early embryonic existence.

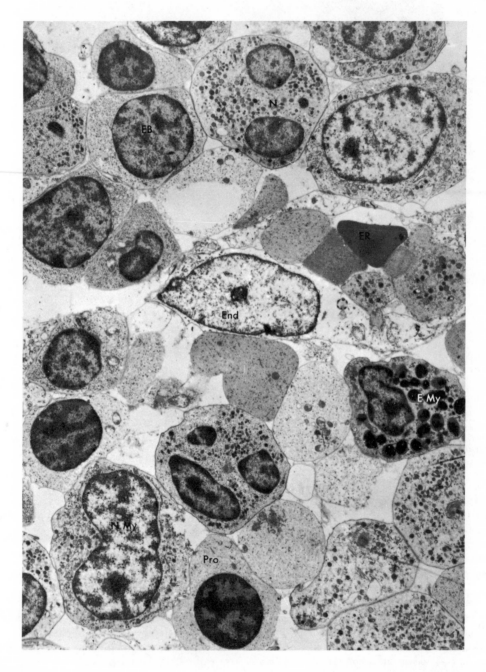

Fig. 7-2
Electron micrograph of bone marrow from cat. **EB,** Erythroblast; **EMy,** eosinophilic myelocyte; **End,** endothelial cell of capillary; **ER,** erythrocyte; **N,** neutrophil; **NMy,** neutrophilic myelocyte; **Pro,** proerythrocyte. (×5,500.)

GERMINAL CENTERS OF LYMPH NODES

In lymphoid tissue there are centers of lymphocyte production. These consist of areas that stain more lightly than the surrounding tissue because they are composed of large, pale cells with vesicular nuclei. These are hematocytoblasts, which differ from the hematocytoblasts of bone marrow in that they are destined to produce one type of corpuscle, the lymphocyte. Some authors prefer to give to them the name lymphoblast on this account. Surrounding such a center of pale cells is a ring of densely packed lymphocytes that, with their deeply stained nuclei and scanty cytoplasm, form a marked contrast of color to the germinal center.

THEORIES OF DEVELOPMENT OF BLOOD

The subject of the development of the different types of blood cells is an extremely complicated one. The red cells, the polymorphonuclear leukocytes, and the platelets are formed in bone marrow; the lymphocytes may develop there also and are certainly found in large numbers in lymphoid tissue scattered throughout the body. The source of the large mononuclears is obscure.

It is clear that the reticular and adipose tissue cells of marrow are derived from mesenchyme, and the hemocytoblasts are thought by some workers to come directly from the same source. Others believe that they develop from reticular tissue cells only. Theories as to the transformation of the hemocytoblast into the corpuscles are various, and the terminology is confused. Only a brief summary of the most widely accepted views will be attempted.

Monophyletic theory

According to the monophyletic theory, hemocytoblasts are present in the bone marrow and in the germinal centers of the lymphoid organs. In bone marrow they give rise to giant cells, lymphocytes, myeloblasts, and erythroblasts. The giant cells produce the platelets; myeloblasts produce the various types of polymorphonuclears; and the erythroblasts are the source of the red blood corpuscle.

Dualist theory

The dualists recognize an intravascular origin of red blood cells derived from the endothelium of the capillaries and sinusoids. The earliest form of erythrocyte was called a megaloblast by Sabin. Megakaryocytes, too, are believed to be of endothelial origin according to this theory. Reticular cells are believed to be multipotential cells that become "primitive" cells capable of developing into myeloblasts, lymphoblasts, and monoblasts, varying with their environment. In the marrow they typically become myeloblasts; in the lymphoid organs, lymphoblasts; and in the spleen, lymphoblasts and monoblasts. The dualist theory differs from the unitarian in three respects: first, in the intravascular origin of red blood cell and megakaryocytes; second, in differentiating the reticular cell from the hemocytoblast; and third, in the independent derivation of mononuclears from the reticular cell instead of from the lymphocyte.

Polyphyletic theory

The polyphyletic theory is based on the recognition of an individual parent blood cell type for each blood cell type. Also, each parent cell is located in a specific locus in the adult.

8
CIRCULATORY SYSTEM

BLOOD VESSELS

Blood and lymph are the carriers of nutritive substances, hormones, and products of metabolism. The circulatory, or vascular, system is the means by which blood and lymph are distributed throughout the body. The system includes the blood vessels, the heart, and the lymphatics.

The blood vessels may be conveniently divided into three main groups for study: the capillaries and sinuses, the arteries, and the veins.

Capillaries

Capillaries have one coat that consists of simple squamous epithelium (endothelium). They are of fine caliber, some of them being so small that only one red blood cell at a time may pass through them. According to some authors the tubule is clasped at intervals by Rouget cells. These are branching cells that are said to be contractile and to cause the constriction of the capillaries. They are not ordinarily seen, however, and it is doubtful whether they should be considered as a regular component of the capillary wall (Figs. 8-1 and 8-2).

Some capillaries do not connect arterioles and venules, and the substances passing through their walls are not oxygen and carbon dioxide. An example of this kind of vessel may be found in the glomerulus of the kidney. The vessel in the glomerulus is, structurally, a capillary; however, blood passing through it gives off nitrogenous wastes but not oxygen. Other vessels consisting of endothelium only are called sinusoids. Their walls are in close apposition with epithelial tissue, from which the blood removes the secretion or to which it gives up substances for storage. Morphologically, sinusoids are enlarged capillaries. Some of them are

lined with an endothelium that exhibits the phagocytic properties of the reticuloendothelial system.

Arteries

Blood is carried from the heart to the capillaries by arteries. The wall of an artery is, in general, characterized by the presence of a coat of smooth muscle circularly arranged and by considerable amounts of elastic tissue. Because of the latter, arteries retain their shape after death and appear circular in transverse section. In this system of vessels there is a gradual change of structure as the caliber of the vessels diminishes. The changes in structure are nowhere abrupt, nor can they be accurately correlated with the size of the vessels. It is convenient, however, to select for study and description certain groups of vessels.

Aorta. In the aorta, the largest of the arteries, the predominant histological feature is elastic connective tissue. The vessel is lined, as are all blood vessels, with simple squamous epithelium (endothelium). This rests on a very thin layer of scattered fibroblasts and collagenous fibers (subendothelial tissue) that in turn covers a thick network of elastic fibers. These three tissues constitute the intima of the aorta.

The second coat, or media, is by far the thickest layer, forming approximately four-fifths of the thickness of the wall. It consists of a mixture of circularly arranged smooth muscle fibers and elastic fibers. The latter predominate and mingle, on the one hand, with the elastic fibers of the intima and, on the other, with those of the outermost layer, or adventitia.

The adventitia is a comparatively thin coat of connective tissue. Elastic fibers are concentrated at the outer border of the media, form-

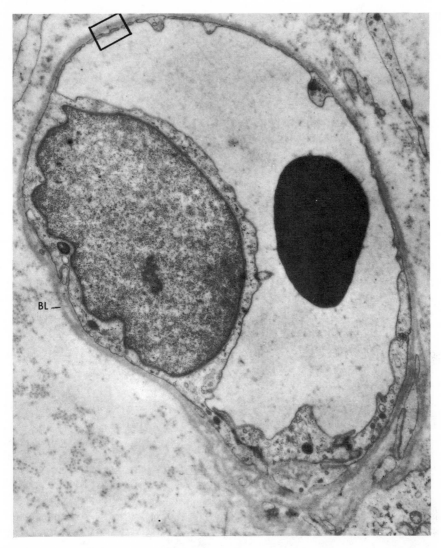

Fig. 8-1

Electron micrograph of a fenestrated capillary cut transversely from human dental pulp. The wall of the capillary consists of an attenuated endothelial cell whose nucleus projects into the lumen. The cytoplasm of the endothelial cell contains many pinocytotic vesicles and is invested by a delicate basement membrane (lamina), **BL.** (×11,000.)

ing the external elastic membrane. Collagenous fibers merge with those of the connective tissue surrounding the vessel. In the adventitia and the outer portion of the media are small nutrient vessels (vasa vasorum) and nerves (nervi vasorum).

The aorta and a few other vessels like it are sometimes called the large arteries, or arteries of the elastic type. The common iliacs, axillaries, carotids, and pulmonaries belong in this group.

Medium-sized arteries. In the group of medium-sized arteries are included most of the vessels observed grossly in dissection to which names have been given. They are characterized by a gradual change, as distance from the heart increases, from the elastic type to vessels having a wall composed mainly of smooth muscle. Arteries of this group is shown in Figs. 8-6 and 8-7. From these arteries one may distinguish the following features: The intima consists of endothelium, a very small amount of subendothelial connective tissue, and

Nucleus of endothelial cell of capillary

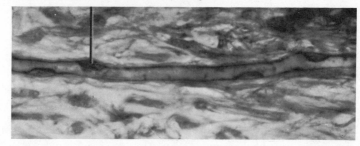

Fig. 8-2
Capillary of human dental pulp, showing alkaline phosphatase localization (black). (×640.) This enzyme is present in the endothelia of all blood vessels. (From Bevelander, G.: Essentials of histology, ed. 6, St. Louis, 1970, The C. V. Mosby Co.)

Capillary

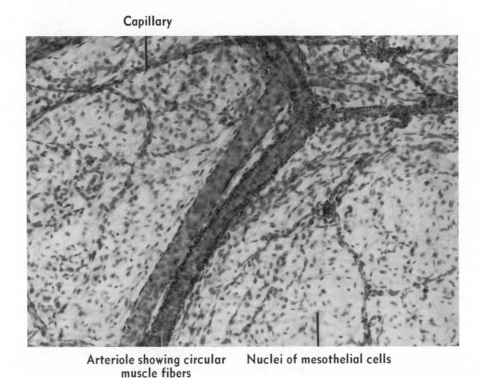

Arteriole showing circular   Nuclei of mesothelial cells
muscle fibers

Fig. 8-3
Surface view of stretch preparation of mesentery. (×40.) (From Bevelander, G.: Essentials of histology, ed. 6, St. Louis, 1970, The C. V. Mosby Co.)

elastic connective tissue. The latter is concentrated in a membrane known as the inner elastic membrane. In cross section this looks like a continuous sheet of elastic tissue, but in surface view it is seen to have open spaces in it (fenestrated membrane). Changes that occur at death cause the smooth muscle to contract, and this contraction throws the elastic membrane and its covering of endothelium into wavy folds. This results in a scalloped appearance of the border of the lumen, as seen in cross section of the vessel.

The media in vessels of this group, like that of the aorta, is the thickest of the three layers. It is composed mainly of smooth muscle circularly arranged. Interspersed among the muscle fibers are isolated strands of elastic tissue, distinguished by their wavy course and their highly refractive quality. The adventitia consists of an external elastic membrane and a layer of collagenous connective tissue, containing small vessels and nerves. In some vessels of this group strands of smooth muscle longitudinally arranged are to be found in the adventitia.

The artery represented in Fig 8-7 is fairly typical of the group. It must be emphasized, however, that a considerable variety of structure is included in the class of vessels that are called medium-sized arteries or arteries of the muscular type. A vessel may have considerably more or considerably less elastic tissue than the one represented and still belong to the same group.

Small arteries and arterioles. Small arteries and arterioles are the types of arterial vessels usually found in sections of organs. They present intermediate forms between the vessels just described and the capillaries or sinusoids, which consist of a tube of endothelium alone. Elements are lost from the wall in the following order: First, the elastic fibers scattered through the media disappear, leaving a middle coat composed entirely of smooth muscle. Second, the external elastic membrane is lost, and the adventitia becomes a covering of collagenous fibers hardly distinguishable from the surrounding connective tissue. From this point on the vessel cannot be said to have the three typical coats—intima, media, and adventitia. In still smaller vessels the inner elastic membrane is first replaced by scattered elastic fibers and then disappears altogether. The muscle of the media also thins out to a few scat-

tered fibers, and finally the blood passes into a tube consisting of endothelium alone. Vessels whose walls consist of endothelium and scattered muscle fibers are called arterioles (Figs. 8-3 to 8-5).

Veins

The walls of the veins, by which blood returns from the capillaries to the heart, are composed largely of collagenous connective tissue, with muscle and elastic fibers much less prominent than they are in the arterial wall. Because of the lack of elastic tissue, veins do not retain their shape after death and appear in sections as irregularly rounded structures. In general, the wall of a vein is not as thick as that of the accompanying artery, but its lumen is larger.

The organization of the tissues in three coats is frequently indistinct. Tracing the system back from the capillaries toward the heart one may observe the following features:

Small veins and venules. Small veins and venules occur in the connective tissue or organs (Figs. 8-3 and 8-6). The first addition to the endothelium that changes the vessel from a capillary to a venule is not muscle but collagenous fibers. These and the accompanying fibroblasts are oriented longitudinally with respect to the vessel. As the caliber of the venule increases, its wall includes, first, muscle and, then, in still larger vessels scattered elastic fibers. The elements are arranged as in arteries but in different proportions. The larger vessels of this group have three coats: The intima consists of endothelium, subendothelial collagenous fibers, and scattered elastic fibers. The latter do not form a membrane and are not present in sufficient number to cause the scalloping of the border of the lumen that is characteristic of arteries. The media is a thin coat of muscle interspersed with collagenous fibers. The adventitia, which consists of white fibrous tissue, is the thickest of the three coats.

Veins of medium caliber. Veins of medium caliber exhibit many of the characteristics just described. The adventitia of collagenous fibers is the thickest of the coats. The muscle of the media and the elastic tissue of the intima increase somewhat in amount, but there is no inner elastic membrane. The intima of many veins of medium caliber, particularly those of the extremities, is extended at intervals in the form of flaps or valves that prevent the reversal of blood flow in the vessels. In some veins of

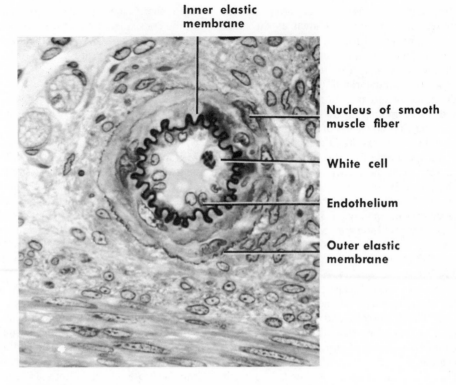

Inner elastic membrane

Nucleus of smooth muscle fiber

White cell

Endothelium

Outer elastic membrane

Fig. 8-4
Transverse section of arteriole. (×640.)

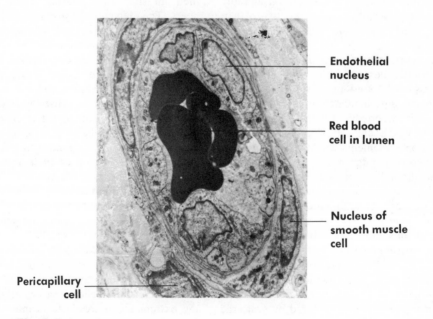

Endothelial nucleus

Red blood cell in lumen

Nucleus of smooth muscle cell

Pericapillary cell

Fig. 8-5
Electron micrograph of transverse section of small arteriole.

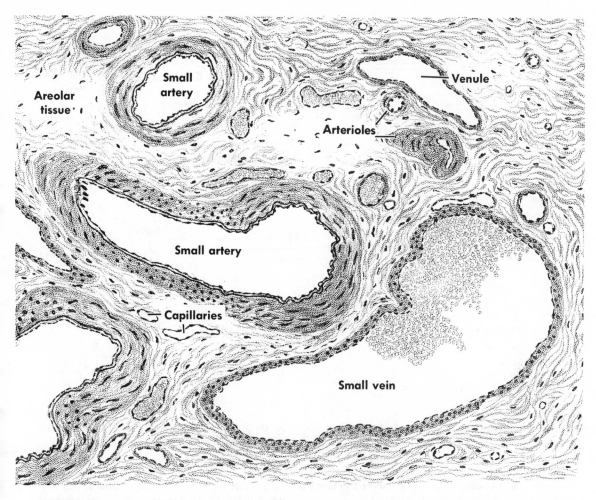

Fig. 8-6
Areolar tissue, capillaries, arterioles, venules, small arteries, and small veins in submucosa of digestive tract.

this group longitudinal muscle fibers occur in the intima and in the adventitia. In the latter coat there may be a complete layer of such muscle fibers placed next to the circular muscle fibers of the media. This is not, however, of common occurrence.

A typical vein of this group is illustrated in Fig. 8-7. As is true of arteries, the group includes a rather wide range of variation in structure.

Large veins. Large veins show an increase in the amount of longitudinal muscle in the adventitia and a slight increase in the amount of elastic tissue in the intima. The elastic tissue, however, is not as prominent even in the largest veins as it is in quite small arteries. The circular

muscle of the media is reduced in veins of this group and is lacking entirely in a few of them.

Comparison of veins and arteries

The difference between the smaller arterial and venous vessels lies in the amount of muscle and connective tissue present in each. Muscle is the predominant tissue in arterioles; in the venules there is little muscle, and the wall consists mainly of endothelium and connective tissue. The larger vessels of the two groups may be distinguished by the following characteristics.

Intima. In arteries the presence of a complete inner elastic membrane is a distinguishing feature. This membrane contracts after death, throwing the intima into small folds and allowing

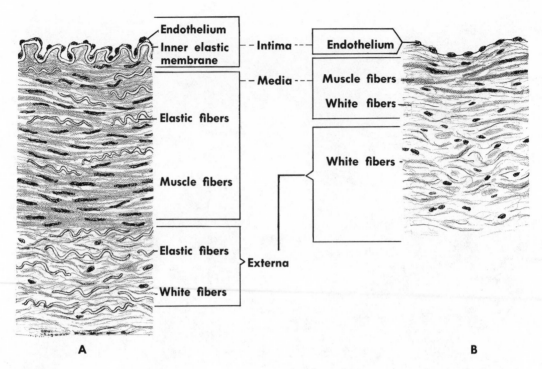

Fig. 8-7
Medium-sized artery, **A**, and vein, **B**.

the endothelial nuclei to project into the lumen of the vessel. In the veins the endothelium remains smooth. The entire intima of some veins extends into the lumen at intervals in large folds or reduplications that serve as valves to prevent the backflow of the blood.

Media. The media is the thickest coat of an artery and consists of muscle interspersed with elastic tissue. In veins the media is a thin coat of muscle; it usually contains all circular, but occasionally longitudinal, fibers. It has more white fibers than the media of an artery and includes elastic tissue only in the largest vessels of the system.

Adventitia. In arteries the adventitia is less important than the media. It contains the outer elastic membrane, and there are seldom any muscle fibers in it. The adventitia of the vein is its thickest coat, and it often contains a large number of longitudinal muscle fibers.

Size of vessels. The lumen of the vein is larger than that of the accompanying artery, but its wall is thinner.

Shape of vessels. Because of the relatively large amount of elastic tissue, arteries retain their round shape in sections more often than

do the veins. The latter are more likely to be collapsed in section.

THE HEART

The heart is a specialized portion of the vascular system that develops from an enlargement of two veins in the embryo. It has three coats.

Endocardium

The endocardium, which corresponds to the intima of the vessels, includes an endothelial lining and a relatively thick subendothelial layer that is made up of connective tissue, smooth muscle, and elastic fibers. The valves of the heart are folds of the endocardium in which the fibroelastic elements are prominent. The annuli fibrosi are rings of elastic tissue that surround the openings from one chamber to another.

Myocardium

The myocardium is a muscular coat that corresponds to the media of the vessels. It is made up of interlacing bundles of muscle. The tissue, however, is not like that of the media of the vessels. It is not smooth muscle but is a specialized type, cardiac, that is found nowhere

Purkinje fibers

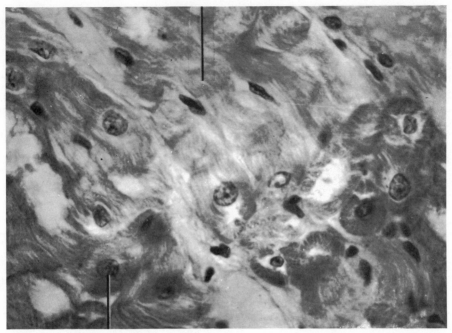

Nucleus of fiber

Fig. 8-8
Purkinje fibers of heart. (×640.)

else in the body. The nature of this muscle has been discussed in Chapter 4.

Epicardium

The epicardium is the visceral portion of the pericardial sac enclosing the heart. Its lining consists of a single layer of flattened mesothelial cells. Subjacent to the mesothelial cells is a fibrous layer containing scattered elastic fibers. The epicardium is attached to the myocardium by a layer of vascularized areolar connective tissue, the subepicardial layer.

Valves of the heart

The atrioventricular valves consist of folds of endocardium subtended on a region consisting of bundles of collagenous fibers. These in turn are continuous with the fibers of the annuli fibrosi and chordae tendinae. The semilunar valves are similar in structure to the atrioventricular valves except that they lack muscle fibers.

Purkinje's fibers

In addition to the foregoing elements the heart includes a peculiar group of fibers known as the atrioventricular bundle of His and a similar collection called the sinoatrial node. These fibers are larger and paler in color than the cardiac muscle fibers. They were described by Purkinje and hence are often called Purkinje's fibers (Fig. 8-8). It is believed that this system of fibers correlates the contraction of different parts of the heart.

LYMPHATIC SYSTEM

The lymphatic system consists of lymph capillaries and vessels but is unlike the blood vascular system in that it does not form a complete circuit through which the fluid leaves and returns to a central propelling organ. Lymph capillaries begin in the connective tissues, from which they collect tissue fluid. The latter passes as lymph from the capillaries to larger vessels that join together, forming ultimately the thoracic duct and the right lymphatic dict. The thoracic duct is the larger of the two, since it alone receives lymph drainage from the abdomen. It empties its contents into the bloodstream at the junction of the left internal jugular and left subclavian veins. In some cases there is a right lymphatic duct opening into the corresponding veins on the right side of the body, but the single duct on this side is often replaced by several smaller lymphatics.

Lymphatic vessels are thin walled and less conspicuous than the blood vessels. The structure of the larger lymphatics most nearly resembles that of the veins, but instead of containing blood they are filled with a granular coagulum containing a few lymphocytes. The large lymphatics are with granular coagulum containing a few lymphocytes. The large lymphatics are composed of three coats: (1) an intima of endothelium and subendothelial tissue, (2) a media of circular muscle with little elastic tissue, and (3) an adventitia of loose connective tissue with scattered bundles of longitudinal muscle. They have numerous valves and are distinguishable from veins chiefly through the absence of blood in them.

9
LYMPHOID ORGANS

The lymphoid organs include the lymph nodes, the spleen, the tonsils, and the thymus. Of these four organs the first three are composed of lymphoid tissue and form part of the defensive mechanism of the body. The thymus is placed with them tentatively because of a morphological similarity that may be deceptive. Lymphoid tissue consists of reticular tissue infiltrated with lymphocytes. The reticular tissue is evenly distributed throughout the organs, but the lymphocytes are more concentrated in some regions than in others, such concentrations being known as nodules. These are to be found in the lymph node, the tonsil, and the spleen and are also widely distributed along the digestive tract, occurring singly or in groups.

Before considering the distribution and arrangement of lymphoid tissue in the organs just mentioned it seems appropriate to point out that this tissue is widely distributed throughout the digestive and respiratory tracts and other parts of the body in a form not sharply differentiated from the rest of the surrounding connective tissue. This is usually referred to as a diffuse lymphoid tissue in contrast to the denser form, such as the lymph nodules, in which the lymphocytes are more closely aggregated.

LYMPH NODE (Fig. 9-1)

A lymph node, or gland, is a mass of lymphoid tissue, the function of which is to filter lymph and to form new lymphocytes. There are many such nodes scattered along the course of the lymph vessels of the body. They are small bean-shaped organs, whitish in color in the fresh specimen. When stained with hematoxylin and eosin, a section of a node appears as a mass of purple tissue enclosed in a connective tissue capsule. The capsule sends trabeculae toward the center of the node from various points along its convex surface, and a group of branching trabeculae extends inward from the indented surface or hilum. Under the low power of the microscope it may be seen that the lymphocytes which give the organ its dark color are not evenly distributed. In the peripheral portion, or cortex, dense aggregations of lymphocytes, known as nodules, appear (Fig. 9-2). When lymphocyte production is active, the primary nodule has at its center a light area, the secondary nodule or germinal center. In the medulla of the lymph node the lymphocytes are collected in uneven clumps with no germinal centers. Between these central masses (medullary cords) there are areas of reticular tissue that are almost entirely free from lymphocytes. These are the medullary sinuses through which the lymph flows. Each sinus intervenes between a medullary cord on the one hand and a trabecula on the other. In a similar fashion one may see that there is a sinus interposed between the capsule and the cortex and that this peripheral sinus courses down along the trabeculae to join the system of anastomosing medullary sinuses. The cortical nodules are not sharply separated from each other or from the cords at the border of the medulla.

Afferent lymph vessels approach the convex surface of the node and pierce the capsule, opening into the cortical sinuses. From there the lymph passes to the medullary sinuses and is eventually collected at the hilum in the efferent vessels. Valves in both sets of vessels prevent the lymph from reversing its direction. Arteries enter the node of the hilum, run for varying distances in the trabeculae, and give off branches that break up into capillaries in the reticular tissue of the node, thus supplying nutriment to the organ. Veins return in the trabeculae and leave at the hilum.

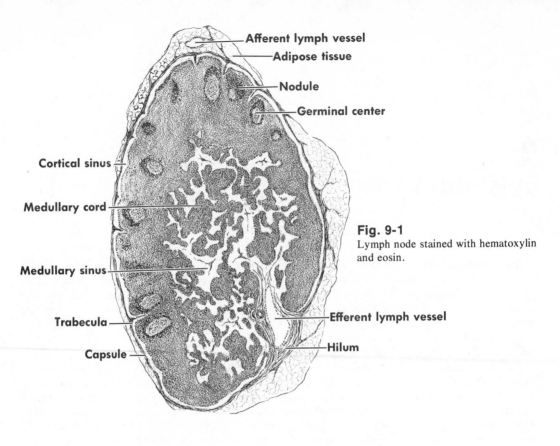

Afferent lymph vessel

Adipose tissue

Nodule

Germinal center

Cortical sinus

Medullary cord

Medullary sinus

Trabecula

Capsule

Efferent lymph vessel

Hilum

Fig. 9-1
Lymph node stained with hematoxylin and eosin.

Capsule

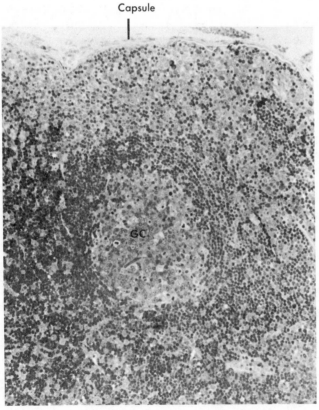

GC

Fig. 9-2
Photomicrograph (plastic section) of the cortex of a cat lymph node, showing germinal center, **GC.** (×160.)

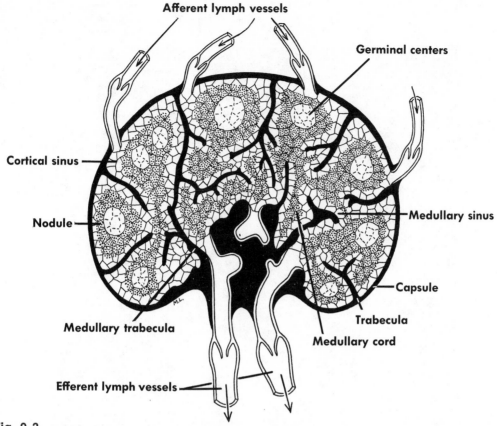

Fig. 9-3

Diagram showing relationship of lymph node to lymphatic vessels. Arterial and venous supply of lymph node are not indicated in this diagram. (Redrawn from Maximow-Bloom.)

The organization of the lymph node is illustrated in Fig. 9-3.

The basic structure of the node consists of a meshwork of reticular fibers that makes up the framework in which free cells occur. The cells are predominantly lymphocytes and may be either large, medium, or small. The small lymphocytes are the most numerous type in the germinal centers. The large lymphocytes are least numerous, and they have a more extensive cytoplasm, which is basophilic, and a large vesicular nucleus. The reticular cells, members of the reticuloendothelial system, have an irregular shape and extensive cell processes. They may on occasion become free macrophages. Plasma cells are usually quite numerous, too. Blood cells, both white and red, also may be found in the node.

Cortex

Capsule and trabeculae. The capsule and trabeculae are composed of dense white fibrous tissue, with occasional elastic and smooth muscle fibers. In the capsule one may usually see the afferent lymph vessels, while the trabeculae contain small blood vessels.

Cortical sinuses. Cortical sinuses, and those that course inward along the sides of the trabeculae, are not definite vessels enclosed in an endothelium. They are merely open spaces in the reticular framework of the node, containing primitive reticular cells and macrophages but relatively few lymphocytes. The lymph seeps through the meshes of the reticular tissue in the sinuses.

Nodules. The nodules have a groundwork of reticular tissue like that of the sinuses. If secondary nodules are present, they appear as regions of closely packed pale cells.

Blood vessels. In addition to the vessels already mentioned as located in the trabeculae, the substance of the cortex contains numerous capillaries. These are so small that they do not form a prominent feature of the cortex.

93

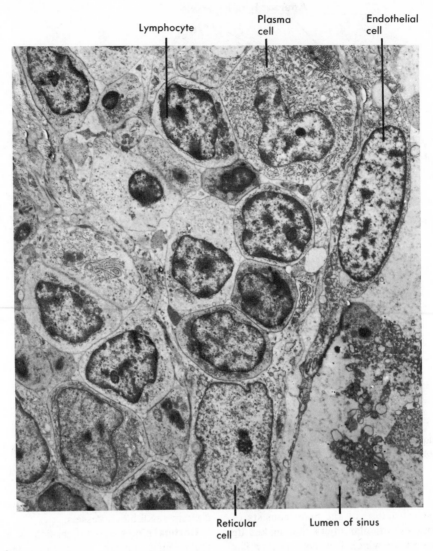

Fig. 9-4
Electron micrograph of part of medullary cord of lymph node of a cat in region of medullary sinus. (×4,800.)

Medulla

Medullary cords. The medullary cords are like the cortical nodules in the great number of lymphocytes present in them. They differ from nodules, however, in their irregular shape and because they do not at any time possess germinal centers. They are accompanied and surrounded by medullary sinuses (Fig. 9-4).

Medullary sinuses. Medullary sinuses are like the peripheral sinus in structure and lie between the cords and the trabeculae of the medulla.

Medullary trabeculae. Medullary trabeculae are composed of dense white fibrous tissue and form a branching system radiating from the hilum that is part of the framework of the gland. Like the trabeculae of the cortex they include blood vessels. Efferent lymph vessels are prominent in the connective tissue of the hilum.

• • •

The lymph node has a dual function. It is a center for the production of lymphocytes, and it is a phagocytic organ in which lymph is purified. The latter function is performed by the fixed macrophages of the reticular stroma.

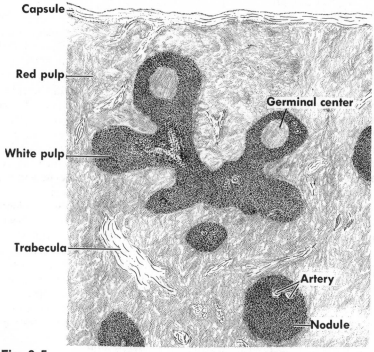

Capsule

Red pulp

Germinal center

White pulp

Trabecula

Artery

Nodule

Fig. 9-5
Spleen stained with hematoxylin and eosin.

SPLEEN (Fig. 9-5)

The spleen is the largest of the lymphoid organs. In man it is a mass of lymphoid tissue 5 to 6 inches long and 4 inches wide. It has been shown that the lymph node consists essentially of a mass of lymphoid tissue placed in the path of one or more lymph vessels, serving as a filter for lymph. In a similar manner the spleen is interposed in the blood vascular system to remove impurities from the blood. Under low-power magnification the spleen is seen to be lighter in color and not as purple as the lymph node. The greater part of a section of spleen is reddish in color when stained with hematoxylin and eosin. Scattered through this reddish tissue, or pulp, are nodules of deep purple. This is the white pulp that contains nodules. There is no regular arrangement of nodules about the periphery of the organ and no division into cortex and medulla (Fig. 9-5). The nodules are pierced by small arteries and lack germinal centers in adult man. The general arrangement of capsule and trabeculae is like that in the lymph node; that is, a series of trabeculae run in from the surrounding capsule on the convex surface, and a system of strands of connective tissue radiates inward from the hilum. Since sections of the spleen are usually prepared from small pieces of the organ, this arrangement of trabeculae is not seen in them.

Blood enters the spleen at the hilum, and the arteries run in the trabeculae for some distance. They enter the pulp, however, while they still have the coats common to small arteries—intima, media, and adventitia. In the pulp the vessels ramify, and it is usually at the point of branching that the nodules are to be found. After passing through the nodules the arteries emerge into the red pulp as the penicilli, in which three parts may be distinguished. The first part (arteriole of the pulp) is of fine caliber and the longest division of the penicillus. This divides into a number of vessels called the sheathed arteries, and these, in turn, divide into two or three branches of the structure of arterial capillaries that may connect with the venous sinuses of the red pulp.

There are several theories concerning the course of the blood after it passes through the arterial capillaries. According to one view it goes directly into the reticular meshwork of the red pulp instead of passing by way of a continuous endothelial tubule to the venules. This is the "open circulation" theory. Other workers believe that no such "dumping" of corpuscles into the reticulum occurs and that the arterial capillaries lead to capillaries that in turn connect with the venules. This is the "closed circulation" theory. The third view is that some arterioles open directly into the pulp, while others connect with venules through capillaries.

The venous circulation begins with the splenic sinus, which is composed of an open-work endothelium through which corpuscles may pass readily. From the splenic sinuses venules lead away and join each other, running back to the trabeculae. Blood leaves at the hilum. The circulation of the spleen is diagramed in Fig. 9-6.

Capsule and trabeculae

The capsule and trabeculae consist of dense white connective tissue with scattered fibers of smooth muscle, much like the corresponding structure in the lymph node. The capsule of the spleen, however, since the organ borders on the body cavity, is covered by the mesothelium, which appears as a layer of squamous epithelium. This is often destroyed in preparing the specimen.

Red pulp

The framework of the pulp is reticular tissue. Since the blood circulation opens directly into it, it contains all types of blood cells in the reticular meshwork. The numerous erythrocytes give the pulp its red color, both in the fresh and in the stained specimen (Fig. 9-7).

Among the reticular cells and corpuscles will be found free macrophages. These cells have vesicular nuclei and stain readily with eosin. They ingest fragments of worn-out erythrocytes, which may be seen in their cytoplasm. The macrophages are distributed throughout the red pulp but are most easily distinguished among the blood cells in the lumen of a sinus. The name splenic cells, which is sometimes given to them, is misleading, as they are not different from other free macrophages found in organs other than the spleen.

Two kinds of blood vessels in the red pulp are of unusual structure. The more prominent of these are the splenic sinuses. These vessels are the beginning of the venous system. They may be recognized as small spaces in the pulp surrounded by a ring of endothelium-like cells whose nuclei project into the lumina of the vessels. Ordinarily, endothelial cells are closely joined, and their nuclei are flattened so as to project only slightly into the lumen of the vessel they surround. In the splenic sinus these cells are loosely grouped, and the lack of tension of the cytoplasm permits the nuclei to extend into the vessel. These cells are surrounded by a loose arrangement of reticular tissue forming a latticework through which the corpuscles may pass. They are phagocytic and belong to the reticuloendothelial system.

The other type of blood vessel peculiar to the red pulp is the sheathed artery (second portion of the penicillus). Sheathed arteries are of capillary diameter and consist of endothelium plus a thin covering of concentrically placed cells that are probably reticular. The vessels are inconspicuous elements of the red pulp in human beings and require special stains for adequate demonstration.

White pulp

The white pulp, like the red, has a groundwork of reticular tissue, but differs from it in containing large numbers of lymphocytes as well as monocytes and plasma cells. It thus resembles the medullary cords of a lymph node. It surrounds the arteries from the point where they leave the trabeculae to their division into penicilli, actually invading and replacing the adventitial connective tissue of the vessels. Elastic fibers belonging to the walls of the arteries are scattered through the white pulp.

At various points, particularly where the vessels branch, the white pulp contains nodules that form extensions of its substance asymmetrically placed with respect to the artery. In fetal life and childhood the nodules contain germinal centers, and these persist into adult life in some animals but not in man.

It will be remembered that all kinds of red and white blood cells are formed in the spleen during embryonic life. One would therefore find in embryonic spleens the precursors of the corpuscles, including giant cells. These, like the germinal centers of the nodules, may persist into adult life in some forms.

Functions of the spleen

The spleen is known to have four functions: First, it is of importance in the metabolism and distribution of the erythrocytes. It acts as a

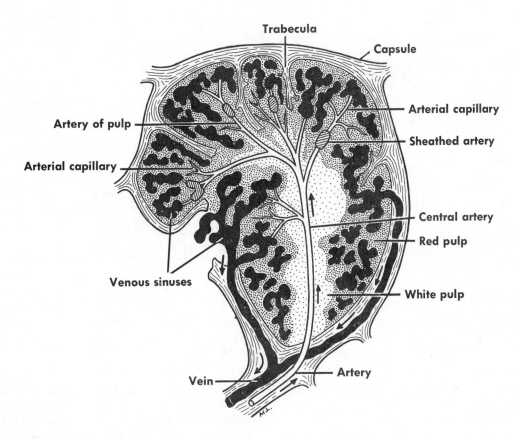

Fig. 9-6
Diagram showing circulation of blood in spleen. (Redrawn from Maximow-Bloom.)

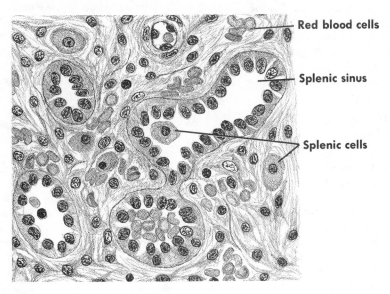

Fig. 9-7
Spleen, high magnification.

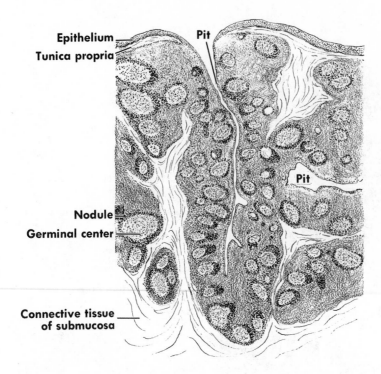

Epithelium
Tunica propria
Pit
Pit
Nodule
Germinal center
Connective tissue of submucosa

Fig. 9-8
Tonsil stained with hematoxylin and eosin.

storehouse for healthy corpuscles, retaining varying numbers of them according to the demands of the body as a whole. The free macrophages of the red pulp ingest fragments of worn-out red blood cells, and the hemoglobin set free by the disintegration of corpuscles is stored in reticular cells. Second, it purifies the blood, since its phagocytes destroy infective agents. Third, it produces new blood cells. In this respect the human spleen is most active during infancy and childhood. Fourth, it produces antibodies that are derived from plasma cells and are concerned with immunological processes.

TONSILS (Fig. 9-8)
Palatine tonsil

The tonsils are masses of lymphoid tissue embedded in the lining of the throat between the arches of the palate. Their arrangement is best understood by reference to the structure of the wall of the pharynx. This consists of a layer of stratified squamous epithelium resting on a tunica propria of reticular or fine areolar tissue. Beneath this lies the submucosa of coarser areolar tissue, which contains scattered mucous glands. The tonsil develops between the tunica propria and the submucosa; as it enlarges it elevates the former and depresses the latter.

The epithelium of the mucosa does not go smoothly over the surface of the tonsil but dips down in numerous deep pits, or fossae. Under low magnification the tonsil appears as a mass of lymphoid tissue, bordered on one side by stratified squamous epithelium and surrounded on the other sides by areolar tissue, which forms a tough capsule immediately around it. The mucous glands sometimes found in the areolar tissue outside the capsule are not part of the tonsil but belong to the pharyngeal wall. Noticeable features of the organ are its deep pits lined with stratified squamous epithelium and the presence of numerous germinal centers. The latter are usually grouped around the pits, but there is no division into cortex and medulla.

The pits (crypts) surrounded by lymphatic tissue are partially separated from each other by connective tissue derived from the capsule. Lymphocytes, mast cells, and plasma cells occur in this connective tissue; also, heterophilic leukocytes may be present, which indicates a mild inflammatory condition. In the deeper regions of the crypts an infiltration of lymphocytes displaces the epithelium of the crypts to a considerable degree. Some of these cells pass through the epithelium and are eventually found in the saliva as the salivary corpuscles.

The lumina of the crypts often contain ac-

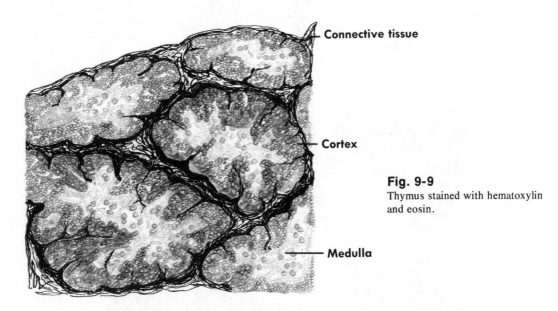

Connective tissue

Cortex

Fig. 9-9
Thymus stained with hematoxylin and eosin.

Medulla

cumulations of living and degenerating lymphocytes, desquamated epithelial cells detritus, and microorganisms. These latter are said to cause inflammation and suppuration.

Pharyngeal tonsil

The pharyngeal tonsil is a median aggregation of lymphoid tissue that lies in the wall of the nasopharynx. In this region the epithelium, as is characteristic of the nasopharynx, is chiefly of the pseudostratified ciliated columnar variety. Patches of stratified squamous epithelium also occur and become more numerous in the adult. The lymphoid tissue is similar to that of the palatine tonsil. The capsule of this organ is thin and contains many fine elastic fibers that radiate into the core of the folds.

The tonsils generally reach their highest state of development in childhood and then usually undergo involution. Unlike the lymph nodes the tonsils do not possess lymphatic sinuses, and hence lymph is not filtered through them. They do, however, possess lymph capillaries that end blindly about the outer surface of the tonsil. The only established function of the tonsils is the formation of lymphocytes.

THYMUS (Figs. 9-9 to 9-11)

The thymus develops as an outgrowth from the pharyngeal wall of the embryo and has a groundwork of epithelial (endodermal) rather than connective tissue (mesenchymal) origin. In later development the groundwork is in-

filtrated with cells closely resembling lymphocytes in appearance that are probably derived from mesenchyme. It is claimed by some investigators that these small, darkly staining cells develop from the cells of the supporting framework and are, therefore, also endodermal in origin. The small cells are generally called thymocytes, a name that does not commit one to either view as to their origin.

The fully developed thymus resembles the other members of the lymphoid group, with which it is here placed, in having a groundwork of relatively large, branching cells, infiltrated with small, deeply staining elements. It differs from them in that it contains neither sinuses nor germinal centers, so that there is no morphological evidence that it serves either as a filter or as a source of new lymphocytes.

Under the low magnification (Figs. 9-9 and 9-10) the thymus appears as a mass of purple and reddish tissue, embedded in a loose investment of connective tissue. The capsule and trabeculae are less definitely organized than those of the lymph node and spleen. The organ is much lobulated and is divided into a cortex and medulla. Of these, the former is the more dense and is a deeper purple in color than the medulla, which is pink when stained with eosin. The medullary substance extends from a central core into each lobule. Often a lobule is so cut that the connection of its medullary substance with the central core is not apparent, and it seems as if a mass of the lighter tissue were completely

Capsule

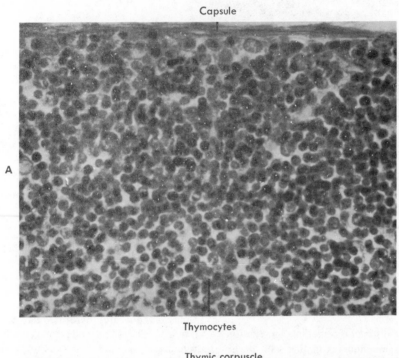

A

Thymocytes

Thymic corpuscle

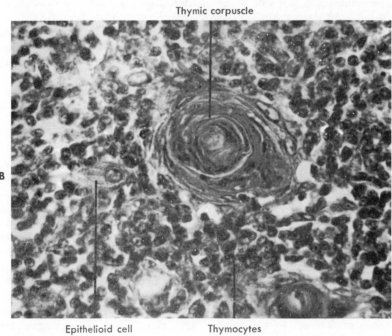

B

Epithelioid cell   Thymocytes

Fig. 9-10
A, Section of cortex of thymus. (×640.) B, Section of medulla of thymus. (×640.)

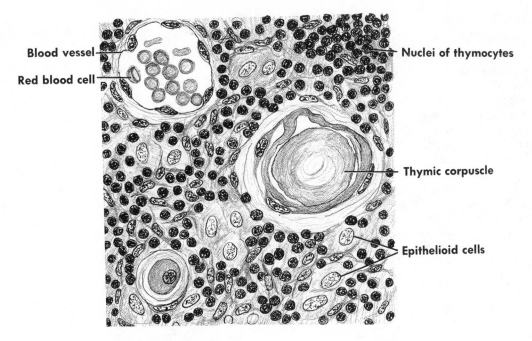

Blood vessel — **Red blood cell** — **Nuclei of thymocytes** — **Thymic corpuscle** — **Epithelioid cells**

Fig. 9-11
Thymus medulla. Dark nuclei in thymocytes.

surrounded by cortical substance. If the lobule is small, it may look like a nodule with a germinal center, an appearance that is deceptive, since there are no centers in the thymus.

Under the high magnification (Fig. 9-11) two types of cells may readily be distinguished in the medulla. They are (1) epithelioid cells, which have an irregular branching form like that of reticular tissue cells but are somewhat larger than the reticular cells of the lymph node, and (2) the thymocytes, which closely resemble small lymphocytes; they have dark nuclei and hardly any visible cytoplasm.

Some investigators believe that the thymus also contains true reticular cells, which are found together with reticular fibers, in the neighborhood of blood vessels. In other parts of the stroma there are, few, if any, fibers. Another feature of the medulla of the thymus is the thymic corpuscle (Hassall's corpuscle). This is a group of cells ranging from 12 to 180μ in diameter. It has a hyaline center, staining red with eosin, that seems to be derived from degenerating cells, since it may contain several pyknotic nuclei. Around this center there are compressed cells concentrically arranged in a sort of whorl. Except for the hyaline center with

its degenerating nuclei, the corpuscle somewhat resembles the small arteries that ramify through the thymic medulla. The cortex of the thymus consists of epithelioid cells and thymocytes, but in this region the latter are so concentrated as to obscure the former.

It will be seen from the foregoing description that a section of the thymus stained with hematoxylin and eosin presents an appearance much like that of a section of a lymphoid organ lacking sinuses and germinal centers. When the organ is studied from the point of view of the origin and behavior of its cells, however, it seems doubtful whether it is, in fact, lymphoid.

SUMMARY AND COMPARISON OF THE LYMPHOID ORGANS
Lymph node

The lymph node consists of cortex and medulla. The cortex contains nodules that may have germinal centers, peripheral sinus, and sinuses in addition to the trabeculae. The medulla is composed of cords, sinuses, and trabeculae. The capsule and trabeculae are of dense connective tissue, with scattered fibers of smooth muscle in the former. The lymph node filters lymph and produces new lymphocytes.

101

Spleen

The spleen has neither cortex nor medulla. It is composed of pulp with many red blood cells in the meshes of the reticular tissue. It has open blood circulation with sheathed arteries and venous sinuses. The nodules contain no germinal centers in the human adult but surround small arteries. The capsule of connective tissue is covered by mesothelium. The spleen filters the blood.

Tonsil

The tonsil is a mass of lymphoid tissue embedded in the wall of the pharynx. It is covered by stratified squamous epithelium that dips into the substance of the organ, forming the pits. Lymph nodules with germinal centers are grouped around the pits. There are no sinuses. The tonsil forms lymphocytes.

Thymus

The thymus is divided into cortex and medulla and is composed of epithelioid cells and thymocytes that resemble lymphocytes. The medulla contains thymic corpuscles. The cortex is a dense mass of thymocytes and epithelioid tissue.

The thymus produces a humoral agent that is effective in stimulating the production of lymphocytes in lymphoid organs. It is also responsible for establishing and regulating immunological reactions.

10
GLANDS

Glands are a prominent feature of each of the several organs to be considered. Accordingly, a general survey and orientation of typical characteristics of glands will be discussed here.

Glands are composed of epithelial cells that perform the highly specialized function of producing *secretions*. These cells remove raw materials from tissue fluid or lymph and from them synthesize substances that ordinarily are not utilized by the gland cell itself to any great degree. The secretory products are released upon free surfaces or into the blood-lymphatic complex of vessels for distribution to sites where the secretion products are utilized. Some glandular secretions are stored until the demands of the organism require the substance involved. In others the secretions are elaborated and released either continually or intermittently.

Excretion, sometimes used interchangeably with secretion, is a process by means of which the end products of carbohydrate, fat, protein, and mineral metabolism are removed from the internal medium of the organism. Thus, liver cells can remove decomposition products of hemoglobin from the blood and convert them into bile salts and bile pigments, which are then passed into the bile system and eventually into the small intestine. Bile salts utilized in lipid absorption and digestion are resorbed and reutilized a number of times. Bile salts may accordingly be considered as secretion products. The bile pigments, by contrast, not utilized in the body are eliminated with the fecal mass. These pigments may be considered to be excretions produced by a secretory mechanism. Certain cells in kidney tubules are capable of adding substances to urine by secretory processes. The sweat glands secrete a modified tissue fluid that serves several functions, one of them at least being excretory. Even the salivary glands are partially excretory by virtue of their ability to

remove salts, the thiocyanate ion, and urea from the body fluid. *Elimination* is the process by which excretions, secretions, and undigested food residue are expelled by the organism.

ENDOCRINE GLANDS

The endocrine glands, or glands of internal secretion, may have ducts in the embryonic state, but in the adult they are absent. They are accordingly classed as ductless glands. The secretions of endocrine glands may be stored or carried directly into blood capillaries, and it is by means of the latter that they are transported throughout the body to so-called target organs. The secretions of endocrine cells are called *hormones,* and in concert with the nervous system they regulate and coordinate the activities of all the cells in the body. In some instances hormones stimulate or suppress the activities of one or more specific glands or organs. In others, as in the case of thyroxin, they regulate the activities of *all* the cells of the body.

Hormones have a varied chemical composition. Some are proteins (insulin), some are modified amino acids (thyroxin), while others are modified sterols (cortisone-like substances, estrogens, androgens, etc.). Most endocrine glands have a dual function. The pancreas, for example, elaborates the hormone insulin as well as pancreatic fluid, which contains a mixture of enzymes and sodium bicarbonate and is accordingly classed as one of the *mixed glands* (that is, both endocrine and exocrine in function).

In glands with known endocrine function there are three major cell arrangements: clumps, follicles, and cords.

Clumps

In the clump type of arrangement, secretion and utilization are of approximately the same order of magnitude. The secretion is stored within the epithelioid cells themselves and is released upon demand into the abundant capillary network that permeates the clump. Examples of this type are the islands of Langerhans in the pancreas and the so-called interstitial cells in the testes. Clumps may be composed of small or large groups of irregularly shaped cells, but they do not form hollow spheres or tubes.

Follicles

A follicle consists of a cylinder or sphere of cells enclosing a cavity containing the stored secretion product. In the thyroid, consisting of many follicles, the cells are usually cuboidal, exhibiting a deeply staining secretion in the lumen called the colloid substance. Increased demand for the secretion results in a transfer from the lumen to the abundant capillary network surrounding each follicle. Depletion of the colloid reserves results in collapse of the follicle followed by the crowding of cells that appear columnar in transverse section. Since it is believed that a depleted reserve results in active secretory activity by the cells, the columnar form is associated with the active or secretory phase of these glands. In the embryo the follicles originate as clumps of epithelioid cells. These cells produce more secretion than can either be utilized or stored within the cells. The secretion is accordingly stored in cavities formed between the cells and thus gives rise to the space known as the "lumen" of the follicle.

Cords

In the cord arrangement the epithelioid cells are arranged in rows. The liver cords consist of two plates of cells closely aligned, while the adrenal cortex exhibits many subparallel rows of cells. Secretions are stored within the cells and transferred to the abundant capillary network as required.

Epithelioid cells

By definition epithelia line cavities. With the exception of the follicular arrangement, endocrine gland cells do not line cavities. Prominent cuboidal or polygonal cells may occur in small or large irregular masses or in cords but invariably lack a cavity. For this special situation the term *epithelioid* (epithelium-like) was introduced. When epithelioid cells occur, one is led to suspect an endocrine function; however, physiological demonstration of endocrine activity is necessary before an endocrine role can definitely

be ascribed to these cells. Cases in point are the thymus gland and the juxtaglomerular apparatus in the kidneys of rodents.

EXOCRINE GLANDS

Exocrine glands, or glands of external secretion, retain connections with surfaces. Unicellular glands (for example, mucous cells) discharge their secretions directly on a free surface. Multicellular glands (for example, the salivary glands) discharge via a system of simple or branching ducts.

Ducts

There are several types of ducts: secretory, excretory, and intercalated.

Secretory ducts. One kind of secretory duct is lined by the glandular cells that produce the secretion (Fig. 10-1, *C* to *E*). In the salivary glands another type of secretory duct is found that contains glandular cells supplying additional substances to the secretion produced at some distance removed from the main gland cells. Special techniques demonstrate the presence of basal striations in these cells, and hence they are frequently called *striated ducts*.

Excretory ducts. Excretory ducts are formed of simple epithelium that presumably conducts secretions without taking part in the elaboration of major secretory components (Fig. 10-1, *D*, *F* to *H*).

Intercalated ducts. Intercalated ducts are interposed between the glandular units and their conducting portions (for example, striated or excretory ducts). The intercalated ducts are lined with flattened cells that presumably do not produce a secretion. The latter are found only in the larger glands (for example, pancreas and salivary glands).

Classification

The simplest glandular unit is the unicellular gland, which consists of a cell that forms part of a lining epithelium and also elaborates a secretion. The goblet cells scattered along the lining of the intestine and respiratory tract are of this type.

The next simplest type is the intra-epithelial gland, consisting of a strip of consecutive glandular cells forming a slight thickening or pocket entirely within the limits of the epithelium. The lining epithelium of the gut contains fingerlike or tubular projections of glandular cells that are below the level of the epithelium in the under-

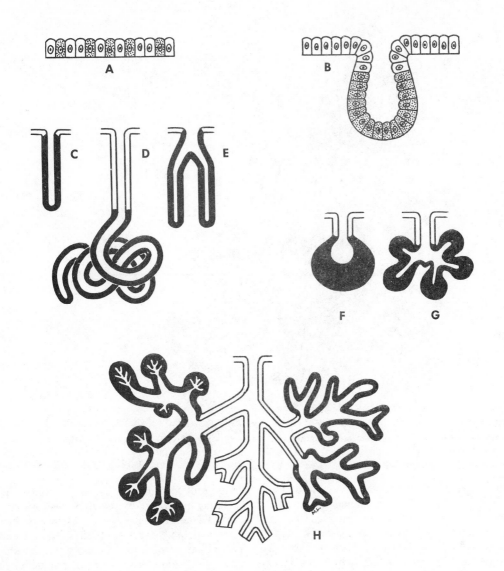

Fig. 10-1

Diagram showing different types of arrangement of glandular tissue. **A,** Glandular cells (granular) scattered among common epithelial cells (clear). **B,** Glandular cells forming saclike invagination into underlying tissue. **C,** Simple tubular gland. **D,** Simple tubular gland coiled. **E,** Simple branched tubular gland. **F,** Simple alveolar gland. **G,** Simple branched alveolar gland. **H,** Compound gland. (Redrawn from Maximow-Bloom.)

lying connective tissue (Fig. 10-1, *B*), maintaining their connection to the surface by means of a duct.

Another means of classifying glands is by the manner and degree to which branching of the excretory or striated ducts occurs. If the ducts are absent (Fig. 10-1, *C*) or unbranched (Fig. 10-1, *D*), the glands are termed *simple.* If the ducts branch (Fig. 10-1, *E*), the gland is called a *compound gland.*

Simple and compound glands are further sub-divided according to the shapes of the secreting portions as follows: tubular, alveolar (acinar), and tubulo-alveolar. The name tubular is self-explanatory; an alveolar gland has secreting portions that are spherical or flask shaped, whereas the tubulo-alveolar variety may exhibit glandular portions intermediate between the two types already mentioned (Fig. 10-1, *H,* left side). Another variety of tubulo-alveolar gland consists of tubular units and alveolar units attached to the same excretory duct. The simple

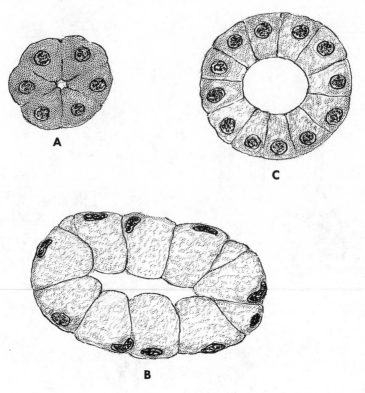

Fig. 10-2
Types of serous and mucus-secreting epithelium. **A,** Serous alveolus. **B,** Alveolus secreting thick mucus. **C,** Alveolus secreting thin mucus.

tubular gland is further differentiated into tubular, coiled tubular, or branching tubular (Fig. 10-1, *C* to *E*). Also illustrated in Fig. 10-1, *G,* is the branching alveolar type. Other kinds of glands have been described, such as those in the eyelid, but because of their highly specialized function and limited distribution they will not be discussed here. Other classifications depend on the mode of secretion (holocrine, merocrine, apocrine) and on the product of secretion (mucous, serous, mixed, zymogenic, etc.).

Secretions

The secretions of exocrine glands are varied, but at present none of these has been identified as a hormone. (The case for parotin has not been confirmed as yet.) Mucigen, for example, is an inadequately characterized mixture of carbohydrate and protein; zymogen (a precursor of enzymes) is in part protein and forms an important component of many serous secretions; sebum and cerumen contain protein, carbohydrate, and much lipid; in addition, secre-

tions produced by the sweat, lacrimal, and lactating glands are extremely varied and complex. Glands, such as the testes, ovaries, and lymphoid and myeloid tissues, are usually classed as *cytogenous glands,* since the chief activity of these glands is the production of living cells.

As we have just mentioned the modes of secretion are utilized in classifying certain glands. In the case of *holocrine* secretion the secretory product is stored in the gland cell, and the entire gland cell is extruded and destroyed in the process of secretion. The sebaceous glands are of this type. In *apocrine* secretion the secretory product accumulates in one or more large vacuoles below the free surface of the cell. During secretion a thin film of surface cytoplasm is removed with the secretory globules; the cell itself, however, is not usually destroyed in the process. In *merocrine* secretion there is a cyclic increase and decrease of the secretory product, which is more or less continually released into the lumen of the gland without, however, destroying the cell or depleting the cytoplasm. Typical of this variety are the glands of the oral cavity and digestive tract.

Unicellular glands

The simplest glands are composed of one cell, and the commonest representative of this group is the mucous or *goblet cell*. These cells are found in profusion in the digestive tract and in parts of the respiratory system. They are initially observed as tall columnar cells with elongate elliptical nuclei, distinguishable from their neighbors only by the absence of cilia or striated border. In the supranuclear position, minute granules and then droplets of mucigen appear, which migrate and accumulate at the free border of the cell. As more mucigen droplets accumulate in the cell, the nucleus is forced toward the base with concomitant changes in form from elliptical to a round and deeply staining conical form, until finally it appears as a flattened disc near the base of the cell. In addition, the apex of the cell expands laterally and distorts the neighboring epithelial cells. At this stage the cell looks like a goblet, with a narrow stem containing the nucleus and an expanded goblet cell containing the nonstaining mucigen droplets in what appears to be a large cavity. In many instances the mucigen droplets nearest the surface are gradually released and dispersed in modified tissue fluid to form the viscid fluid known as *mucus*. In other instances the mucigen globules are released en masse; the goblet then collapses and appears as an irregularly outlined tall columnar cell consisting of a narrow strip of cytoplasm containing a deeply staining, incredibly thin nucleus. The process of secretion is cyclic and may be repeated a number of times before the cell is replaced.

The presence of a large mass of nonstaining mucigen in hematoxylin and eosin preparations gives the impression of a large vacuole in cells filled with secretion. The principal ingredient of mucigen is a polysaccharide-containing protein called *mucin*. In addition to its adhesive properties it has the ability to combine with and coagulate in the presence of acids to form a protective coating on surfaces. The para-aminosalicylic acid (PAS) reaction demonstrates the polysaccharide moiety as a red to purplish red staining region. Certain aluminum-containing stain mixtures (micicarmine, mucihematin) stain mucigen droplets a vivid red or blue.

Multicellular glands

The example commonly used to illustrate the multicellular variety is the salivary glands. In these and in other similar glands the cells are grouped into *secretory units*. These are of three types: mucous, serous, and seromucous, or mixed, units. They are usually arranged in alveoli (acini) and branched or straight tubules.

Mucous units are composed of a type of cuboidal epithelium, which is so disposed about a small lumen that the cells take on the form of truncated pyramids and are accordingly called pyramidal cells. At the beginning of a secretory cycle the nuclei tend to be round or ovoid and occupy a position nearer to the base of the cell rather than the center. As the mucigen globules accumulate near the lumen of the gland, the nuclei are displaced toward the base and are compressed to such an extent that they appear as flattened darkly staining rods in contact with the cell boundary. Some authors maintain that mucous units with rounded nuclei secrete thin mucus, but in view of their cyclic activity this contention would be difficult to verify. Since the mucigen takes up so much of the volume of the cytoplasm and does not stain with hematoxylin and eosin, the cytoplasm of these cells does not appear eosinophilic and may on occasion even exhibit a pale bluish color. In certain of the salivary glands the mucous units are easily detected under low power of the microscope as very pale areas. With PAS the mucigen stains such a deep purplish red that all cellular detail may be obscured. Although these cells exhibit cyclic activity, the release of secretion is gradual and typical of the merocrine type of secretion.

Serous units are also composed of pyramidal cells but differ in that their nuclei are always centrally disposed in the cell. Their secretion granules are either slightly or extremely acidophilic and are primarily protein in character. Since these cells frequently elaborate enzymes (which are partly protein), the secretion droplets within the cell are called *zymogen granules*. In many instances the granules are so small and so widely dispersed that the entire apex of the cell appears intensely acidophilic, while in other situations the granules are quite large and evenly distributed throughout the entire cell (Paneth's cells). These cells produce an inactive precursor of the enzyme (zymogen). Zymogens are sometimes transported for a considerable distance before being activated. Since these cells are actively engaged in protein synthesis, the presence of large amounts of ribonucleic acid (RNA) or basophil substance in the perinuclear and subnuclear positions correlates well with their function. The serous cells of the pancreatic acini in well-stained hematoxylin and eosin preparations exhibit acidophilic apices and basophilic bases. The serous units of the salivary glands may be distinguished from the mucous units by the more central position of their nuclei and much greater affinity for dyes.

Mixed units are composed of both mucous and serous cells. The most easily demonstrated mixed units are found in the submaxillary glands of man. In one type of mixed unit the mucous cells form a tubular portion joining the duct, while the terminal portion consists of the more deeply staining serous cells. Cn occasion the mucous cells are so numerous they crowd the serous cells away from the lumen and form a crescentic cap of deeply staining cells or *demilune*. Occasionally, a mucous cell is also extruded into the *demilune* complex. In section it is not always possible to distinguish between a "pure" mucous unit and the tubular portion of a mixed unit. A pure serous unit exhibits a small but distinct lumen in its center. In favorable sections through the terminal part of a mixed unit the serous cells are separated from the lumen by mucous cells. In tangential sections of a demilune one may observe serous cells only; a central lumen is usually lacking, however. The student should be careful to distinguish between the mixed unit and the *mixed gland,* the latter being composed of both mucous and serous glands and sometimes mixed units as well. Mixed glands of the type discussed here are also known as mucoserous or seromucous glands. The term mixed gland is also applied to glands that perform both an endocrine and an exocrine function. (Compare pancreas, ovary, etc.)

Occasionally, certain stellate contractile cells may be found between the secretory unit and its basement membrane. These cells are called basket or myoepithelial cells and contain thin prominent dark-staining crescentric nuclei. They are said to propel secretions into gland ducts as a result of their contraction.

A number of serous or albuminous cells of certain oral glands are slightly PAS positive and from a histochemical point of view are termed mucoserous cells. They are not, however, morphologically distinguishable from serous cells and are accordingly classed with them.

Glands that are neither serous nor mucous do not, as a matter of fact, form a group united by similarities of function or morphology. They are mentioned here merely to point out that many glandular organs exist that are not to be classified as serous or mucous. They are so varied that no general statement regarding them can be made, and they will be discussed individually in later chapters.

11

DIGESTIVE TRACT

The digestive tract is a hollow tube running from the oral cavity to the anus, modified in its various parts but consisting throughout of four coats or layers (Fig. 11-1).

Mucosa

The mucosa is made up of (1) an epithelial lining that borders on the lumen of the tract and rests upon (2) a tunica propria of reticular or fine areolar tissue. The tunica propria may contain glands, scattered fibers of smooth muscle, and lymph nodules. The nodules are often quite large, extending below the mucosa into the adjacent coat of the tract. Fine capillaries and lymphatics are present in the tunica propria. In the greater part of the digestive tube the mucosa includes a third layer (3), the muscularis mucosae, which is a thin coat of smooth muscle fibers.

Submucosa

The second coat of the wall is the submucosa. This is composed of areolar tissue, which contains a plexus of small blood vessels known as Heller's plexus. It also includes numerous lymphatics and a plexus of nerve fibers and ganglia (Meissner's plexus). In the esophagus and duodenum the submucosa has in it the end pieces of mucous glands. In other parts of the tube, lymphoid tissue extends from the mucosa into the submucosa.

Muscularis

The muscularis is a coat composed of two layers of muscle. The fibers of the inner layer are arranged circularly about the tube, while those of the outer layer lie in its long axis. This arrangement is followed throughout the tract, but in the stomach there is a third oblique layer next to the submucosa. Thickenings of the circu-

lar layer form sphincters at various points of the tract. In the upper end of the esophagus and the lower end of the rectum the muscle is striated; elsewhere it is smooth. The two layers of muscle are separated by a thin layer of connective tissue in which may be seen the myenteric (Auerbach's) plexus.

Adventitia or serosa

The fourth layer of the tract is composed of loose areolar tissue, frequently containing adipose tissue. In places where the tract borders on the body cavity the areolar tissue is covered by the mesothelium and is called the serosa; elsewhere it blends with the surrounding fascia and is called the adventitia.

• • •

Table 6 summarizes the coats of the digestive tract. Structures, the names of which are enclosed in parentheses, are present in some but not in all divisions of the tract.

ESOPHAGUS (Fig. 11-2)
Mucosa

The mucosa of the esophagus is distinguished from the remainder of the digestive tract by the fact that it is lined with stratified squamous epithelium, which rests upon a fairly thick tunica propria (Fig. 11-3). In many mammals the epithelium is cornified at its surface. There are two narrow zones of glands in the mucosa of the esophagus, one at its junction with the stomach and the other at the level of the cricoid cartilage. These glands, called superficial glands, are shallow, branching tubules secreting mucus into the lumen of the organ. The mucosa also contains small lymph nodules and scattered lymphoid tissue.

The muscularis mucosa is lacking in the

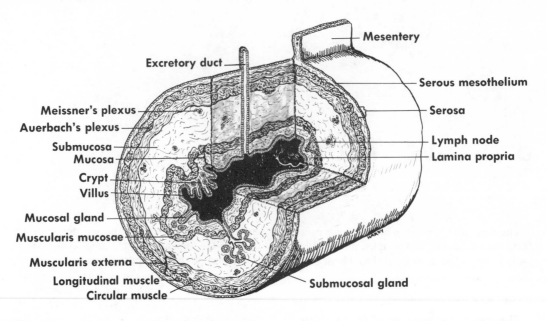

Fig. 11-1
Stereogram of general plan of gastrointestinal tract.

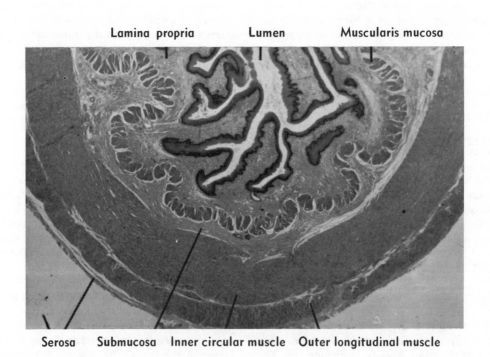

Fig. 11-2
Transverse section of esophagus of dog. (×16.) (From Bevelander, G.: Essentials of histology, ed. 6, St. Louis, 1970, The C. V. Mosby Co.)

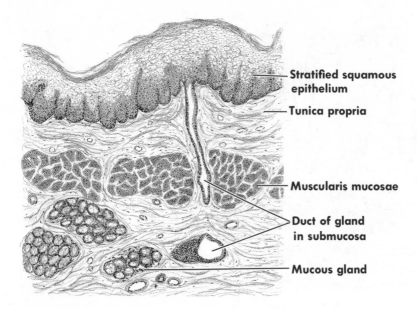

Fig. 11-3
Mucosa and submucosa of human esophagus.

Table 6. Coats of the digestive tract

1. Mucosa
   a. Epithelium
   b. Tunica propria containing
      (Glands)
      (Lymphoid tissue)
      (Scattered muscle fibers)
      Capillaries and small lymphatics
   c. (Muscularis mucosae)
2. Submucosa
   Areolar tissue, containing
      (Glands)
      (Lymphoid tissue)
      Heller's plexus of blood vessels
      Meissner's plexus of nerves
      Lymphatics
3. Muscularis
   a. (Oblique layer)
   b. Circular layer
   c. Connective tissue containing Auerbach's
      plexus of nerves
   d. Longitudinal layer
4. Adventitia or serosa
   Areolar tissue containing
      Adipose tissue
      Blood vessels
      (Mesothelial covering)

Parentheses indicate the structures present in some but not all divisions of the digestive tract.

upper part of the esophagus, its place being taken by a rather indefinite elastic membrane that separates the mucosa from the submucosa. Smooth muscle first appears about a fourth of the way down the tube in the form of scattered bundles longitudinally arranged. Further down the tract these are consolidated in a complete layer. A unique feature of the muscularis mucosa of the esophagus is that it is thicker than in any other part of the digestive tract; also, the fibers run in only one direction.

Submucosa

The submucosa of the esophagus is generally described as a layer of areolar tissue containing throughout its length blood vessels, nerves, and the secreting portion of mucous glands, the ducts of which run through the mucosa to open onto the epithelial surface. As a matter of fact, the glands are not constant in their distribution, and some animals (for example, the monkey) have few in this layer.

Muscularis

In the upper half of the esophagus the muscle is striated like that of the tongue. It is not, however, under the control of the will. In the lower half of the esophagus the muscle changes to the smooth variety; in the middle portion the two kinds may be found intermingled. The arrange-

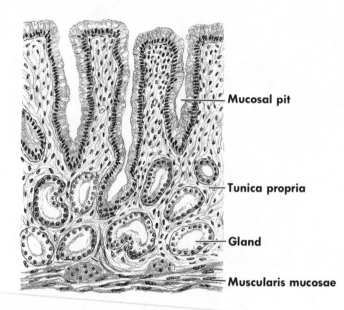

Mucosal pit

Tunica propria

Gland

Muscularis mucosae

Fig. 11-4
Mucosa of cardiac region of
monkey stomach.

ment of the muscular coats of the esophagus is less regular than that of other parts of the digestive tract. Two coats are present, but both may have the fibers obliquely placed, so that the typical orientation in an inner circular and an outer longitudinal layer may not be apparent. This is particularly true in the esophagus of the dog.

• • •

The mucosa and submucosa of the esophagus are illustrated in Fig. 11-3. Particular attention is called to the wide lumina of the ducts that lead from the glands of the submucosa to the surface.

STOMACH
Mucosa

At the junction of the esophagus and stomach the lining epithelium changes abruptly from stratified squamous to simple columnar, the cells of which secrete mucus. The epithelium of the stomach, unlike that of the small intestine, does not have a cuticular border. The surface of the mucosa is thrown into folds (rugae), the height and number of which depend on the degree of distention of the organ. In addition to the rugae the surface of the mucosa is marked by closely set pits, which are lined with the same sort of epithelium. Beneath the epithelium there is a tunica propria of reticular or fine areolar tissue, and below the level of the pits this layer contains glands. The shape and proportionate

depth of the pits and the characteristics of the glands are different in different parts of the stomach. At the junction of the esophagus and stomach the pits are shallow, and the glands, which are lined with a simple cuboidal epithelium, have wide lumina and secrete mucus (Fig. 11-4).

In the fundic region (Fig. 11-5) the mucosa is much deeper than in the zone immediately below the esophagus, and it contains a greater number of glands.

The lamina propria is reduced to a fine interglandular stroma in its deeper portion, and the pits extend only about one-fourth of the distance from the surface to the muscularis mucosae. The glands are called fundic glands, or (since they are found in all parts of the organ except the cardiac and pyloric zones) they may be called gastric glands.

The surface mucous cells cover the entire surface and line the pits. They are columnar cells with nuclei located in the basal region. With routine preparations the apical cytoplasm stains faintly and has a foamy appearance. The electron microscope shows dense elliptical secretory granules in the apical part of the cell. Each gastric gland is composed of four kinds of cells: (1) chief (peptic) cells, (2) parietal or oxyntic cells, (3) neck mucous cells, and (4) argentaffin cells.

The chief cells line the lower part of the gastric glands. They are of the low columnar variety and have the appearance of typical serous cells.

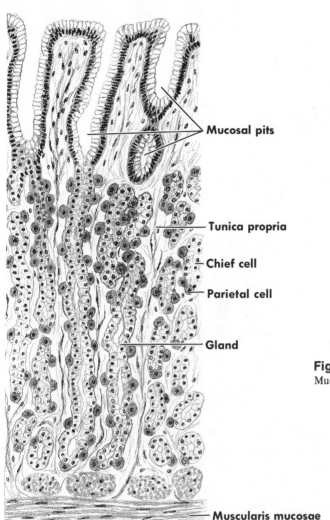

Mucosal pits

Tunica propria

Chief cell

Parietal cell

Gland

Fig. 11-5
Mucosa from fundus of stomach of monkey.

Muscularis mucosae

These cells contain abundant striated basophilic material corresponding to the cisternae of the endoplasmic reticulum. They also exhibit numerous mitochondria and secretory granules containing the precursor of pepsin.

The parietal cells are relatively large and intensely acidophilic. They are most numerous at the neck of the gland. They do not border directly on the lumen but are crowded away from it by the chief cells. The parietal cells appear somewhat oval, with the narrow end directed toward the lumen. These cells elaborate the antecedent of hydrochloric acid. At the electron microscope level it has been shown that the cytoplasm contains numerous mitochondria and surface indentations, the secretory canaliculi.

The surfaces of the canaliculi are lined with microvilli.

The neck mucous cells are relatively few in number, have a wide base, and taper in the apical region. They are smaller than the surface cells and exhibit a considerable amount of basophilia. The mucous droplets in these cells, as shown by the electron microscope, are larger and less dense than those of the surface cells, and they are distributed deep in the cell as well as in the apical region.

The argentaffin cells are few and are scattered between the basement membrane and the chief cells. They contain characteristic granules, which are clearly shown in electron micrographs. The granules are believed to contain serotonin,

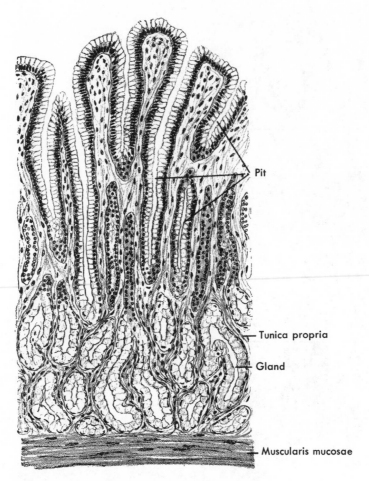

Fig. 11-6

Mucosa from pyloric region of stomach of monkey.

a vasoconstrictor that stimulates the contraction of smooth muscle. The nucleus is markedly infolded.

In the pyloric region the pits are relatively deep, extending at least halfway to the muscularis mucosae (Fig. 11-6). They are V shaped, tapering off into the glands that open into them. The glands in this portion of the stomach are composed of large mucus-secreting cells and have wide lumina. No parietal cells exist in the pyloric glands except in the transition zone, where they merge with glands of the gastric type.

The muscularis mucosae of all parts of the stomach is a complete layer of smooth muscle, which includes both the circular and the longitudinal fibers.

Submucosa

The submucosa is composed of areolar tissue and does not contain glands in any part of the stomach. In a section of the junction of the esophagus and stomach some of the end pieces of deep mucous glands may extend into the submucosa of the stomach; but since their ducts open into the esophagus they should be considered as part of the wall of the latter organ. Small arteries, veins, and lymphatics may easily be seen in the submucosa. Meissner's plexus of nerves and ganglia is less conspicuous.

Muscularis

In the stomach the muscular coat consists of two complete layers (inner circular and outer longitudinal) with an incomplete layer of

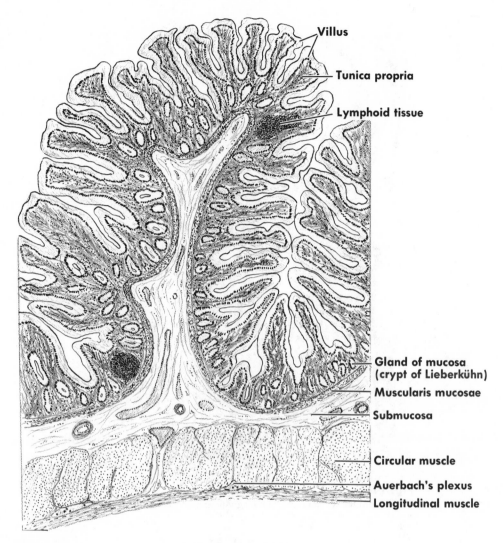

Villus

Tunica propria

Lymphoid tissue

Gland of mucosa
(crypt of Lieberkühn)

Muscularis mucosae

Submucosa

Circular muscle

Auerbach's plexus

Longitudinal muscle

Fig. 11-7
Longitudinal section of monkey jejunum, showing a plica circularis.

obliquely arranged fibers between the circular layer and the submucosa. The circular layer is by far the thickest of the three coats. The arrangement of fibers is somewhat irregular, and the student may have some difficulty in distinguishing the three coats of the muscularis in a microscopic section of this region. Auerbach's plexus is present between the circular and longitudinal fibers.

Serosa

The greater part of the stomach is covered with a layer of mesothelium outside the loose connective tissue that invests the muscle layers. This is, however, usually destroyed in the preparation of the piece of tissue for sectioning, so that all that is seen of the serosa is a coating of areolar tissue containing blood vessels, adipose tissue, and occasional nerve fibers.

SMALL INTESTINE

The inner surface of the small intestine may be seen, on gross examination, to be marked by the presence of ridges that are circularly disposed and extend into the lumen throughout this part of the tract. These ridges are the plicae

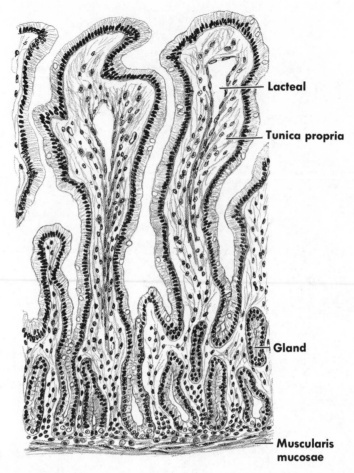

Fig. 11-8
Mucosa of monkey jejunum, showing villi and crypts of Lieberkühn.

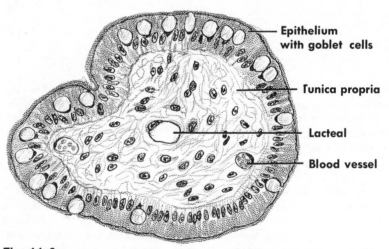

Fig. 11-9
Transverse section of a villus.

circulares. Each consists of a projection of the connective tissue of the submucosa, covered by the mucosa. The plicae circulares provide a greater surface for the absorption of food. The mucosal surface is still further increased by the presence of minute fingerlike projections of epithelium and tunica propria, which cover the surface of each plica. These are the villi, which are hardly visible to the naked eye (Fig. 11-7).

Mucosa

Villi. Under the microscope each villus is seen to consist of a projection of the tunica propria covered by simple columnar epithelium. The tunica propria is made of reticular tissue and contains capillaries, lymphatics, and scattered muscle fibers. In an injected specimen it is apparent that the vessels have a definite plan of distribution. There is, in each villus, a central lymphatic called a lacteal (Figs. 11-8 and 11-9), into which nutriment from the tract is absorbed. An arteriole enters the villus at one side and breaks up into capillaries at the distal end. Blood is collected from the capillaries by a venule that passes out along the side opposite to that occupied by the arteriole. Villi occur in all parts of the small intestine and are its most characteristic feature. In the duodenum they are leaf shaped; in the jejunum they are tall and somewhat enlarged or forked at their distal ends. The ileum has shorter, club-shaped villi. Other parts of the tract have projections that, at first sight, might be mistaken for villi. In the stomach, for instance, the tissue between two pits has somewhat the same form as a villus and consists of a mass of reticular tissue covered by columnar epithelium. Closer examination reveals, however, that the organization of vessels, which is characteristic of a villus, is lacking in the stomach.

The lining cells of the small intestine are of the tall columnar variety, having round or oval nuclei located in the basal part of the cell. With the light microscope it is possible to observe a striated border at the free surface, which has been shown to consist of minute fingerlike extensions, the microvilli, arranged in parallel arrays (Fig. 11-11). This specialization increases the surface and is characteristic of absorptive cells. At or near the free surface are terminal bars. Also present are the Golgi apparatus and numerous mitochondria. The endoplasmic reticulum is abundant and of the smooth variety.

Glands. Between the bases of the villi, glands extend into the lower part of the mucosa (Fig. 11-8). These are the intestinal glands (crypts of Lieberkühn). At the base of each gland is a group of cells, the cells of Paneth, which are somewhat larger than the surrounding cells and have paler nuclei (Fig. 11-11). Their cytoplasm is sometimes darker, sometimes lighter than that of the surrounding cells. They are believed to form a digestive enzyme. Cells similar to the Paneth cells have been found in other parts of the digestive tract, but it is in the small intestine that they are most numerous and, therefore, most easily found.

The rest of the crypt is lined with columnar epithelium somewhat resembling that which covers the villi. Its cells are, however, not quite so tall, and fewer of them are goblet cells. Special stains indicate that some of the lining cells have an affinity for silver stains, but this type (argentaffin cells) is not distinguishable when stained with hematoxylin and eosin. Like the cells of Paneth, argentaffin cells occur in other parts of the gut as well as in the small intestine.

Lymphoid tissue. Lymphoid tissue is widely distributed throughout the mucosa of the small intestine. In the ileum the nodules are gathered into groups (Peyer's patches) and fill not only the mucosa but the submucosa. These groups of nodules will be more fully described.

Muscularis mucosae. The muscularis mucosae consists of two thin layers of smooth muscle: an inner circular and an outer longitudinal layer. It thus repeats in miniature the arrangement of the muscularis coat.

Submucosa

The submucosa layer of the intestinal wall is different in the three divisions of the small intestine. Its basis is the same throughout: a layer of areolar tissue containing the vessels and nerves of Heller's and Meissner's plexuses, respectively. In the duodenum the layer contains, in addition, groups of mucous glands. These are the duodenal glands of Brunner (Fig. 11-12). Their secretion, which is mucus like that formed in the cardiac glands of the stomach, enters the duodenum through the ducts that open on the surface between the crypts of Lieberkühn or into the crypts themselves. In the ileum there are groups of lymph nodules that occupy both mucosa and submucosa (Fig. 11-13). Each group consists of ten to sixty

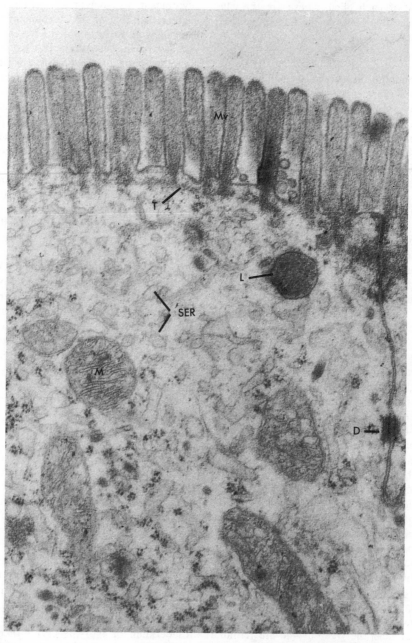

Fig. 11-10
Electron micrograph of a portion of an epithelial cell from small intestine of a mouse. **D,** Desmosome; **L,** lysosome; **M,** mitochondrion; **Mv,** microvilli; **SER,** smooth endoplasmic reticulum; **T,** terminal web. (×48,000.)

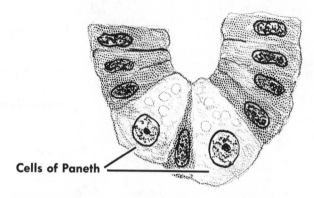

Cells of Paneth

Fig. 11-11
Epithelium at base of crypt of Lieberkühn, showing cells of Paneth.

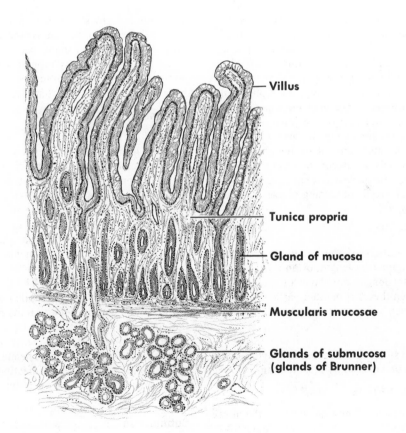

Villus

Tunica propria

Gland of mucosa

Muscularis mucosae

Glands of submucosa
(glands of Brunner)

Fig. 11-12
Mucosa and submucosa of monkey duodenum.

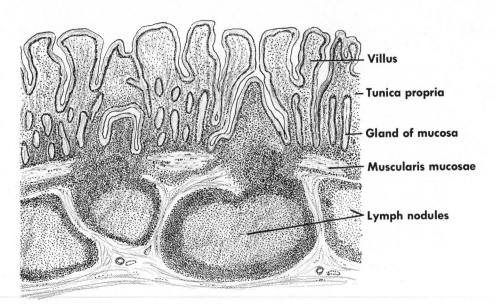

Fig. 11-13

Mucosa and submucosa of ileum, showing Peyer's patches.

nodules with germinal centers, and the groups are so large as to be visible to the naked eye. They not only fill the submucosa and the mucosa but extend a little into the lumen of the intestine, obliterating the villi. They are called Peyer's patches, or the aggregate lymph nodules of the intestine. There may be similar aggregates in the lower part of the jejunum, but the majority of sections from this part of the tract have only a small amount of lymphoid tissue in them. Glands are never found in the submucosa of the jejunum. It is characterized by its exceptionally high, branching plicae circulares and its long villi.

Muscularis

The muscularis of the small intestine consists, throughout its length, of an inner circular and an outer longitudinal layer of smooth muscle. Between these, as in other parts of the tract, lies Auerbach's plexus of nerves.

Serosa

As in the stomach the serosa is a layer of connective tissue covered by mesothelium.

LARGE INTESTINE

In this division of the digestive tract the plicae circulares are replaced by the semi-lunar folds, which include not only the mucosa and submucosa but also the inner layer of the muscu-laris and are grossly visible on the outside as well as the inside of the gut. As the name implies they are crescentic in shape, each one extending about a third of the way around the wall of the large intestine. The four coats of this region have the following characteristics.

Mucosa (Fig. 11-14)

Water is absorbed from the large intestine, and its lining is well supplied with mucus-secreting cells. There are no villi in the mucosa of the colon. In the embryo, villi are present there but disappear during late fetal life. The epithelium is simple columnar with conspicuous goblet cells. The tunica propria contains many glands. These are simple tubular glands, closely set and lined with epithelium like that which covers the surface of the mucosa. They have no cells of Paneth in them. The tunica propria has in it blood and lymph capillaries, but these are not organized in definite units like those of the small intestine. Solitary lymph nodules are present and are often so large as to break through into the submucosa. The muscularis mucosa is here, as in the small intestine, composed of an inner circular and an outer longitudinal layer (Fig. 11-15).

Submucosa

The submucosa of the colon has no glands in it. In addition to the areolar tissue with ves-

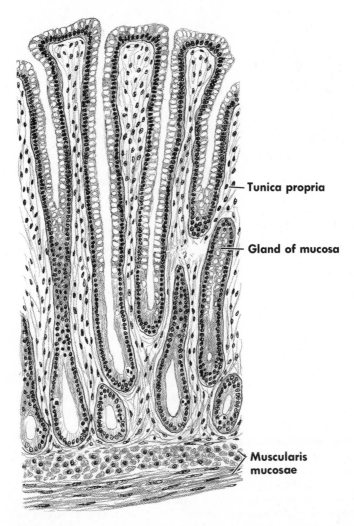

Tunica propria

Gland of mucosa

Muscularis
mucosae

Fig. 11-14
Mucosa and submucosa of dog colon, showing solitary lymph nodule.

sels and nerves, it contains only the solitary lymph nodules mentioned previously (Fig. 11-15).

Muscularis

The inner circular layer of this coat is continuous around the wall and is thrown into folds along with the mucosa and submucosa. The longitudinal layer is in the form of three bands, which run through the length of the large intestine. These are called the taeniae coli. When the taeniae coli are dissected away from the rest of the wall, they are found to be considerably shorter than it is, and this difference in length produces the semilunar fold in the longer parts of the wall. The effect of the taeniae is like that of a drawstring run through a piece of cloth.

Serosa

The serosa contains large deposits of adipose tissues that protrude on the outer surface of the tube and are microscopically visible as the appendices epiploicae.

RECTUM AND ANUS

The rectum is divided into an upper and a lower part. The upper part extends from the third sacral vertebra to the diaphragm of the pelvis. The mucosa of the upper part is similar

121

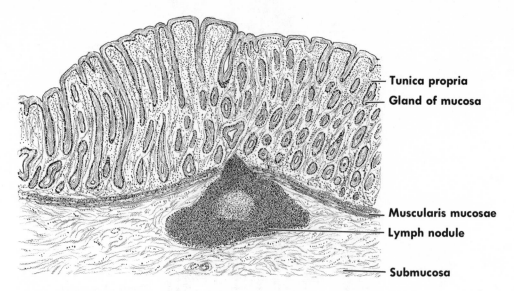

Tunica propria
Gland of mucosa

Muscularis mucosae
Lymph nodule

Submucosa

Fig. 11-15
Mucosa of dog colon.

to that of the colon. The crypts of Lieberkühn are, however, longer and contain many mucous cells. The muscularis mucosa, submucosa, and circularly arranged smooth muscle are also similar to those of the colon. The taeniae coli, however, spread out and form a continuous layer that is much thickened in the dorsal and ventral surface of the viscus.

The surface of the lower part of the rectum (anal canal) is thrown into several longitudinal folds known as the rectal columns (of Morgagni). At the lower termination these folds unite with one another to form the anal valves. At the level of the anal valves the epithelium becomes stratified squamous of a noncornified variety. The noncornified epithelium extends nearly to the anal orifice, where it changes to stratified squamous epithelium, characteristic of the epidermis. At the level of the anal orifice, hairs, sweat glands, and sebaceous glands occur.

The sweat glands are of two types. One type has the structure characteristic of the glands found in various parts of the body; the second type (circumanal) is large and resembles the axillary sweat glands.

At the approximate level of the valves the muscularis mucosa becomes much diminished and eventually is lacking entirely. The submucosa contains an abundant supply of arteries and veins. The inner circular layers of the muscularis of the anal canal are composed of smooth muscle, are relatively thick, and serve as the internal and sphincter. The outer longitudinal layer of smooth muscle continues over the inter-

nal sphincter and attaches to connective tissue. Also present is an external sphincter composed of striated muscle lying internal to another sphincter, the levator ani.

VERMIFORM APPENDIX

The wall of the vermiform appendix resembles that of the colon (Fig. 11-16). It may be described as follows.

Mucosa

The epithelium is simple columnar with goblet cells, forming glands like those of the colon. The tunica propria contains a great deal of lymphoid tissue. Often the nodules are confluent and the number of glands greatly reduced. The muscularis mucosa is interrupted by the lymph nodules, so that in places only a few strands of it are present.

From the preceding description it will be seen that the appendix is composed of the same elements as those that form the colonic mucosa. In the appendix, however, the glands are less numerous, and there is a greater amount of lymphoid tissue (Figs. 11-14 and 11-15).

Submucosa

The submucosa is composed of areolar tissue with vessels, nerves, and lymphoid tissue.

Muscularis

The muscularis is composed of two complete layers as in other parts of the tract.

122

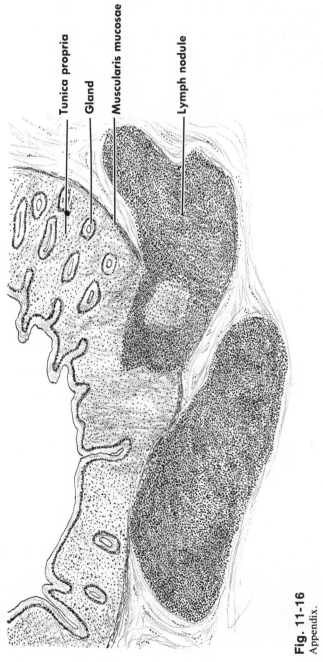

Tunica propria

Gland

Muscularis mucosae

Lymph nodule

Fig. 11-16
Appendix.

123

Table 7. Diagnostic characteristics of the digestive tract

	Mucosa	Submucosa	Muscularis
Esophagus	Stratified squamous epithelium Glands confined to two narrow zones Muscularis mucosae lacking in upper part	Mucous glands	Striated in upper part
Stomach	Pits in surface Glands closely packed and long; made up of chief and parietal cells		Oblique layer of muscle inside circular layer
Duodenum	Villi, leaflike	Mucous glands; plicae are low	
Jejunum	Villi, tall	Tall branching plicae	
Ileum	Villi, club shaped	Large groups of lymphoid nodules	
Colon	No pits or villi Many goblet cells in epithelium		Longitudinal muscle arranged in three bands
Appendix	No pits or villi; much lymphoid tissue	Much lymphoid tissue	
Rectum	Partly like colon; partly stratified squamous		Internal circular muscle forms external sphincter
Anus	Noncornified stratified squamous epithelium		

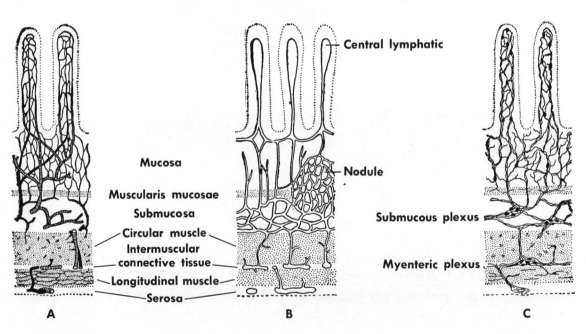

Fig. 11-17
A, Diagram of blood vessels of small intestine; arteries appear as coarse black lines, capillaries as fine lines, and veins are shaded (after Mall). **B,** Diagram of lymphatic vessels (after Mall). **C,** Diagram of nerves based upon Golgi preparations (after Cajal). (From Bremer, J. L., and Weatherford, H. L.: A text-book of histology, New York, 1948, McGraw-Hill Book Co.)

Serosa

The serosa presents no exceptional features.

• • •

Table 7 presents the peculiarities of different parts of the digestive tract, which may be used as diagnostic features in identifying slides.

BLOOD SUPPLY OF STOMACH AND INTESTINES

The arteries that supply the gut pass through the mesentery to reach the serosa, where they branch into smaller vessels. The latter continue through the two coats of the muscularis to the submucosa, where they form an extensive plexus (Heller's plexus). From the plexus of the submucosa, blood passes to the mucosa and to the muscular coat of the gut (Fig. 11-17).

NERVE SUPPLY OF STOMACH AND INTESTINES

The nerve supply of the stomach and intestines consists chiefly of nonmedullated and medullated (preganglionic) fibers of the autonomic system. When the nerves reach the connective tissue between the two layers of the muscularis coat, they are associated with ganglion cells to form the plexus of Auerbach. From the plexus, fibers pass to the submucosa, where they form another plexus, Meissner's plexus.

12

GLANDS ASSOCIATED WITH THE DIGESTIVE TRACT

In addition to the glands situated in the wall of the digestive tract there are large masses of glandular tissue that lie outside the limits of the tube and pour their secretion into it through ducts. These are the salivary glands, the ducts of which open into the oral cavity, and the pancreas and liver from which the secretions go to the intestine. The pancreas resembles the salivary glands and is studied most conveniently in connection with them.

SALIVARY GLANDS (Figs. 12-1 to 12-7)

The salivary glands consist of several glandular structures that secrete a fluid known as *saliva.* There are numerous small glands located in the oral mucous membrane. The secretions of these glands serve to moisten and lubricate the membrane. In addition, three pairs of large glands are situated some distance from the oral cavity. These structures, usually known as the salivary glands proper, are the parotid, submaxillary (submandibular), and sublingual glands. In the human being the parotid has only serous alveoli; the submaxillary and sublingual glands have both serous and mucous alveoli. Accordingly, the parotid glands are classified as serous, the palatine glands as mucous, and the submaxillary and sublingual glands as mixed.

The salivary glands consist of the glandular tissue proper, also known as the *parenchyma,* and a supporting interstitial connective tissue framework, the *stroma.* The connective tissue septa divide the glands into units known as lobes and lobules. Collecting ducts and vascular and nerve elements are located in the septa.

Parotid (Figs. 12-1 and 12-2)

The parotid has excretory, secretory, and intercalated ducts that lead out from serous alveoli. The arrangement of these elements in sequence is not as clear in sections as it is in Fig. 12-1. A number of alveoli with intercalary and secretory ducts are crowded together to form a lobule. A fine connective tissue stroma, often containing fat cells, surrounds the alveoli, and a heavier sheath of the same tissue separates adjacent lobules. A group of lobules forms a lobe, which is in turn covered with a connective tissue sheath that mingles at the outer borders of the gland with surrounding fascia. Within the lobule the alveoli and ducts are cut in various directions, and their connections are not always clear. One may, however, find a group of alveoli through which the plane of section has passed vertically, and in such a case the arrangement is visible.

Several alveoli open together into a fine duct called the intercalary duct. This tubule is composed of flattened cells. Several intercalary ducts open into a tubule lined with columnar epithelium, the secretory (striated) duct. The cells lining this branch of the duct system show, under special treatment, striations in the basal part of the cytoplasm that are supposed to be indicative of secretory activity. These ducts open in turn into excretory ducts that are lined with tall columnar epithelium. As one traces these ducts toward the opening into the oral cavity, the epithelium is seen to change first to pseudostratified and then to stratified squamous.

The end pieces or alveoli are composed entirely of serous cells, which are wedge shaped and grouped about a small lumen. The cell boundaries are usually indistinct. The appearance of the cells varies considerably, depending upon the state of activity. In the resting condition numerous granules appear in the distal portion of the cell. After secretion the number

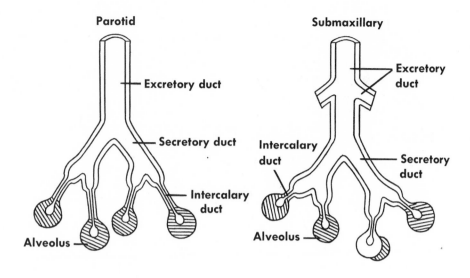

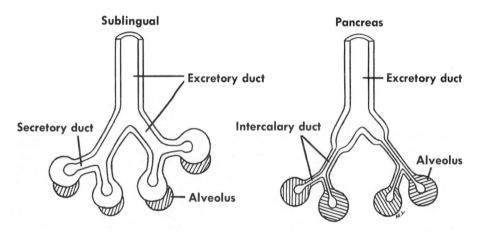

Fig. 12-1

Diagram showing composition of secreting portions and duct systems of salivary glands and pancreas. Alveoli and crescents, which are shaded, are serous cells; those unshaded are mucous cells.

of granules is reduced, and they occur in the apical region of the cell. These granules, which are refractile, are known as *zymogen granules* and are concerned with the elaboration of the enzyme produced by the cell.

In addition to mitochondria and a Golgi apparatus, common to secreting cells, a constituent of the cytoplasm known as the *chromophilic material* (ergastoplasm), appearing as a group of parallel filaments adjacent to the nuclei, is also an important cytological component of the serous cells. The filaments are strongly basophilic and are composed of ribonucleoprotein. They are associated with the synthesis

of proteins within the cell such as the zymogen granules.

With the aid of special techniques, delicate *intercellular secretory canaliculi* may be demonstrated in serous alveoli. These canaliculi appear to penetrate the cells themselves and are known as the *intracellular secretory canaliculi.* They are common to serous alveoli. An additional element demonstrated by special methods is a peculiar stellate-shaped cell occupying a position between the secreting cells and the basement membrane. Closely associated with the secreting cells, their processes form a basketlike structure around the alveolus. The function of

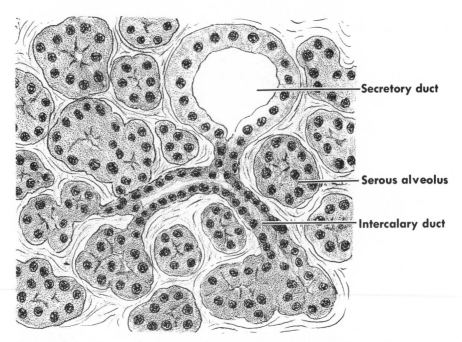

Fig. 12-2
Parotid gland.

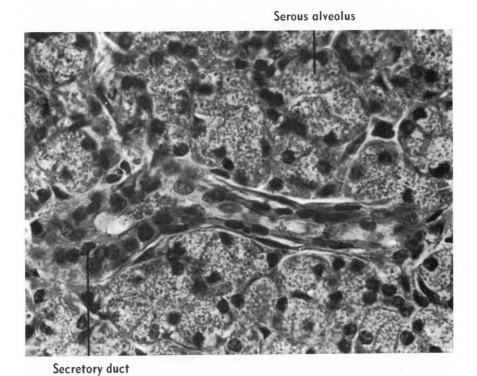

Fig. 12-3
Human parotid gland. (×640.) (From Bevelander, G.: Essentials of histology, ed. 6, St. Louis, 1970, The C. V. Mosby Co.)

Salivary
duct

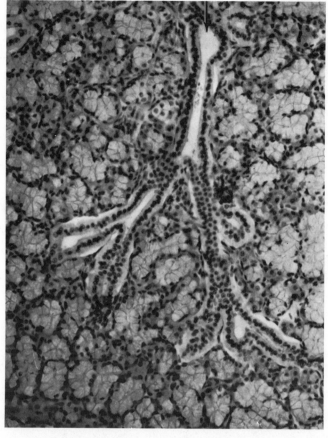

Fig. 12-4
Mixed sublingual salivary gland of dog, chiefly of mucous alveoli together with ducts in septa. (×200.) (From Bevelander, G.: Essentials of histology, ed. 6, St. Louis, 1970, The C. V. Mosby Co.)

these *basket,* or myoepithelial, cells is not well established.

Submaxillary

As in the parotid gland, there are excretory, secretory, and intercalary ducts in the submaxillary gland (Fig. 12-7), but the last named are short and difficult to find. The alveoli are of two kinds. Many are pure serous, like those of the parotid; others are mixed serous and mucous. The mucous cells of a mixed alveolus are grouped around the lumen and are distinguished from the serous cells by their paler cytoplasm and their basal, flattened nuclei. The serous cells are arranged in the form of a cap outside the mucous cells. They do not border on the lumen of the alveolus but pour their secretion into it through minute channels between the mucous cells. Such groups of serous cells are often crescent shaped in sections and are called demilunes of Heidenhain. In the submaxillary gland, which has many purely serous alveoli, the demilunes of the mixed alveoli are small.

The mucous cells occurring in either the mixed or pure mucous alveoli are modified cuboidal or low columnar cells and, when stained with hematoxylin and eosin, appear as follows: The cells rest upon a fine reticular basement membrane, and in this resting condition their nuclei appear flattened and occupy a position near the base of the cell. The cytoplasm appears pale blue in contrast to the deeper blue or purple coloration of the serous cells. The

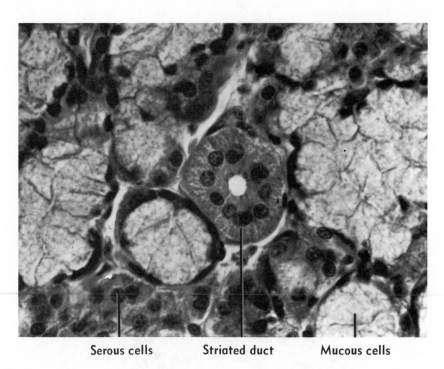

Serous cells   Striated duct   Mucous cells

Fig. 12-5
Mixed sublingual salivary gland in dog. (×640.) (From Bevelander, G.: Essentials of histology, ed. 6, St. Louis, 1970, The C. V. Mosby Co.)

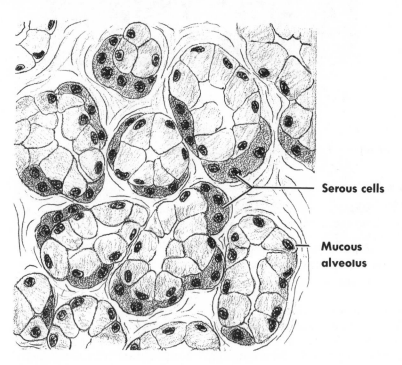

Serous cells

Mucous
alveolus

Fig. 12-6
Mixed salivary gland.

Serous alveolus

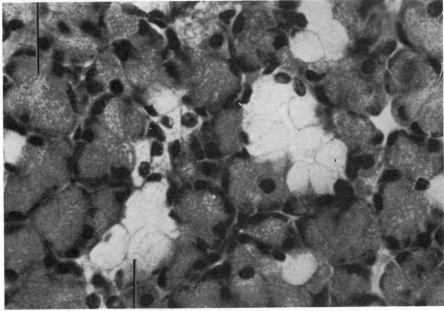

Mucous alveolus

Fig. 12-7
Mixed submaxillary salivary gland of cat, chiefly serous alveoli. (×640.) (From Bevelander, G.: Essentials of histology, ed. 6, St. Louis, 1970, The C. V. Mosby Co.)

cytoplasm contains a basophilic network and numerous granules. In the active condition the granules enlarge and become droplets, which may occupy a considerable portion of the cell. During secretion the droplets of mucin are discharged, and the cell returns to the resting state. Mitochondria and the Golgi apparatus are not prominent features of these cells, and intracellular canaliculi are lacking.

Sublingual

The duct system of the sublingual differs from that of the other salivary glands in that it lacks intercalary ducts. The alveoli open directly into short secretory channels. All the alveoli are of the mixed type, consisting of mucous cells bordering on the lumen and large serous crescents (Fig. 12-6).

The salivary glands have a relatively rich blood supply consisting of arteries, veins, and lymphatics that run in the connective tissue septa along with the ducts. The arteries branch into capillary networks where they eventually surround the alveoli.

Physiology of salivation

The flow of saliva is regulated by nerves of the autonomic nervous system. Both sets of nerves, parasympathetic and sympathetic, are able to effect the secretory process, which occurs reflexly. The primary centers of secretion are the salivary nuclei located in the medulla oblongata. Higher regions of the central nervous system can excite or inhibit the medullary reflexes as shown by the classical studies of Pavlov on conditioning this reflex in dogs. Mechanical stimulation of the oral cavity and the presence of most types of food or highly seasoned substances evoke salivation reflexly. Since saliva can be secreted against pressure, it is now generally agreed that saliva formation is the result of some metabolic process. Electrolytes presumably are transported from the plasma to saliva by duct cells, and some ions are selectively resorbed along the ducts. Water, mucus, and protein are probably contributed by the acinar portions of the gland. The secretory process is very complex, and there is little evidence at this time that specific histological cell types have selective functions.

Blood and nerve supply

The salivary glands have a relatively rich blood supply consisting of arteries, veins, and lymphatics, which run in the connective tissue septa along with the ducts. The arteries branch

131

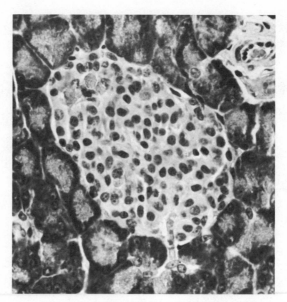

Fig. 12-8
Photomicrograph of island of Langerhans of squirrel monkey, surrounded by acinar cells. (×400.)

into capillary networks where they eventually surround the alveoli. The innervation of the salivary glands is complicated and involves fibers of the sympathetic and parasympathetic systems.

PANCREAS (Figs. 12-8 and 12-9)

The pancreas is really a union of two organs having entirely different functions—the pancreatic tissue proper and the islands of Langerhans. The former tissue makes up a gland of external secretion; the latter are endocrine in function.

The pancreas has long intercalary ducts that lead directly into excretory ducts without the intervention of a secretory portion. The alveoli are shorter and rounder than those of the parotid and are composed, like them, of serous cells. With careful preparation some of the cells may show dark granules in the portion toward the lumen. These are zymogen granules, which are transformed into the secretion of the gland.

A peculiar feature of the pancreatic alveoli is the presence of centroalveolar cells. These are small cells that are situated in the lumen of the alveolus, often filling it completely. The centroalveolar cells may be recognized by their dark, oval nuclei as well as by their position. They are derived from the cells of the intercalary duct, which they resemble in form.

The islands of Langerhans are collections of cells that arise as outgrowths from the walls of the ducts of the pancreas during embryonic life. Although they are thus connected developmentally with the ducts, they do not secrete into the tubules. They may become entirely detached from them or retain a connection through a cord of cells that has no lumen. They consist of coiled anastomosing cords of cells, penetrated by a network of capillaries into which they secrete. The cells are pale in color and polygonal in shape, containing vesicular nuclei. With special treatment three kinds of cells, alpha, beta, and gamma, may be distinguished, but they are not differentiated by the ordinary fixatives and stains.

If the entire pancreas is removed from an animal, diabetic symptoms occur that indicate a disturbance of the carbohydrate metabolism. If, however, the pancreatic duct is ligated, the alveoli degenerate, but the islands of Langerhans are unharmed. In this case there is no disturbance of carbohydrate metabolism. It is thus clear that the two kinds of tissue have entirely different functions.

The alveoli compose a gland of external secretion, forming an alkaline fluid containing enzymes used in digestion (trypsin, amylase, lipase). The islands are glands of internal secretion (endocrine glands) producing two hormones: insulin and glucagon.

Serous alveoli   Fat cells

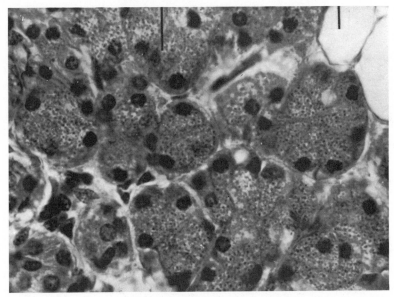

Fig. 12-9
Section of human pancreas; serous cells show zymogen granules. (×640.) (From Bevelander, G.: Essentials of histology, ed. 6, St. Louis, 1970, The C. V. Mosby Co.)

Insulin is associated with carbohydrate metabolism. In its absence the cells of the body are unable to utilize available glucose. The condition resulting from insulin deficiency, known as diabetes mellitus, is characterized by hyperglycemia and glycosuria. The specific cells responsible for the production of insulin are the beta cells.

Glucagon is believed to be derived from the alpha cells. Although the function of this hormone is not as clearly defined as is that of insulin, it is believed that its action is antagonistic to that of insulin by elevating the blood sugar as a result of glycogenolysis in the liver.

Blood supply

The blood supply to the pancreas is derived chiefly from the superior and inferior pancreaticoduodenal arteries and also from divisions of the splenic artery. As in the case of the salivary glands, the arteries pass in the connective tissue septa to end in capillaries among the acini and islands of Langerhans. Corresponding veins return the blood to the superior mesenteric and portal veins.

Nerve supply

The nerves that supply the pancreas are derived from the splanchnic and the vagus nerves.

SUMMARY OF SALIVARY GLANDS AND PANCREAS

It is sometimes difficult for the student to distinguish the four glands just described, and to aid him in doing so the following facts may be emphasized. Of the four, two contain no mucous cells. These are the parotid and the pancreas, which are alike in that the cells of their alveoli are all serous. They are differentiated by the presence of islands of Langerhans and centroalveolar cells in the pancreas. In differentiating between the submaxillary and sublingual glands, one should look for purely serous alveoli in the former. It must be remembered, however, that the large serous crescents of the sublingual may be so cut that their relation to the mucous alveoli is not seen, and they appear to be separate alveoli. Such instances are, however, isolated, and if more than half the cells in a section are serous, it is certainly from the submaxillary gland. Some specimens are difficult to identify, especially as the proportions of serous and mucous cells vary in different animals and even in different parts of the same gland.

LIVER

The liver develops embryologically as an outgrowth from the wall of the gut, lying in the pathway of the vitelline veins. It later intercepts

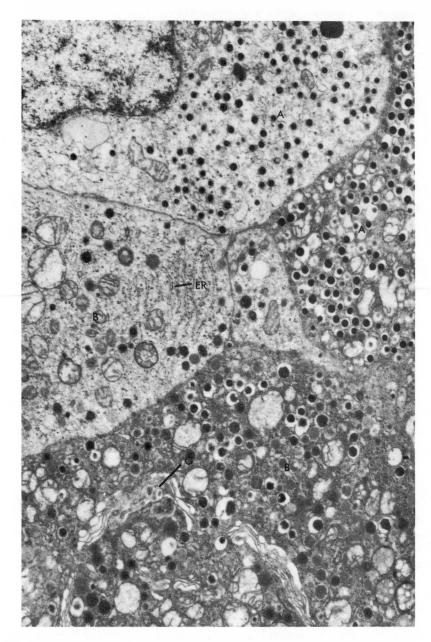

Fig. 12-10

Electron micrograph of islet cells of Rhesus' pancreas. The character and size of the granules are the most important distinguishing features of these cells. **A**, Alpha cell; **B**, beta cell; **ER**, endoplasmic reticulum; **G**, Golgi apparatus. (×11,500.)

the umbilical veins, and all four vessels are broken up by the glandular tissue into a multitude of small sinusoids. The liver tissue is divided into lobules, each of which is surrounded by a connective tissue sheath. These sheaths are continuous with the superficial covering of the

whole liver, and the aggregate of connective tissue is known as Glisson's capsule.

Under the low power of the microscope a section of a piece of the liver of a pig appears as a group of lobules that are, roughly, six sided (Fig. 12-11). Each is surrounded by connective

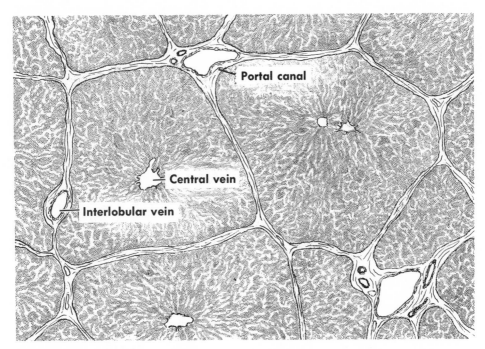

Fig. 12-11
Pig liver, low magnification, showing relations of lobules to portal canal, central vein, and interlobular vein.

tissue that, at certain of the angles of the lobules, forms a conspicuous island containing blood vessels and ducts. These islands are the portal canals. Along some of the straight sides of lobules, vessels, which are the interlobular veins, may be seen. The same arrangement of vessels is present in human liver, but the connective tissue capsules surrounding the lobules are much thinner and therefore less easy to see. The tissue of the lobule is made up of radiating cords of cells alternating with sinusoids. The sinusoids converge to a vessel in the center of the lobule (central vein). Under higher magnification the arrangement of cords and sinusoids is much clearer, and the following details may be seen.

Liver cells and sinusoids

The parenchyma of the liver is composed of large epithelial cells supported by reticular fibers (Fig. 12-13) and apparently arranged in irregular interconnecting plates known as the hepatic cords. The plates are arranged in a radiating fashion around the central vein (Fig. 12-16). The hepatic plates form the secretory part of the liver and are accordingly analogous to the secretory tubules of other glands. Special technique is required to demonstrate the capil-

laries by which the bile, secreted by the liver cells, is carried to the larger ducts in the portal canals. Each cell has, in the side adjacent to its neighboring cell, a minute groove. Two grooves fitting together form a duct known as the bile canaliculus.

The hepatic cells are relatively large, are polyhedral in shape, and usually exhibit clear cell boundaries. The appearance of the cytoplasm is variable depending on the physiological state of the cell. The usual cytological components consist of a centrally placed nucleus with a prominent nucleolus. Occasionally, the cells are binucleate. The mitochondria are fairly numerous. The Golgi apparatus is situated adjacent to the bile canaliculus. Scattered basophilic material corresponding to rough endoplasmic reticulum or dispersed ribosomes is abundant. The various kinds of observable granules are glycogen, lipid, and bile pigment. The cords of cells anastomose freely, forming a spongy network that radiates from the central vein. The meshes of the network of secreting cells contain the sinusoids, which are lined with an endothelium, part of which belongs to the reticuloendothelial system. In an ordinary preparation stained with hematoxylin and eosin, the lining of these vessels appears to be composed

135

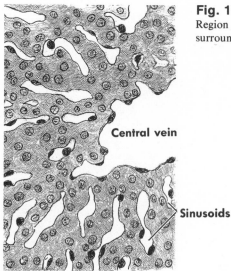

Fig. 12-12

Region of liver lobule immediately surrounding a central vein.

Central vein

Sinusoids

of cells that lie flat along the sides of the liver cells. The nuclei of these endothelial cells are small and dark, and their cytoplasm forms a thin film along the border of the sinusoid. Such cells are the undifferentiated lining cells. With special methods a second type of cell may be demonstrated, the stellate cell of Kupffer. When these cells are properly stained, they appear to be in the bloodstream anchored to the wall of the sinusoid by cytoplasmic processes. Their reaction to vital dyes is characteristic of other reticuloendothelial cells (Fig. 12-12).

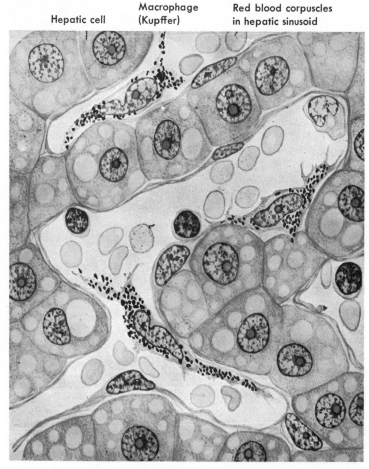

Hepatic cell   Macrophage (Kupffer)   Red blood corpuscles in hepatic sinusoid

Fig. 12-13

Hepatic sinusoids, showing endothelial cells and macrophages lining them. (×1,200.) (From Nonidez, J. F., and Windle, W. F.: Textbook of histology, New York, 1953, McGraw-Hill Book Co.)

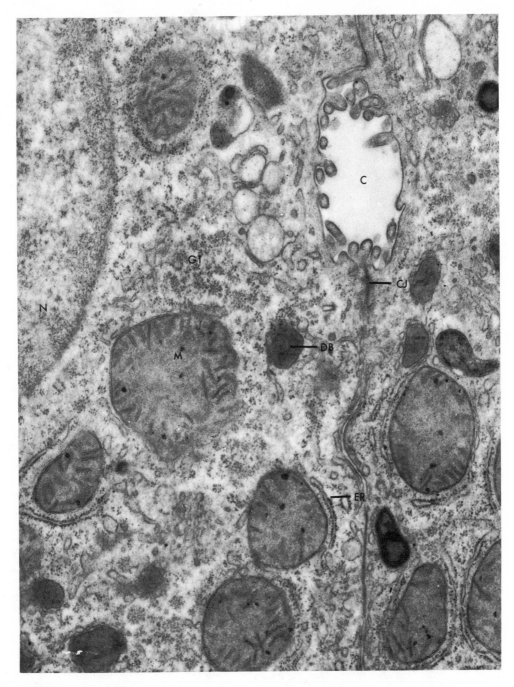

Fig. 12-14
Electron micrograph of parts of two adjacent cells of rat liver, showing bile canaliculus, **C. Cj,** Cell junction; **DB,** dense body; **ER,** rough endoplasmic reticulum; **Gl,** glycogen; **N,** nucleus; **M,** mitochondrion. (×15,000.) (Courtesy Dr. S. Luse, New York, N. Y.)

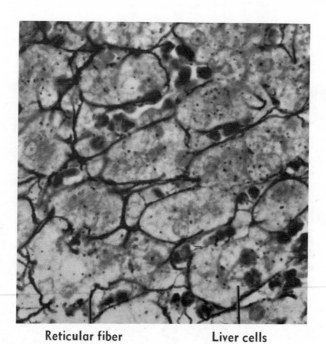

Reticular fiber   Liver cells

Fig. 12-15
Section of human liver showing reticular fibers. (Bielschowsky method; ×640.) (From Bevelander, G.: Essentials of histology, ed. 6, St. Louis, 1970, The C. V. Mosby Co.)

Portal canal

The portal canal consists of an island of connective tissue that is approximately triangular in shape. It contains a branch of the hepatic artery, a branch of the portal vein, and a bile duct. Of these the vein is by far the largest. The bile duct is readily distinguished from the blood vessels by its lining of columnar epithelium (Fig. 12-16).

Circulation

The circulation of the liver is peculiar in that it is derived from two sources: (1) arterial blood from branches of the hepatic artery and (2) venous blood by way of the portal vein (Fig. 12-17). The hepatic artery is chiefly concerned with nourishment of the liver tissue.

The portal vein carrying venous blood from the intestine, together with branches of the hepatic artery, enters the liver at the porta. These vessels divide and run through the connective tissue septa of the lobes as the interlobar vessels. The interlobar veins give off branches that run between the lobules and are known accordingly as interlobular veins. These vessels encircle the lobule, eventually penetrate it, and break up into fine capillaries, the hepatic

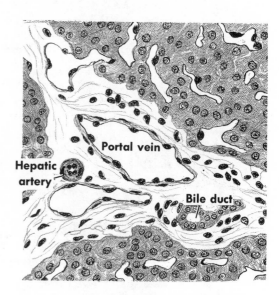

Fig. 12-16
Portal canal containing a branch of portal vein, a branch of hepatic artery, and a bile duct. Note in upper left-hand part a small vein opening into a sinusoid.

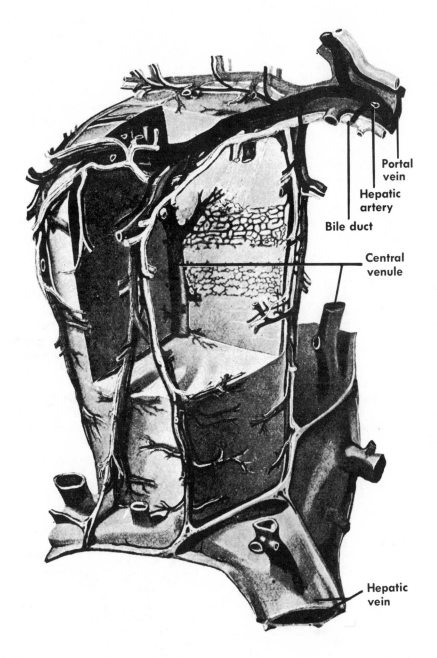

Fig. 12-17
Reconstruction of liver lobule of pig, showing relation of blood vessels and bile ducts to liver parenchyma. (Modified from Braus, H.: Anatomie des Menschen, vol. 2, Berlin, 1924, Verlag Julius Springer; from Nonidez, J. F., and Windle, W. F.: Textbook of histology, New York, 1953, McGraw-Hill Book Co.)

sinusoids. The sinusoids empty into the central vein, which is considered to be the first part of the efferent system of the hepatic vessels. The central veins passes down through the lobule, collecting blood from many sinusoids and eventually uniting with other central veins that lead into the sublobular vein. Blood from these veins is eventually collected by the hepatic vein and is finally carried to the vena cava.

It is this circulatory arrangement that enables the liver to perform one of its functions, namely, the storage of glycogen. The blood of the portal vein comes from the intestine and is laden with nutriment. Through the arrangement of sinusoids it easily reaches the liver cells, which store glycogen obtained from the blood. The same arrangement serves to return the nourishment to the circulation when it is needed.

Another function of the liver is the formation of bile for the digestion of food in the intestine. This substance is apparently secreted by the same cells that store the glycogen. The bile ducts of the right and quadrate lobes form the right hepatic duct. Those of the left ducts unite to form the common hepatic; this receives the cystic duct and then continues to the duodenum as the common bile duct.

In addition to the functions mentioned the liver also plays an important role in intermediate carbohydrate metabolism as well as in the metabolism of amino acids and lipids. It produces numerous phagocytic cells and is known to be concerned with the elaboration or storage of certain hormones and enzymes. Finally, the liver is also involved in the mechanism of blood clotting by virtue of its ability to form or store fibrinogen and heparin.

Nerve supply

The nerves that supply the liver are chiefly nonmedullated fibers derived from the sympathetic system. They accompany the blood vessels and ducts, terminating in these structures and among the liver cells.

GALLBLADDER

The gallbladder is a hollow, pear-shaped organ closely adherent to the posterior surface of the liver. It consists of a blind end known as the fundus, a body, and a neck, which continues as the cystic duct.

The four layers common to other parts of the digestive tract are poorly developed and more or less intermingled in the gallbladder (Fig. 12-18). It is lined with a columnar epithelium in which the cell walls are distinct. This epithelium rests on a connective tissue layer (lamina propria), which represents the tunica propria and submucosa of other parts of the tract. The connective tissue and epithelium are irregularly folded, forming numerous elevations and pockets. Often the latter are tangentially cut, so that they appear as closed sacs that look like glandular follicles. There is, however, no secretion in the gallbladder except that of a small group of mucous glands near its neck.

Outside the connective tissue there is a layer of smooth muscles that consists of intermingled groups of circular, longitudinal, and oblique

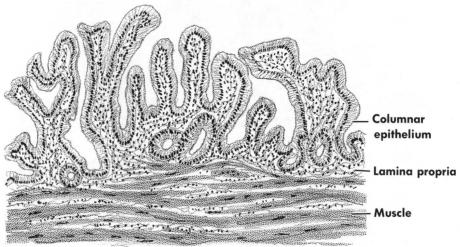

Fig. 12-18
Monkey gallbladder.

— Columnar epithelium

— Lamina propria

— Muscle

fibers. The muscular coat is thin and has much connective tissue combined with the muscle fibers. There is a fairly thick serosa of loose connective tissue covered by the mesothelium.

Blood supply

The gallbladder is supplied by the cystic artery, and the venous blood is collected by veins that empty into the cystic branch of the portal vein. The gallbladder is richly supplied by lymphatics, and many plexuses occur in this organ.

Nerve supply

Branches of both the vagus and splanchnic nerves supply the gallbladder.

13
RESPIRATORY TRACT

For the purpose of presentation the respiratory tract is arbitrarily divided into an upper part, extending from the nose to the larynx, and a lower part, which includes the trachea and its branches within the lung. Strictly speaking, this division is not anatomically accurate.

The upper part of the respiratory system (Fig. 13-1) is composed of two nasal passages, the nasopharynx, laryngopharynx, and larynx. The lower part consists of the trachea, two primary bronchi that enter the lungs and branch repeatedly to form a system of bronchi, bronchioles, and finally alveolar sacs. The oral cavity and thoracic rib cage are secondarily included as part of the respiratory system, as is the diaphragm, which separates the thoracic and abdominal cavities.

Aside from its respiratory function (which involves the exchange of gases between the tissue fluids, plasma, and air spaces in the lung), the air in the respiratory system must be moistened, filtered, and warmed to permit proper functioning of the parts. The mucus supplied by goblet cells in pseudostratified epithelium and by the submucosal glands serves to entrap dust particles and bacteria and also to supply enzymes that lyse certain bacteria. The same secretion moistens the air and also dissolves certain molecules that are perceived as odors with the aid of the olfactory organ in the nasal passages. The coordinated beating of cilia on cell surfaces moves the secretions from the nasal passages through the nasopharynx to the oropharynx, while similar activity of ciliated cells located in the bronchioles, bronchi, and trachea propels mucus to the epiglottis. From this locus the secretions are either expectorated or pass into the esophagus. An abundant supply of venous blood vessels in the submucosal tissues of the nasal passages warm the air. Several

of the functions mentioned are facilitated by an abundant surface area in each nasal passage by virtue of (1) four accessory sinuses (frontal, ethmoidal, sphenoidal, and maxillary, named for the bones that enclose them) and (2) the presence of three conchae containing the twisted turbinate bones. Certain phagocytic cells called "dust cells" are located in the lung tissues. They remove and store foreign particles that enter the lungs. The olfactory organ serves to warn the organism of the presence of noxious substances in the air. The specialized respiratory epithelium of the lung alveoli is admirably suited for its function of gas exchange. The conducting tubules are constructed so as to maintain open passageways for gases under the widely fluctuating pressures produced in the ventilation process. These tubules gradually change in structure from thick-walled, rigid tubes to increasingly thinner and softer ones, a change similar to that occurring in blood vessels.

UPPER PARTS OF RESPIRATORY TRACT
NASAL PASSAGES

The nose consists of two passageways separated by the cartilage-containing *nasal septum*. Each passageway begins at the *external nares* as an inflection of the keratinized stratified squamous epithelium of the wings (alae) of the nose. The inflected portion forms the *vestibule* of the nose and is covered by numerous hairs (vibrissae). Large sebaceous glands and numerous sweat glands are also found in this region. The connective tissue papillae are deep, and scattered mixed serous and mucous glands may be observed. In the posterior region of the vestibule the epithelium becomes nonkeratinized or forms only small patches of nonhairy

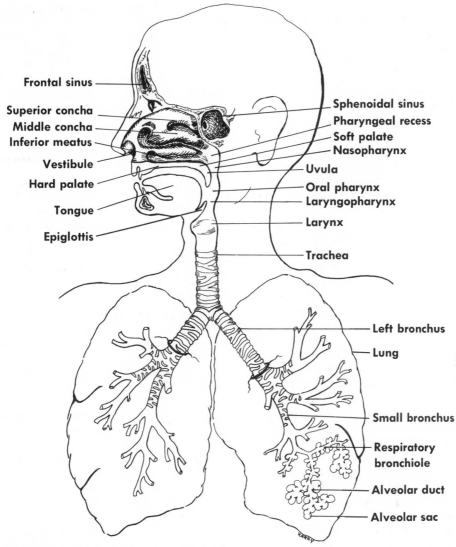

Fig. 13-1
Topographic representation of respiratory apparatus.

keratinized epithelium. The latter indicates the beginning of the so-called *respiratory part* of the nasal passage, which in turn terminates in a small orifice called the *choana* leading into the nasopharynx.

The respiratory portion of each nasal passage includes the sinuses, olfactory organ, the three conchae, including the meati, and the upper surface of the hard palate. In general the epithelium of this region is ciliated pseudostratified, usually exhibiting four or five rows of nuclei containing goblet cells. The under-

lying lamina propria, composed of both elastic and collagenous fibers, is usually adherent to a nearby periosteum or perichondrium. A basement membrane containing elastic fibers occurs irregularly.

The sinuses indicated are located in certain bones of the head and are usually viewed in decalcified sections of the head of an embryo or fetus. They are usually identified by their location rather than by histological characteristics. The epithelium is ciliated pseudostratified, of approximately one-half the thickness of other parts of the tract, exhibiting two or three rows of nuclei and very few goblet cells. The basement membrane is very thin and is rarely observed. The lamina propria is also thin, mainly collagenous, and closely adherent to the periosteum. It has few glands but is frequently supplied with lymphoid aggregations and other leukocytic forms.

The superior, middle, and inferior conchae are usually observed in frontal sections through the head of the human fetus as coiled and re-curved projections arising from the walls oppo-site the septa (paraseptally). In animals like the pig only parts of the conchae are visible because the head is prolonged into a snout. The space inferior to each concha is, in se-quence, the superior, middle, and inferior meatus.

The middle and inferior conchae bear the usual thick type of pseudostratified epithelium, containing many goblet cells. The basement membrane is thick and is readily demonstrated. The lamina propria exhibits both serous and mucous alveoli as well as a large number of prominent venous passages. The latter may be either engorged with blood or collapsed, and their walls contain both circular and longi-tudinal bands of smooth muscle. Each meatus bears a thin epithelium containing a few goblet cells that rest upon a very thin basement mem-brane. The superior concha as well as parts of the roof of the nasal passage and adjacent sep-tum form part of the olfactory organ. The epithelium is extremely thick, and since the pro-cesses are almost impossible to trace in hema-toxylin and eosin preparations, its appearance is like that of stratified columnar epithelia. The surface cells contain pigment granules when properly preserved, and the cilia present are covered by a coagulated secretion which gives the impression that the tissue is covered by a cuticle.

NASOPHARYNX

In the parts of the nasopharynx that do not come into contact with surfaces of other tissues the epithelium is ciliated pseudostratified, and the lamina propria contains mixed or seromu-cous glands. In certain transitional zones strati-fied columnar epithelium may occur but is not easily distinguished from the pseudostratified variety. In the superior and posterior portions of the nasopharynx there are many aggrega-tions of lymphoid cells that may be extensions of the pharyngeal tonsils or adenoids. Similar aggregations forming the tubal tonsils are found surrounding the entrance of the eustachian tubes into the nasopharynx. The posterior wall of the nasopharynx, at about the lower level of the tonsils, is covered by a nonkeratinized stratified squamous epithelium with numerous low papillae. The superior surface of the soft palate and uvula also bear a nonkeratinized stratified squamous epithelium.

LARYNX (Fig. 13-2)

The uppermost portion of the larynx is known as the epiglottis. The lingual or anterior surface of the epiglottis is covered by a non-keratinized stratified squamous epithelium and bears many seromucous glands in the lamina propria, especially near its connection with the base of the tongue. The upper part of the poste-rior surface of the epiglottis is covered by nonkeratinized stratified squamous epithelium, which merges into a transition zone that appears irregularly as ciliated stratified columnar epi-thelium. The lower part of the posterior surface bears ciliated pseudostratified epithelium with goblet cells, and near the base one may observe scattered taste buds. The lamina propria in-cludes some mucous and serous units. The zone between the two surfaces is occupied by a large piece of cartilage containing a number of thick elastic fibers, the so-called elastic cartilage. In the epiglottis of some animals the cartilage may contain a central zone invaded by fat cells. No perichondrium, however, occurs in the invaded zone.

The epithelium of the true vocal cords is of the nonkeratinized stratified squamous variety and does not contain mucous glands in the lamina propria. Above and below the true vocal cords the epithelium is ciliated pseudo-stratified with goblet cells, and many mucous glands are present in the lamina propria. Patches of the stratified squamous epithelium are some-times found in this region.

LOWER PARTS OF RESPIRATORY TRACT

Morphologists have divided the lower parts parts of the respiratory tract on the basis of gross dissection and by the injection of low melting point alloys into the passageways. Thus, there are lobes and lobules of the lung, with their attendant blood and lymphatic circulation con-taining various air tubules. Ordinarily, one does

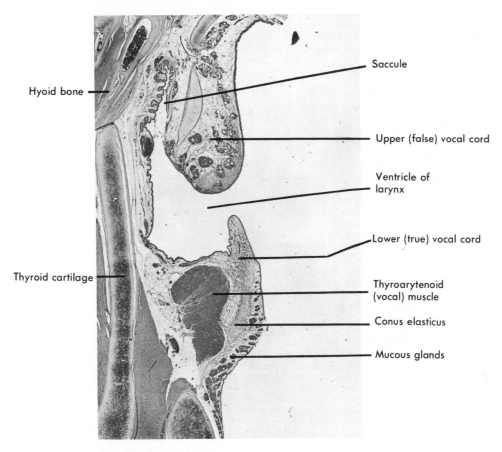

Hyoid bone —

Thyroid cartilage —

Saccule

Upper (false) vocal cord

Ventricle of
larynx

Lower (true) vocal cord

Thyroarytenoid
(vocal) muscle

Conus elasticus

Mucous glands

Fig. 13-2
Half of frontal section of the larynx of a monkey. (×10.)

not utilize more than a small portion of a lobule for study. In addition, the former tendency to utilize the diameter of a tubule as a criterion for identification is no more valid here than it is for blood vessels. In routine histology the salient features to observe in the tubules and lungs are (1) the epithelial makeup, (2) the presence or absence of cartilage and its disposition (that is, location, shape, and extent), (3) the glands and their disposition, (4) the disposition of the muscles, and (5) the relation of the parts to each other at the microscopic level. The student should attempt to visualize how each component appears in cross section and longitudinal section.

TRACHEA

The trachea consists of (1) mucosa, (2) submucosa, and (3) a layer of cartilage and muscle that corresponds to the muscularis of the diges-

tive tract (Fig. 13-3). External to the perichondrium of the cartilage is a fibrosa, or adventitious layer, of connective tissue that fuses with the tissue of the mediastinum and the similar layer enclosing the esophagus. This layer is usually destroyed during dissection of the trachea.

The mucosa consists of (1) a ciliated pseudostratified epithelium with numerous goblet cells bounded by (2) a prominent basement membrane that is part of (3) the lamina propria (tunica propria), consisting mainly of reticular or fine areolar tissue containing a number of elastic fibers. At the outer edge of the lamina propria coarse elastic fibers are oriented longitudinally to form (4) a relatively compact elastic membrane or lamina, which is said to be comparable to the muscularis mucosae of the digestive tract and the similar elastic layer in the upper part of the esophagus. In the epithelium small patches of the stratified squamous

145

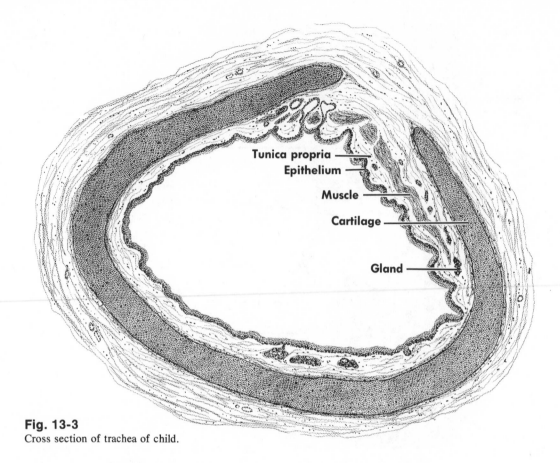

Fig. 13-3
Cross section of trachea of child.

variety are encountered, especially in older animals or those with chronic inflammations.

The submucosa is areolar tissue. It contains fat cells and the secreting portions of mixed glands with some units exhibiting prominent serous crescents. In longitudinal sections dense clusters of these glands are seen in the triangular regions between the adjacent cartilage rings, to be described.

In cross sections of the trachea the cartilages appear as a single C-shaped or U-shaped crescent with the open end or prongs directed posteriorly towards the esophagus. The prongs may branch so that more than one piece of cartilage may appear near the open side of the crescent. Bands of smooth muscle fibers transversely arranged appear between the prongs and at times may be observed inserting in the perichondrium either inside or outside the crescent. External to this muscle band one may observe the cut ends of longitudinally and obliquely arranged muscle fibers and their associated elastic fibers. The tracheal glands fre-

quently penetrate the muscle layers. In longitudinal sections the cartilages appear as two rows of ovoid bodies. Occasionally, two adjacent cartilages may fuse or be connected by a small longitudinal bar of cartilage. In the region between cartilages there are longitudinal bands of tough, dense connective tissue that merge with the perichondria of the cartilages. In older animals some cartilages may appear to contain fibers or to be partly calcified.

BRONCHI

The extrapulmonary or primary bronchi are histologically identical with the trachea in almost all details except size. In the lungs the cartilages of the bronchi are arranged in a series of overlapping crescentic plates that completely encircle these structures. Deeper in the lung these soon give way to irregular masses of cartilage with more or less rounded edges (Fig. 13-4) that may or may not overlap when viewed in cross section. The intrapulmonary bronchi differ from the trachea as follows: (1) The elastic

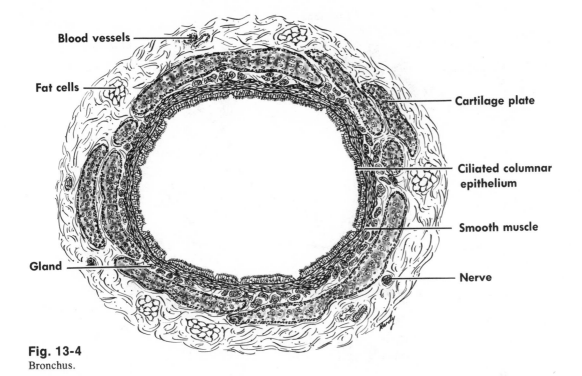

Blood vessels

Fat cells

Gland

Cartilage plate

Ciliated columnar epithelium

Smooth muscle

Nerve

Fig. 13-4
Bronchus.

membrane of the tracheal lamina propria is replaced by a layer of smooth muscle that completely encircles both the epithelium and the elastic, fiber-containing lamina propria. (2) Mucous and seromucous glands are more numerous and more generally distributed in the bronchi than in the trachea and often extend through the muscle and between adjacent cartilage plates. (3) The single crescent-shaped cartilage is replaced by a concentric ring of overlapping crescents. These eventually give way to smaller irregular masses of cartilage that continue to diminish in size until the tubules are completely devoid of cartilage. In the smallest bronchi only glands may be seen, and the cartilage is completely absent (Fig. 13-5). As the tubules become smaller the muscle bands that encircle the lumen become more prominent, with the concomitant reduction of the other structures. The muscles are arranged, however, as two opposing spirals that tend to form looser helices as the tubule branches and narrows. In cross section the looser spirals in smaller tubules appear as gaps between muscle bands at the same level. Upon death, contraction of the spiraling circular muscles throws the pseudostratified epithelium into longitudinal folds, carrying with it folds of elastic lamina propria. Classifi-

cation of large, medium-sized, and small bronchi on the basis of definitely overlapping crescentic plates of cartilage, circles of nonoverlapping plates, or no cartilage at all introduces as many problems as it solves and is not a satisfactory criterion to use for identification.

BRONCHIOLES

In bronchioles there are neither glands nor cartilages (Fig. 13-5). The lumen is lined by ciliated simple columnar epithelium that lacks goblet cells. The lamina propria is elastic and very thin and is surrounded by the same type of loosely spiraling smooth muscle bands found in the bronchi. It is interesting to note that ciliated cells are found beyond the point where glands are no longer in evidence. It has been postulated that this is a protection against the accumulation of mucus in the respiratory portion of the lungs. Subdivision of bronchioles into different types according to size is not histologically feasible and accordingly is not elaborated upon in this text.

RESPIRATORY BRONCHIOLES

In the first part of the respiratory bronchiole the epithelium is of the ciliated low columnar or cuboidal type. Distally the epithelium becomes

147

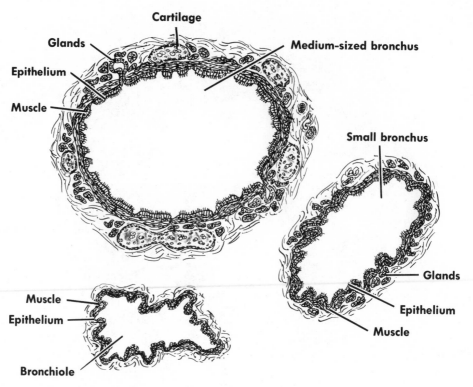

Fig. 13-5
Terminal intrapulmonary passageways of respiratory tract.

nonciliated cuboidal. The lamina propria is a very thin layer of diffuse reticular, collagenous, and elastic fibers. The spiraling muscle bands are quite prominent, but between adjacent muscle bands in the region where the lamina propria is not in evidence one can observe thin walls composed of simple cuboidal epithelium supported on a few helical elastic fibers. Some authors consider this to be respiratory epithelium, and from the appearance of these flattened plates the name respiratory bronchiole has arisen. It should be noted that in some sections the cells are so attenuated that the nuclei in these plates are not visible. In addition, pulmonary alveoli may arise directly from the walls of the respiratory bronchiole so that they appear as pockets in the tubule wall. Near their termini, respiratory bronchioles flare out and give rise to two or more alveolar ducts.

ALVEOLAR DUCTS

The alveolar ducts are similar to the respiratory bronchioles from which they branch. The walls of the ducts are provided with so many openings into the alveoli that the wall appears discontinuous. Small bits of the branching, spiraling muscle fibers are seen around the openings into the alveoli or the chambers that lead into the alveoli.

In the alveoli of the lung there are respiratory epithelium and elastic tissue. To understand the arrangement of the former one must remember that all the tubules of the fetal lung are lined with cuboidal epithelium and are embedded in embryonic connective tissue. When respiration begins, at birth, some of the epithelium is stretched into the form of thin plates described previously in this discussion. They remain, however, at the angles between alveoli areas where the cells are not flattened. The surrounding connective tissue is reduced to a network of elastic fibers and a few fibroblasts between the alveoli. One may see, therefore, in a section of lung regions where the cells are reduced to a mere line and other regions where they are polygonal and evidently nucleated.

In human beings the atria are rare, and in other animals they are an inconstant feature, so we may well consider this term to be superfluous.

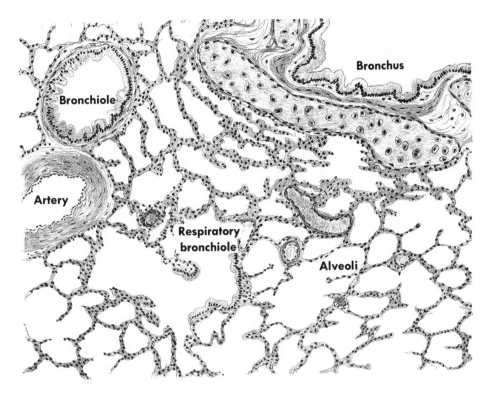

Fig. 13-6
Section of dog lung.

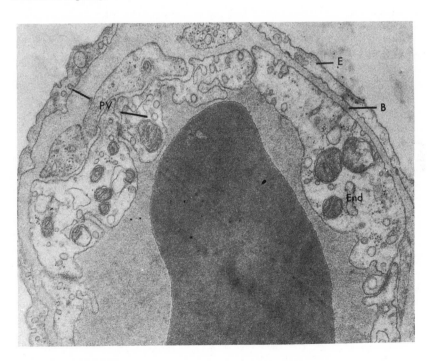

Fig. 13-7
Electron micrograph of alveolar membrane of mouse. The alveolar air is separated from the blood by a thin epithelium, **E;** a basement membrane, **B;** and the capillary endothelium, **End.** Pinocytotic vesicles, **PV,** are present in epithelium and endothelium. (×28,000.)

149

The original shape of each alveolus, or air sac, is round. The mutual pressure of adjacent sacs, however, alters the shape, and they appear as irregular polygonal spaces open on one side. They are so grouped that a number of them open into a common central space, or atrium, which in turn opens into an alveolar duct.

The true relation of the parts described is not often clear in a section of the lung. Occasionally, one may have the good fortune to see an area in which the relations of respiratory bronchioles, alveolar ducts, atria, and alveoli appear.

With the light microscope one may observe that there are capillaries and some connective tissue between the air spaces of adjacent alveoli. The fine structure of the alveolar wall has now been resolved, and it has been shown that it consists of three basic cell types. (1) The most numerous cells of the alveolar wall are the *endothelial cells* of the capillaries. The nuclei of these cells are usually smaller and more elongated than those of epithelial cells. (2) Thin attenuated epithelial cells *(squamous alveolar epithelial cells)* fit together and form a continuous lining of the alveolar spaces. This lining is so thin that it is not observable at the light level. The cytoplasm is devoid of an endoplasmic reticulum but contains a variety of other organelles. (3) *Great alveolar cells* seem to be epithelium. These cells are cuboidal or rounded and are less numerous than the squamous alveolar cells. They usually occur at the junction of the walls of several alveoli but may make up part of the air sac. In light microscopy the cytoplasm appears vacuolated, and the nuclei are large and vesicular. These cells have microvilli on the borders, and the cytoplasm contains osmiophilic inclusions known as cytosomes. They are variable in appearance, especially in regard to the microvilli and organelles.

The barrier between alveolar air and blood is extremely thin and consists of the capillary endothelium, connective tissue space, basement membrane, and the alveolar epithelium (Fig. 13-7). In the thicker regions of the alveolar wall, the basal laminae are separated by reticular and elastic fibers. Fibroblasts and other cells occur in the regions where the connective tissue space is thickest.

BLOOD SUPPLY OF LUNGS

The lungs have a dual blood supply, (1) the *pulmonary arteries* and (2) the *bronchial arteries*. The pulmonary arteries carry deoxygenated blood from the right ventricle to the lungs to be purified. The pulmonary artery gains access to the lung with the corresponding chief bronchus. It follows the branching of the bronchus, and on reaching the alveolar duct, the artery divides into a capillary plexus located in the alveolar walls. Veins arise from these capillaries, which pass first through the septa, then along the bronchioles to the root of the lung.

The *bronchial arteries* arise from the aorta. They accompany the bronchi and supply them, as well as the connective tissue of the lung, with oxygenated blood. These vessels terminate in capillaries, which anastomose with capillaries of the pulmonary plexus. Part of the blood carried by the bronchial arteries reaches the pulmonary veins through this anastomosis, the remainder via the bronchial veins.

LYMPH SUPPLY OF LUNGS

Two groups of interconnected lymphatic vessels are present in the lung. One, a superficial or pleural group, occurs in and drains the pleura; the other deep group follows the bronchi, pulmonary artery, and vein. All drain centrally to the hilum, where they communicate with the efferent vessels of the superficial group.

NERVE SUPPLY OF THE LUNGS

The lungs are supplied by branches of the vagus and also fibers of the thoracic ganglia. The fibers that supply the constrictor elements are derived chiefly from the vagus. Those that innervate the dilators of the bronchi are mainly sympathetic in character; they are said to arise from the inferior cervical and upper thoracic ganglia.

14
UROGENITAL SYSTEM

URINARY SYSTEM
KIDNEY

In mammals the main excretory pathways are the respiratory, integumentary, and urinary systems. The urine formed in the kidneys is transported with the aid of peristalsis through the ureters to a urinary bladder. As the sphincters leading out of the bladder relax, the whole bladder contracts, and the urine is forced out through the urethra.

The kidney offers two unusual opportunities to the student. (1) The gross structure of the dissected kidney correlates well with the pattern observed microscopically. (2) Instead of a vague mass of unnamed blood vessels, each one is named and exhibits definite microanatomical relations easily recognizable by beginning students. Because of its simplicity we will describe the rodent kidney first, then the human kidney.

Gross structure of the unilobar kidney

The kidney of a rodent, such as a rabbit, is a bean-shaped gland covered by a fibrous tunic or *renal capsule,* which involutes into the kidney parenchyma along the medial aspect to form the *kidney sinus.* The external orifice of the sinus is called the *hilum,* or hilus. The ureter expands into an *extrarenal pelvis,* which enters the kidney sinus and gives rise to an *intrarenal pelvis.* The distal portion of the latter is expanded into a trumpet-shaped cup or *calyx.* The lateral walls of the calyx fuse with the tissue lining the sinus. In addition to the ureter the renal sinus contains a prominent fat pad, nerves, lymphatics, and branches of the renal artery and vein. (The highly vascularized perirenal fat body in the abdominal cavity functions to cushion and support the kidney.)

If one slices a rabbit kidney lengthwise, it is seen to be composed of a single large mushroom-shaped lobe (unilobar kidney). The cap of the structure appears granular and is known as the kidney *cortex.* The stemlike portion appears triangular and striated and in three dimensions resembles a *pyramid* (from which it derives its name). The tip of the pyramid is called the *papilla,* and it is this part that projects into and is received by the calyx. In the unilobar, unipyramidal kidney the term *medulla* applies to the pyramid itself, whereas the region near the base of the pyramid in the cortex is called the juxtamedullary region. Examination of the *juxtamedullary region* reveals fine strands of medullary substance penetrating and subdividing the cortical parenchyma. The former are called *medullary rays* (rays of Ferrein), and the latter are the *cortical labyrinths.* Also found in the juxtamedullary region are arched blood vessels running parallel to the base of the pyramid, which give rise to radial, branches supplying and draining the cortical labyrinths.

Each lobe is subdivided into *lobules.* Most authors describe a lobule as centered about a medullary ray and bounded by *interlobular arteries* running parallel to the ray in all the adjacent cortical labyrinths. Smith and others give valid reasons for supporting the idea that the artery located in the cortical labyrinth should be considered the center of the lobule, which is then bounded by the centers of adjacent medullary rays. In the vascular lobule the artery becomes a *lobular artery,* which is synonymous with the interlobular artery of the previous system.

Gross structure of the multilobar kidney

Examination of the external aspect of the kidney of a 6-month-old infant reveals remnants

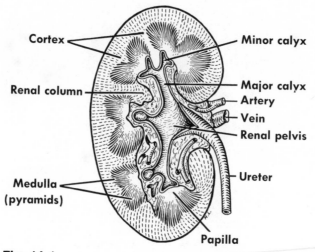

Fig. 14-1

Diagram showing topography of kidney. (Redrawn after Bailey.)

of a number of lobes (twelve to eighteen). With maturation the external evidence of lobation in man is obliterated. In the larger mammals (for example, ox, elephant, seal, etc.) the lobes are externally visible, and each one appears to act like a separate kidney. Man has a multilobed, multipyramidal kidney.

In man the intrarenal pelvis branches into three anterior and posterior tubes called the *major calyces,* which in turn branch to form a total of eight *minor calyces* (Fig. 14-1). Each minor calyx receives a papilla from a single pyramid or a papilla formed by the fusion of two or more pyramids. As a result of fusion there are fewer papillae (four to thirteen) than pyramids (eight to eighteen). In multipyramidal kidneys, trabeculae of the cortical parenchyma fill in the spaces between adjacent pyramids and are called the *renal columns* or columns of Bertini, or Bertin. The physiologist considers only the renal pyramids and medullary rays to constitute medulla and the cortical labyrinths and renal columns to constitute the cortex of the kidney.

Circulation

Each kidney is supplied by a single *renal artery,* which divides in the renal sinus into two sets of *secondary renal arteries.* One set supplies the anterior two-thirds of the kidney, whereas the other supplies the posterior one-third. As they pass through the fat body of the sinus they divide again prior to penetrating between adjacent pyramids or between a pyramid and an adjacent renal column. The latter are called *interlobar arteries* (a term obviously not suited to unilobar kidneys). Each lobe is supplied by a number of interlobar arteries (six to fourteen), which curve abruptly in the juxtamedullary region to form incomplete arterial arches known as *arciform arteries* (arcuate arteries). Along their entire path over the base of the pyramid the arciform arteries give rise to radial or perpendicular *lobular arteries* (interlobular arteries) that supply the cortical labyrinths. In the cortical labyrinths the lobular arteries give rise to numerous short straight *afferent arterioles* that supply small tufts of blood vessels called *glomeruli.* The lobular arteries become progressively smaller and terminate in the subcapsular region in a plexus of arterioles and capillaries that supply part of the capsule.

The blood flow leaving the glomeruli differs according to the location of the latter. Each of the *cortical glomeruli* (outer two-thirds of the cortex) gives rise to an *efferent arteriole* of a diameter equal to that of the afferent vessel. The efferent arterioles divide shortly to form a *peritubular capillary network* within the cortical labyrinths and medullary rays found in the cortical region. Each *juxtamedullary glomerulus* (located in the inner one-third of the cortex) gives rise to an efferent arteriole whose diameter is equal to or larger than the afferent vessel. The efferent arterioles of these glomeruli penetrate the pyramid and divide there into a series of long straight parallel blood vessels passing into the papilla and are collectively referred to

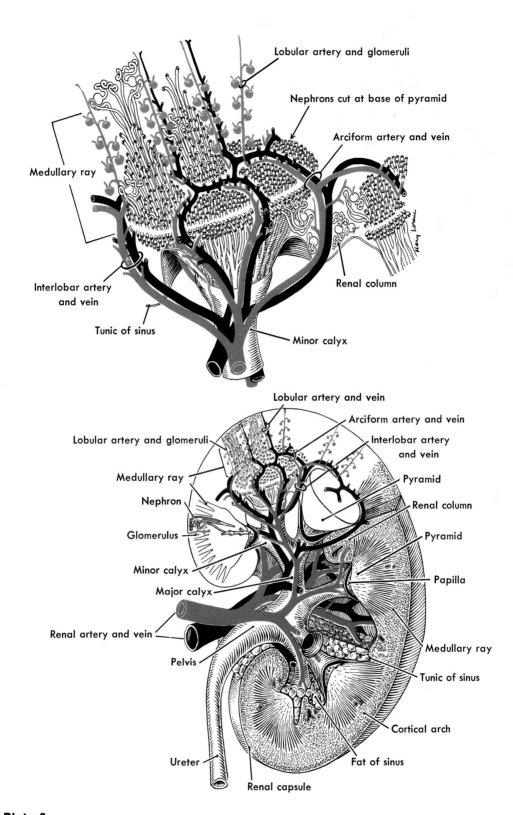

Plate 3

Circulatory plan of kidney. (From Smith, H. W.: Principles of renal physiology, New York, 1956, Oxford University Press, Inc.)

as the *vasa recta*. Their diameter is roughly equal to that of the efferent vessels, and the presence of intermittent circularly arranged smooth muscle elements indicates the source of the name *arteriolae rectae*. Careful observation is necessary to differentiate these from ordinary capillaries. An incomplete inner elastic membrane may occur in afferent arterioles but not in the efferent or glomerular vessels. The smooth muscle elements of the efferent arterioles may be lacking or replaced at intervals by groups of contractile pericytes or Rouget cells.

If the renal capsule is stripped away carefully, one may observe that a series of subcapsular blood vessels merge at certain points. These give the impression that the kidney surface is covered by a number of star-shaped blood vessels. These are the so-called *stellate veins,* and the central point of fusion marks the beginning of the *lobular vein* (interlobular vein). The lobular veins pass through the cortical labyrinths in company with the lobular arteries. The freely anastomosing peritubular capillaries drain into short cortical veins (intralobular veins), which in turn join the lobular veins. In the juxtamedullary region the lobular veins join the *arcuate veins* (arciform veins). In contrast with the arcuate arteries the arcuate veins form complete arches over the surface of the pyramidal base. The papilla is drained by a series of straight blood vessels, *venae rectae.* The walls of these veins contain smooth muscle spirally arranged. The venae rectae drain directly into the arcuate veins in the juxtamedullary region.

The renal artery sends a branch to the adrenal gland as well as much smaller branches to the ureter, renal pelvis, adipose tissue, and nerves of the sinus, calyces, and vasa vasorum of the larger blood vessels entering the kidney parenchyma. The collateral circulation of the kidney is described in more advanced texts.

Finer structure of the kidney

The urinary functions of the kidney are carried out by three groups of structures. These are (1) the glomeruli, (2) the nephrons, and (3) the collecting tubules and papillary ducts. It is by the activity of nephrons that urine is formed, and nephrons are described as the functional units of the kidney. There are about one million nephrons in each human kidney.

Glomeruli. In tissue sections each glomerulus is observed as an oval or rounded body consisting of a mass of capillaries containing many red blood cells and bounded by a small space (Figs. 14-2 and 14-4). The space is the cavity of Bowman's capsule, formed by invagination of the capillary into an enlargement of the end of the nephron. Thus, Bowman's capsule is a double-layered structure composed of simple squamous epithelium, with nuclei bulging into the capsular space. The inner layer of Bowman's capsule is known as the *visceral layer* and is in intimate contact with all the exposed surfaces of the glomerular tuft. The parietal layer forms the outer boundary of the capsule. A prominent basement membrane is visualized by the PAS technique and is located around the *parietal layer* of the capsule and between the visceral layer and the glomerular capillaries.

The side of the glomerulus where the afferent and efferent arterioles enter and leave and approximate each other forms the vascular pole of the glomerulus. The end directed toward the tubular portion of the nephron is known as the urinary pole of the glomerulus (Fig. 14-4).

As the afferent arteriole approaches the vascular pole it gives rise to the juxtaglomerular apparatus (Fig. 14-4). As it enters Bowman's capsule the afferent arteriole loses its inner elastic membrane and gives rise to from four to eight primary capillaries, which branch and form a number of anastomosing secondary capillaries. They in turn merge to form primary capillaries draining into the efferent arteriole. As a result of this arrangement of capillaries the glomerulus is described as *lobulated.* In section, however, the mass of capillaries observed in glomeruli rarely appear lobulated.

The glomerulus and its enveloping Bowman's capsule form the *malpighian corpuscle,* or renal corpuscle. Although there is considerable variation in size, the juxtamedullary glomeruli appear to be larger and in man may average approximately 0.2 mm. in diameter. Glomeruli are limited to the cortical labyrinths and renal columns and are not ordinarily found in the medullary rays or pyramidal tissue of the kidney. *Note:* Many lower chordates (for example, certain fishes) possess aglomerular kidneys.

Nephron. On an anatomical basis the nephron consists of four parts: Bowman's capsule, proximal convoluted tubule, loop of Henle, and the distal convoluted tubule (Fig. 14-3). Bowman's capsule has been described previously as an invaginated dilation of the nephric

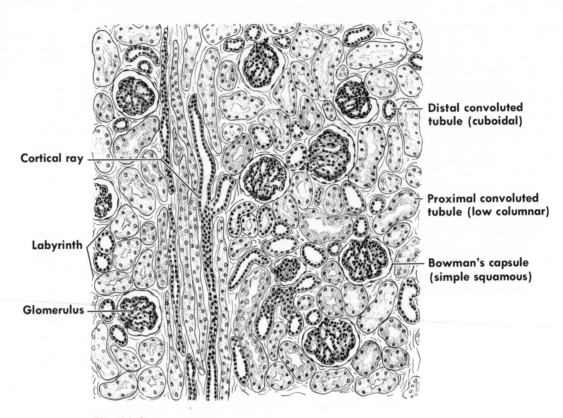

Fig. 14-2
Section of part of cortex of human kidney.

Labels on figure:
- Cortical ray
- Labyrinth
- Glomerulus
- Distal convoluted tubule (cuboidal)
- Proximal convoluted tubule (low columnar)
- Bowman's capsule (simple squamous)

tubule. The parietal layer leads into a small neckline constriction that contains ciliated cells in submammalian forms but not in human beings. The tubule leading from the capsule almost immediately begins a twisted and tortuous path through the cortical labyrinth and is accordingly named the proximal convoluted tubules. In sections this is indicated by tubules cut in several planes (Fig. 14-2); most, however, appear in transverse or in tangential section.

The proximal tubule enters a medullary ray at the site where it bends toward the papilla and forms a relatively straight tube, the *descending arm* of Henle's loop, which extends for a variable distance and then reverses its direction to form the so-called *ascending arm* of Henle's loop, which is approximately parallel to the descending arm. In the region of the actual curvature the tubule becomes extremely thin, giving rise to the *thin segment* of Henle's loop. The thin segment is a variable structure, since it may be located on the ascending side, the descending side, or both. Thin segments of nephrons arising from cortical glomeruli are abbreviated or are lacking entirely, whereas nephrons originating in the juxtamedullary region bear long thin segments penetrating deeply into the pyramids. In summary, the loops of Henle are located entirely within the medullary rays and pyramids. They consist of a thick descending limb, a thin segment that varies in location and length, and a thick ascending limb.

The ascending limb enters the cortical labyrinth slightly below the level of the glomerulus of origin and passes between the afferent and efferent vessels and makes tangential contact with the vascular pole of the glomerulus. The region of tangential contact gives rise to the *macula densa* (Fig. 14-4). The portion of tubule extending beyond the vascular pole is known as the *distal convoluted tubule*. It is less convoluted than the proximal tubule. The distal tubule leads to an arched tubule that enters the medullary ray to join the system of collecting tubules.

On a cytological-physiological basis only four

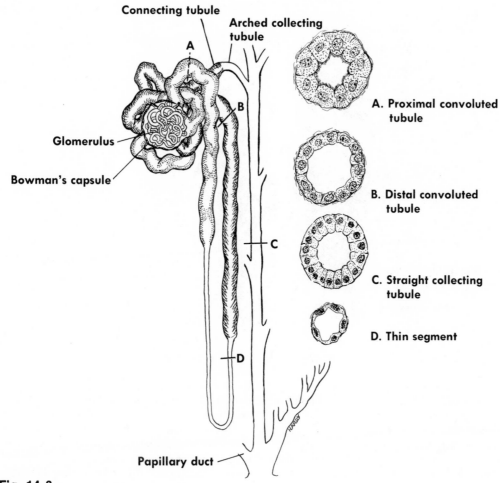

Connecting tubule

Arched collecting tubule

A

B

Glomerulus

Bowman's capsule

C

D

Papillary duct

A. Proximal convoluted tubule

B. Distal convoluted tubule

C. Straight collecting tubule

D. Thin segment

Fig. 14-3

Diagram of essential structures of nephron.

subdivisions of the nephron are designated: Bowman's capsule, a proximal segment, a thin segment, and a distal segment.

Bowman's capsule. The *parietal* layer of Bowman's capsule consists of squamous epithelium with prominent nuclei that protrude into the capillary space (Fig. 14-4). The inner or *visceral* epithelium forms a thin sheet over the loops of the glomerular capillaries. This fact was not clearly demonstrated until observed by electron microscopy. Studies utilizing the electron microscope have shown that the cells comprising the visceral epithelium are branching cells called *podocytes* (Fig. 14-5). Each cell consists of a central mass containing a nucleus and several radiating processes, which in turn give rise to smaller processes known as *pedicles*.

The pedicles make contact with the basal lamina of the capillary. Pedicles from adjacent cells interdigitate and leave slits (filtration slits) that communicate with the larger spaces between major extensions. They all empty into the capsular (urinary) space.

The endothelial cells of the capillaries are thin flattened cells with a mass of cytoplasm in the area of the nucleus. In the thinner portions of the cells they exhibit a specialization that consists of numerous round openings (fenestrations), which are regularly arranged and close to one another.

Another component of the glomerulus consists of cells and intercellular matrices occupying a position between the capillary loops known as the *mesangium*. The mesangial cells have

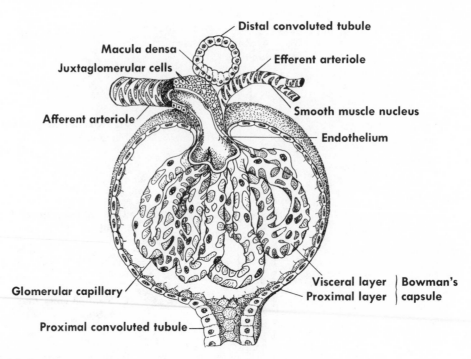

Fig. 14-4
Representative drawing of renal corpuscle. (Redrawn and modified from Bailey.)

been described as having a dense cytoplasm and radiating cytoplasmic processes and tonofilaments.

Proximal segment. The proximal segment consists of tubules with low columnar epithelium (Fig. 14-3) bearing a brush border at the free surface and basal striations in the subnuclear position. The latter represent infoldings of the cell membrane along which mitochondria may be visualized by special methods. Inasmuch as adjacent cells interdigitate freely, the cell outlines are rarely seen in cross sections of the tubule. The coarsely granular eosinophilic cytoplasm bulges into the lumen, and the nuclei are basally located. The brush border is not ordinarily well preserved, and accordingly, the free edge of the cell appears rounded and slightly ragged. Similarly, mitochondria and basal striations are not well preserved in routine preparations and are not usually apparent to the novice. The basal striations become less distinct as the thin segment is approached. Despite considerable postmortem degeneration, these cells are considerably more eosinophilic than those found in adjacent tubules.

The proximal segment consists of a convoluted portion in the cortical labyrinth and a straight descending limb in the medullary ray and pyramid.

Thin segments. The thin segments are tubular structures consisting of squamous cells. The cytoplasm appears agranular, and the nucleus is slightly compressed. In cross section they may be confused with capillaries and arteriolae rectae, especially since red blood cells are sometimes forced into the thin segments during preparation of the tissue. They are distinguished from capillaries by (1) the more extensive protrusion of nuclei into the lumen and (2) the greater number of cells visible in cross section through a tubule.

Thin segments are demonstrable in profusion in the deeper portions of the pyramids, since they extend almost to the papillae. Thin segments of the kind described are lacking in reptiles, most birds, amphibians, and fishes.

Distal segment. The thin segment joins the distal segment, the latter being composed initially of low cuboidal cells with indistinct boundaries. As the ascending limb approaches the cortex the cells are taller but are still cuboidal and bear irregular projections into the lumen. Upon entering the cortical labyrinths the tubule passes the vascular pole of the glomerulus of

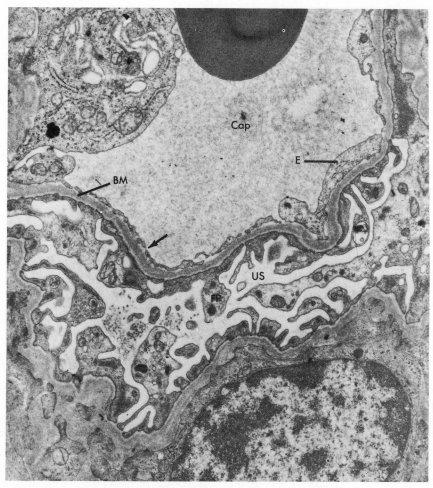

Fig. 14-5

Electron micrograph of part of the glomerulus of a monkey's kidney. The capillary, **Cap,** is lined with endothelium, **E,** which at intervals contains pores (arrow). The outer walls of the capillaries are invested by the cytoplasm of podocytes, whose fingerlike processes, called pedicles, **FP,** extend from the capillary into the lumen of the urinary space, **US.** The cytoplasm of the basal portions of the endothelial cells and the podocytes are separated by a prominent basement membrane, **BM.** (× 10,000.)

origin and makes tangential contact with the afferent arteriole. At the point of contact the cuboidal cells become more closely packed so that the cells appear taller (sometimes columnar), and many nuclei are visible and crowded together to form the *macula densa.* Beyond this structure the tubule becomes convoluted, consisting of smaller cuboidal cells, the free surfaces of which are smooth. These cells are less eosinophilic (or more basophilic) than those found in the proximal tubule. The cells do not bear a striated border or brush border or basal striations, nor do they exhibit definite cell

boundaries in sectioned material. The basement membrane is prominent along all parts of the tubule except in the region of the macula densa. Since the convoluted portion is short, fewer sections through this segment are seen in the cortical labyrinths.

Collecting tubules and papillary ducts. At the termination of the distal convoluted tubule one may sometimes observe a short connecting tubule. It contains a mixture of the cuboidal cells characteristic of the distal segment and occasional isolated large granular cells (intercalated cells). This is supposedly the region of embryonic fusion between the nephron and the collecting tubule.

The connecting tubule is continuous with the *arched collecting tubule,* which passes into the medullary ray, where it joins the *straight collecting tubule.* The straight tubules, along with Henle's loops, lie in parallel bundles and occupy most of the medulla, with the exception of the papilla. The cells of the collecting tubules are noted for their distinct boundaries, spherical nuclei at approximately the same level in the cell, and relatively agranular cytoplasm. Eventually, the straight tubules reach the papillary region and fuse to form relatively large ducts, the *papillary ducts* (ducts of Bellini). These consist of tall columnar cells. In each papilla sixteen to twenty papillary ducts develop that penetrate the apex of the papilla to form a sievelike region, or *area cribosa.* From this site the urine formed in the nephrons is drained into a minor calyx.

Juxtaglomerular apparatus. At the vascular pole of the glomerulus (Fig. 14-4) the media and adventitial reticulum of the afferent arteriole are replaced by cells that vary from cuboidal to columnar. These form a thickening or cuff around the arteriole (periarteriolar pad). A number of cells may spill over into the cleft between the afferent and efferent vessels to form an asymmetrical cap (polkissen, or polar cushion). This complex of cells is referred to as the *juxtaglomerular apparatus.* The polkissen and periarteriolar pad both may be in contact with the macula densa, and their region of contact is marked by the absence of a PAS-positive basement membrane. The polkissen cells of certain rodents exhibit some large epithelioid cells containing brilliant fuchsinophil granules. In canines and man the cells are small and agranular. In addition, the juxtaglomerular apparatus is not demonstrable in man for the first 2 years of postnatal life. The presence of epithelioid cells similar to those found in certain endocrine organs suggests an endocrine function. Physiological experiments have failed to produce consistent changes in the juxtaglomerular apparatus, and thus, the status of this structure remains to be elucidated.

Lymphatic circulation. The lymphatic plexi are found in three main regions as follows: (1) A network of lymphatic capillaries permeates the cortex and renal columns; these capillaries form an anastomosing network around blood vessels, especially the larger arteries; the plexus drains into the lymphatic vessels, leaving the hilum of the kidney, and then goes into the lateral aortic nodes (2) beneath the renal capsule in intimate association with the stellate veins and subcapsular plexus of blood capillaries. This group communicates with (3) the lymphatics draining the perirenal fat body. The perirenal lymphatic plexus drains into the lateral aortic nodes.

Lymphatics are lacking in the renal pyramids and glomeruli and do not enter the tubules. No specific function has been demonstrated for the kidney lymphatics.

Connective tissue. The renal capsule is formed of a dense fibrous connective tissue, which is primarily collagenous with some elastic fibers and a few scattered smooth muscle cells. A thin inflexion of this capsule lines the renal sinus and fuses with the adventitia of the blood vessels and epineurium of the larger nerves. It also disperses into fine strands in the fat body of the renal sinus. The renal capsule is easily stripped from normal kidneys because of a lack of trabeculae from the capsule.

The basement membrane entirely envelops all parts of the nephron and collecting tubules except as noted previously. The ground substance of the basement membrane is PAS positive, and the reticular fibers are typically argyrophil and quite fine. In the pyramids the reticular fibers form an extensive network, binding ducts and blood vessels together.

URETER

Urine collects in the pelvis of the kidney and passes out through the ureter. This is a thin duct, composed of the following layers:

Mucosa

The mucosa includes an epithelium of the transitional type, resting on a tunica propria of reticular and fine areolar tissue. There is no muscularis mucosae.

Submucosa

The submucosa consists of loose areolar tissue and blends with the tunica propria on one side and with the intermuscular connective tissue of the muscularis on the other.

Muscularis

The muscularis reverses the usual arrangement of coats, having an inner longitudinal and an outer circular layer. In the lower portion of the ureter there is a third layer of muscle,

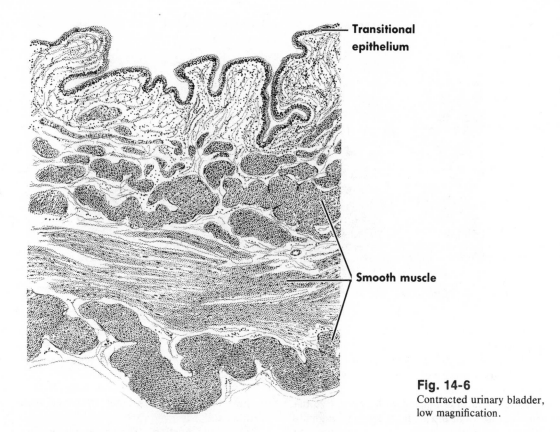

— **Transitional epithelium**

Smooth muscle

Fig. 14-6
Contracted urinary bladder, low magnification.

longitudinally disposed, outside the circular layer. All three layers are somewhat loosely arranged, with a great deal of areolar tissue among the muscle fibers.

Adventitia

The adventitia is formed of loose connective tissue.

URINARY BLADDER (Figs. 14-6 and 14-7)

The wall of the urinary bladder is composed of the same elements as that of the lower part of the ureter (namely, transitional epithelium, tunica propria, submucosa, three layers of muscle, and adventitia). In the bladder the epithelium varies in thickness according to the degree of distention of the organ. The muscular layers of the bladder are not as regular in their arrangement as those of the ureter, but they form a thicker layer.

URETHRA

The urethra of the female serves as an outlet for urine from the bladder, while that of the male functions also as the terminal portion of the ducts of the reproductive system. The organ is, therefore, somewhat different in the two sexes.

Female urethra

In the female the tube is composed of an epithelial lining, a connective tissue layer, and a muscular coat. The epithelium of the proximal part is like that of the bladder. This type is replaced, farther down the tube, first by stratified columnar or pseudostratified epithelium and later by stratified squamous epithelium toward the distal end.

The connective tissue layer contains elastic fibers and a rich plexus of veins that may be compared with the corpus cavernosum of the male urethra (see later), although it is much less extensive. The lumen of the organ is irregular, since the connective tissue and epithelium are thrown into longitudinal rugae. There are also small diverticula from the lumen (lacunae), into which open the mucus-secreting glands of Littre.

The muscularis consists of two sets of smooth

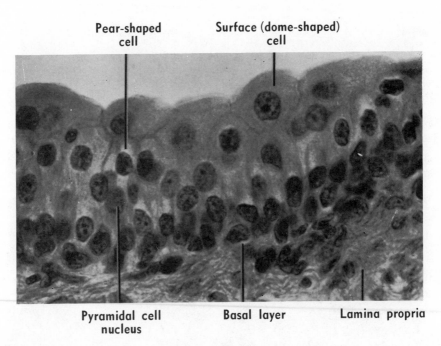

Pear-shaped cell **Surface (dome-shaped) cell**

Pyramidal cell nucleus **Basal layer** **Lamina propria**

Fig. 14-7
Section of mucosa of urinary bladder of dog, showing transitional epithelium. (× 640.) (From Bevelander, G.: Essentials of histology, ed. 6, St. Louis, 1970, The C. V. Mosby Co.)

muscle fibers intermingled with connective tissue. The fibers of the inner set are longitudinally placed; the outer have a circular direction. At the distal end of the urethra there is, in addition, a sphincter of striated muscle.

Male urethra

The male urethra shows modifications of the structure described. It is divided into three portions.

Prostatic portion. The proximal end of the prostatic urethra is homologous to the female urethra and resembles it in structure as well as in function. As the tube passes through the prostate gland it receives the openings of the ducts from the testes and numerous small ducts from the prostate.

Membranous portion. The membranous portion of the urethra, which passes through the urogenital diaphragm, is also somewhat like the female urethra. The epithelium changes in or about this region from transitional to stratified columnar or pseudostratified, but the location of the change varies considerably in different individuals. Glands are more common than in the female urethra. The bulbourethral (mucous) glands of Cowper are situated in the muscle near the distal part of the membranous

urethra, but their ducts enter the cavernous urethra.

Cavernous portion. The cavernous portion is the longest segment of the urethra, lying in the penis. The tissues surrounding it will be discussed more fully in the section on the male reproductive system. The epithelial lining of the urethra changes at the distal end to stratified squamous with well-developed connective tissue papillae. The tunica propria contains an extensive plexus of blood vessels that forms the corpus cavernosum urethrae, and the glands of Littre are most numerous in this portion of the tube. The muscular coat is broken up into scattered groups of fibers.

BLOOD VESSELS AND NERVES OF THE EXCRETORY PASSAGES

The blood supply of the ureter, bladder, and urethra comes from arteries that penetrate the muscular coats of the organs and form plexuses in the deeper layers of the tunica propria. From here vessels continue inward, forming the other plexuses just below the epithelium. The deeper layers of the connective tissue and probably the muscular layers have a rich lymphatic supply.

Plexuses of medullated and nonmedullated

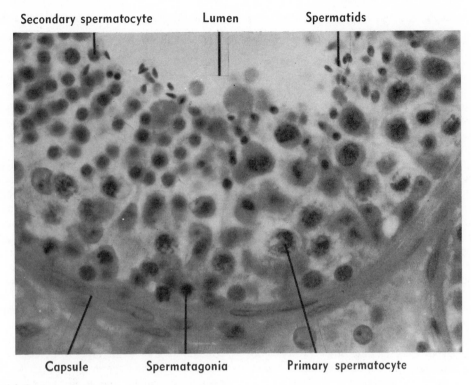

Secondary spermatocyte   **Lumen**   **Spermatids**

Capsule   **Spermatagonia**   **Primary spermatocyte**

Fig. 14-8

Section of portion of human seminiferous tubule. (×640.) (From Bevelander, G.: Essentials of histology, ed.6, St. Louis, 1970, The C. V. Mosby Co.)

nerves occur in the walls of the ureter and the bladder. The nonmedullated nerves supply the muscles; the medullated, the mucosa. Numerous ganglia are present in the connective tissue.

MALE REPRODUCTIVE SYSTEM
TESTIS (Fig. 14-8)

The testis in the adult lies in the scrotum, partly surrounded by a serous sac, the tunica vaginalis, which is a diverticulum from the peritoneum. This gland is covered by a two-layered connective tissue capsule. The outer layer, or tunica albuginea, is composed of dense white fibrous tissue; the inner layer, or vasculosa, is of looser areolar tissue, richly supplied with blood vessels. From the capsule, trabeculae extend inward to a central mass of connective tissue, the mediastinum, which contains the proximal portions of the duct system. The parenchyma of the testis is thus divided into many pyramidal lobules, which contain the closely packed coils of the seminiferous tubules and a stroma of interstitial connective tissue.

In the connective tissue there are blood vessels and groups of endocrine cells called the interstitial cells of the testis.

The convoluted, seminiferous tubules are lined with germinal epithelium, which may contain as many as five layers of cells. Each layer represents a different stage in the development of the spermatozoa, or male sex cells. Nearest the outside of the wall of the tubule lie the spermatogonia, or primordial germ cells. These are small cuboidal or rounded cells with vesicular nuclei. Next to them, toward the lumen, are the primary spermatocytes, larger cells in the nuclei of which the chromatin is collected in dense clumps. Then follow the secondary spermatocytes, similar in appearance but somewhat smaller than the primary spermatocytes. Superimposed on these are the spermatids, which are much smaller cells with vesicular nuclei; bordering on the lumen are the fully formed spermatozoa. These have dark, elongated nuclei and flagella.

The process involved in the development of the spermatozoa consists of, first, a rearrangement of the chromatin material of the nucleus and, second, the formation of motile cells. In ordinary mitoses, or cell divisions, the chromatin condenses into a number of small bodies, the chromosomes. Each chromosome divides, so that half of it goes to one daughter cell and half to the other. The number of chromosomes formed at each mitosis is constant and characteristic for each species of animal (probably forty-six in man). This number also appears in the divisions of the spermatogonia. When, however, the primary spermatocytes divide, the individual chromosomes do not split. Half of them go undivided to one secondary spermatocyte, half to the other. This is known as maturation, or the reduction of chromatin. A similar process takes place in the development of the ovum, or female sexual cell. Its result is obvious: The spermatozoon, containing twenty-three chromosomes, unites with the ovum, which also contains twenty-three chromosomes; the resulting new individual is thus provided with forty-six of these bodies, half of which are derived from each parent. Since the chromosomes are the bearers of hereditary characteristics, their distribution is of great interest to geneticists. The details of maturation, however, are not to be observed in ordinary slides. This is true also of the second part of the development of the spermatozoa, that is, the formation of motile cells from nonmotile cells. The stages mentioned may be identified in most slides of the testis.

The process of spermatogenesis is not in the same stage in all parts of the tubule at a given time. The completion of spermatozoa occurs in a series of waves that pass down the tubule. For this reason a lobule of the testis, when sectioned, will show some portions of the tubules in which all five stages are present and others in which only three or four can be demonstrated.

Spermatogenesis is the maturation of the spermatid to form spermatozoa. The spermatid exhibits a large centrally located nucleus, numerous mitochondria, and a pair of centrioles. The prominent supranuclear Golgi apparatus consists of numerous lamellae and vesicles. Granules that appear in these vesicles coalesce to form the *acrosome* within the acrosome vesicle (Fig. 14-9). The acrosome and its vesicle lie between the Golgi apparatus and nuclear membrane. The acrosomal vesicle enlarges and eventually envelops approximately half of the

surface of the nucleus; it finally collapses and forms a closely applied membrane covering the acrosome, known as the *head cap*. During the formation of the acrosome at one pole of the nucleus, one of the centrioles becomes modified into a slender flagellum at the opposite pole. Further differentiation consists in the application of a filamentous sheath around the axial filaments of the flagellum. Meanwhile, the other centriole migrates toward the surface of the cell and gives rise to the annulus encircling the longitudinal axial filaments. The nucleus decreases in size, becomes flattened and elongated, and is then known as the sperm head. Development of the tail consists in a shift of the cytoplasm and a rearrangement of the mitochondria to the region between the basal centriole and the annulus. In this region the mitochondria become aligned in helical fashion and make up the mitochondrial sheath of the middle piece of the developing sperm. As differentiation continues the excess cytoplasm is shed as the residual body; thus, eventually the spermatozoon is covered by a very thin layer of cytoplasm.

The mammalian sperm is comprised of three main components; the head, neck, and tail. The head mainly consists of a dense nucleus that is surmounted by a small crescentic acrosome. The neck, or connecting piece between the head and the tail, contains linear fibrils surrounded by a mitochondrial sheath. The middle piece of the tail consists of two central filaments and nine doubled peripheral ones. External to the latter are nine outer coarse fibers of uneven size enclosed by a helical mitochondrial sheath. The main segment of the tail has two central and nine peripheral filaments and except in the terminal portion is enclosed by a thin layer of cytoplasm.

It will be noticed that the germinal epithelium of the testis, although it is stratified, is not to be classed with any other type of epithelium. In those types already studied the stratification has as its purpose the formation of a protective layer. In the germinal epithelium it is simply the accidental result of the piling of one stage of development on another. The tissue differs from other epithelia also in the relation of the cells to each other. In stratified squamous epithelium, for instance, the cells are closely applied to each other and are held together by cement substance. In germinal epithelium the cells are so loosely piled that many of them retain their spherical shape.

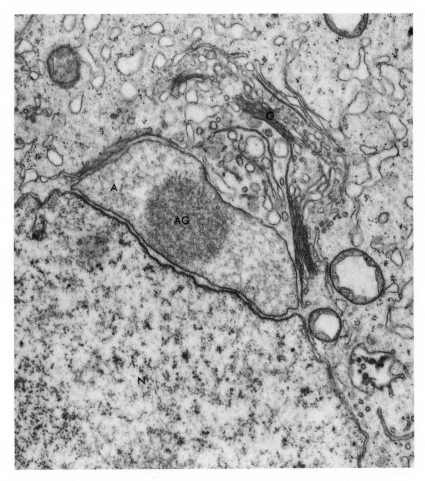

Fig. 14-9
Electron micrograph of developing spermatid of mouse, showing relation of Golgi apparatus, **G**, to acrosome. **A**, Acrosomal vesicle; **AG**, acrosomal granule; **N**, nucleus. (×28,000.)

In addition to the cells that represent stages of spermatogenesis, the seminiferous tubule has in its wall a number of supporting cells—the sustentacular, or Sertoli, cells. These are irregular elongated elements, the bases of which lie against the basement membrane, while their apices border on the lumen. Because of the pallor of their cytoplasm and the crowding of the germinal cells, it is difficult to see the outlines of a sustentacular cell. Its nucleus may be identified by its elongated shape and lack of chromatin; it is much paler than the nucleus of any of the stages of spermatogenesis. When mature spermatozoa are present, they tend to gather in groups with their heads (nuclei) embedded in the free end of the Sertoli cell, and this fact will aid the student, since the groups of sper-

matozoa are easily seen. It is supposed that the sustentacular cells furnish nourishment to the spermatozoa as well as form a supporting framework for the other germinal cells.

The spermatogenic tubules lie coiled in a stroma of loose connective tissue in which, entirely separated from the tubules, are groups of cells that are not concerned with the formation of spermatozoa. These are the interstitial cells, or cells of Leydig, which produce the male hormone known as testosterone as well as a large proportion of the female hormone estrogen. These cells are fairly large and are ovoid or polygonal. The nucleus is large and eccentrically placed. The cytoplasm near the nucleus is dense and granular; peripherally it is vacuolated and stains lightly. These cells may also exhibit

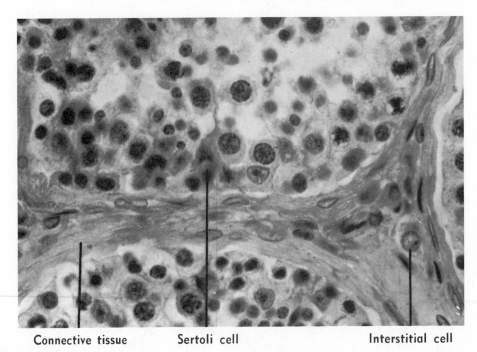

Connective tissue   Sertoli cell   Interstitial cell

Fig. 14-10
Section of human seminiferous tubules. (×640.) (From Bevelander, G.: Essentials of histology, ed.6, St. Louis, 1970, The C. V. Mosby Co.)

Cavernous space

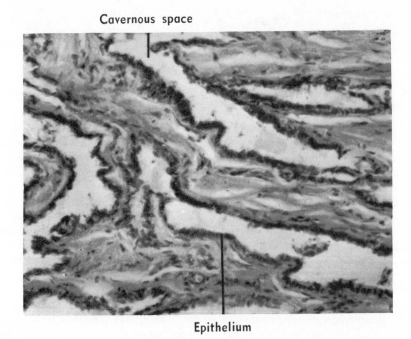

Epithelium

Fig. 14-11
Section of rete testis of dog. (×200.) (From Bevelander, G.: Essentials of histology, ed. 6, St. Louis, 1970, The C. V. Mosby Co.)

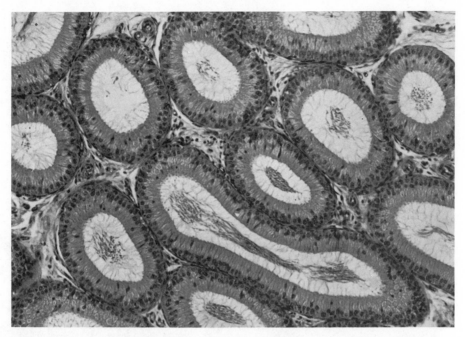

Fig. 14-12
Section of epididymis of dog, showing several sections through ductus. (×160.) Stereocilia are prominent, and lumen contain spermatozoa. (From Bevelander, G.: Essentials of histology, ed. 6, St. Louis, 1970, The C. V. Mosby Co.)

pigment granules and crystalloids (Fig. 14-10).

The action of testosterone, the male hormone, has been ascertained by direct observation and by many experimental procedures involving castration at various stages of sexual maturity. In brief, it has been shown that the male hormone is necessary for the appearance of the so-called secondary sex characteristics in the developing mammal. If castration is performed after sexual maturity has occurred, the effect on already-established secondary sex characteristics is less pronounced than in the developing individual. In the latter situation, involution of the epithelium of the genital ducts and accessory glands is the most constant feature observed.

From the convoluted tubules the spermatozoa pass into the proximal part of the duct system of the testis, which lies in the mediastinum of the organ. They go through the tubuli recti, or straight tubules, into the rete testis, which is a network of fine tubules occupying a part of the mediastinum (Fig. 14-11). The walls of the tubuli recti and the rete testis consist of low cuboidal epithelium. From the rete testis a number of spiral tubules lead to the epididymis. These are called tubuli efferentes and are lined with

a peculiar epithelium in which groups of ciliated columnar cells are interspersed among the cuboidal elements, giving the border of the lumen an irregular outline.

EPIDIDYMIS

The epididymis lies near the testis, partly surrounded by a fold of the tunica vaginalis and enclosed in a connective tissue capsule (Fig. 14-12). The epididymis contains one tubule, the ductus epididymidis. It is, however, much coiled so that a slide made from a piece of this organ presents a great number of sections of it, cut longitudinally, transversely, or tangentially. The duct is lined with ciliated epithelium, described as pseudostratified by some and as stratified columnar by others. The epithelium is surrounded by smooth muscle, circularly arranged.

DUCTUS DEFERENS

The ductus deferens is a continuation of the ductus epididymidis. It is lined with a somewhat lower epithelium without cilia. This rests on a well-developed tunica propria. The muscularis has three layers: a thick circular one, with thin

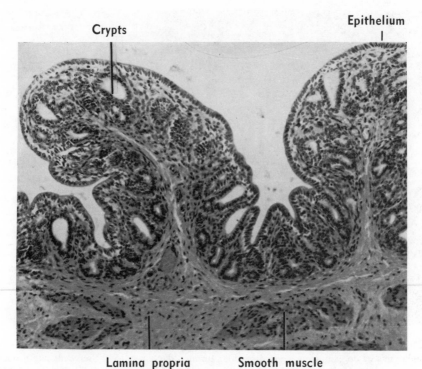

Crypts   Epithelium

Lamina propria   Smooth muscle

Fig. 14-13
Mucosa of seminal vesicle of cat. (×160.) (From Bevelander, G.: Essentials of histology, ed. 6, St. Louis, 1970, The C. V. Mosby Co.)

layers of longitudinal fibers on both sides of it. Just before reaching the prostate gland the ductus deferens is dilated to form the ampulla. As it passes into the substance of the prostate, it is constricted again to form the narrow ejaculatory duct that opens into the prostatic part of the urethra.

SEMINAL VESICLE

The seminal vesicle is an elongated saccular organ lying near the ampulla of the ductus deferens and opening into the latter at the point where it narrows to form the ejaculatory duct. The most striking histological characteristic of the seminal vesicle is the folding of its mucosa (Fig. 14-13). This produces a great number of projections and pockets, and since the latter are often tangentially cut there appear to be follicles in the mucosa. The appearance is much like that of the gallbladder. The epithelium of the seminal vesicle is, however, pseudostratified or stratified columnar, and it has a thinner muscular coat than that of the gallbladder.

PROSTATE

The prostate is a much-branched follicular gland that surrounds the urethra as the latter emerges from the bladder. Its secreting portions are lined with columnar epithelium and have large irregular lumina (Fig. 14-14). They may contain lamellar bodies, which stain red with eosin and are called prostatic concretions. If a follicle is somewhat distended by such a mass, the epithelium is flattened to the cuboidal type. A characteristic feature of the prostate is the presence of scattered fibers of smooth muscle in the connective tissue surrounding the follicles. The muscle does not form layers about the glandular portions but is distributed in groups of a few fibers running in various directions.

PENIS

A section of the penis shows, under the low magnification, three large masses of erectile tissue, each of which contains a great number of anastomosing blood vessels (Fig. 14-15). The

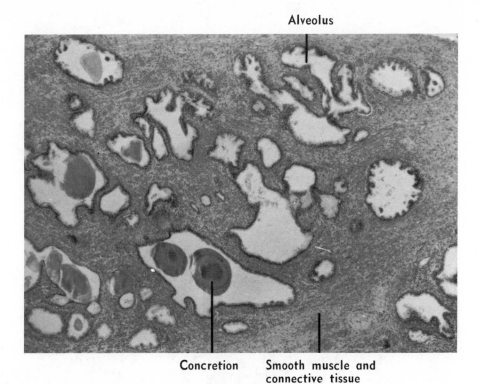

Alveolus

Concretion

Smooth muscle and
connective tissue

Fig. 14-14
Section of human prostatic urethra. (×40.) (From Bevelander, G.: Essentials of histology, ed. 6, St. Louis, 1970,
The C. V. Mosby Co.)

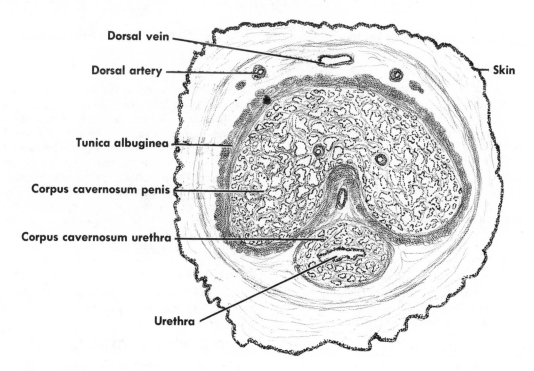

Dorsal vein

Dorsal artery

Skin

Tunica albuginea

Corpus cavernosum penis

Corpus cavernosum urethra

Urethra

Fig. 14-15
Transverse section of penis of newborn infant.

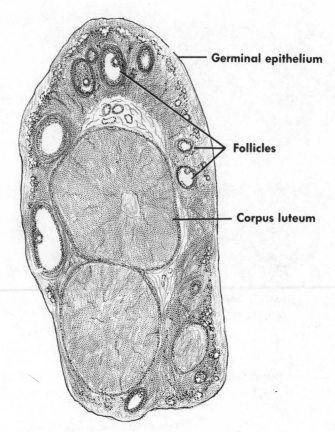

Fig. 14-16
Cat ovary, low magnification.

Germinal epithelium

Follicles

Corpus luteum

two dorsal masses, connected by a bridge of the same kind of tissue, are the corpora cavernosa penis. The smaller ventral mass surrounding the urethra is the corpus cavernosum urethrae, called also the corpus spongiosum.

The cavernous bodies are surrounded by a sheath of dense connective tissue, the tunica albuginea. Outside this is a stroma of loose connective tissue containing blood vessels, nerves, and lamellar corpuscles. There is no well-defined corium of the skin covering the penis, and it has a thin epidermis.

Blood is brought to the penis by the arteria penis, which branches to form the dorsal artery and the paired deep arteries. The dorsal artery sends branches to the tunica albuginea and to the large trabeculae of the cavernous bodies. Such branches break up into capillaries, from which blood passes into the lacunae of the erectile tissue and thence to a plexus of veins in the albuginea. The deep arteries run lengthwise, giving off branches that open into the cavernous

spaces. During times of sexual excitement the flow of blood into the cavernous spaces is greatly increased, especially that coming from the deep arteries. The veins that drain the blood spaces leave at an oblique angle. The central spaces are filled first, and their distention compresses the peripheral spaces and obstructs the flow of blood through the angular openings into the veins, thus producing rigidity of the penis. In the flaccid condition of the organ the incoming flow of blood is less and the passage into the veins remains open.

Nerve supply

The penis has an abundant supply of spinal, sympathetic, and parasympathetic fibers and many sensory end organs.

FEMALE REPRODUCTIVE SYSTEM

The female reproductive system consists of the ovaries, the fallopian tubes (oviducts), the uterus, and the vagina. Because of its functional

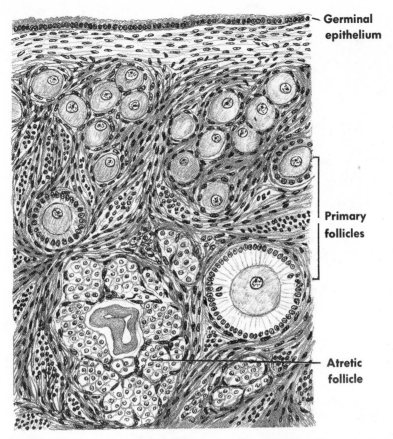

Germinal epithelium

Primary follicles

Atretic follicle

Fig. 14-17

Cortex of ovary, showing germinal epithelium and primary follicles in various stages of development. An atretic follicle is also shown.

relation to the reproductive tract, the mammary gland is discussed with the group of genital organs.

OVARY

The ovary differs greatly from the testis in its appearance, although it has the functions of forming sexual cells and of maintaining secondary sexual characteristics. In the testis the germinal epithelium forms the lining of a series of tubules, and the process of maturation is completed within the organ. In the ovary, on the contrary, the germinal epithelium forms the outer covering of the whole organ, and the only part of the development of ova that takes place in this part of the tract is growth. Maturation of ova occurs in most forms only after insemination, while the egg is passing from the ovary to the uterus.

The ovary is a small ovoid body, consisting of a mass of cellular connective tissue covered by germinal epithelium (Fig. 14-16). In the adult it contains interstitial cells and various stages of development and atrophy of the ova and their follicles. The entire organ is very vascular.

During embryonic life the germinal epithelium forms a many-layered mass at the periphery of the ovary, proliferating cells downward into the underlying connective tissue. Some of these cells are destined to develop into oogonia, while others are to form the follicles. The mass of cells is broken up by invading connective tissue into smaller clumps, the egg nests, or cords of Pflüger. Later the nests are subdivided into units, in each of which one may recognize a large central cell, the ovum, and a surrounding group of flat follicular cells (Fig. 14-17). Such units are called primary follicles and are found in the ovary at birth. The connective tissue

169

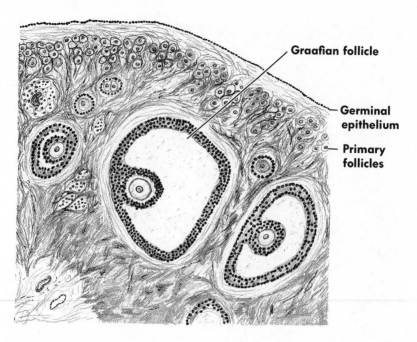

Fig. 14-18
Cortex of ovary.

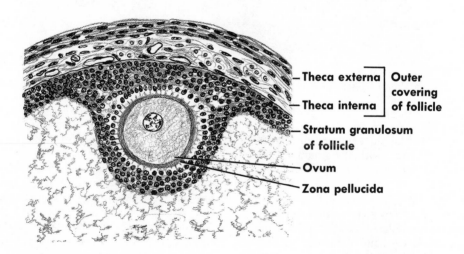

Fig. 14-19
Part of a graafian follicle, showing ovum and surrounding structures.

forms a thick sheath, the tunica albuginea, just beneath the germinal epithelium, and the latter is reduced to a single layer of cells that are columnar at first and cuboidal later.

At this stage of development the ovum is a spherical cell about 50μ in diameter. It contains a vesicular nucleus, and the granular cytoplasm stains red with eosin. The flattened cells of the follicle multiply and change in form from a squamous to cuboidal and then to columnar. Finally, a layer of stratified columnar epithelium surrounds the ovum. The latter enlarges, and the outer part of its cytoplasm is modified to form a hyaline coating called the zona pellucida.

Later stages involve chiefly the development of the follicle; the ovum attains a diameter of about 100μ, but its appearance is otherwise unchanged.

As the follicle sinks still deeper into the cortex of the ovary, its cells come to form a many-layered covering for the ovum. This is, at first, solid; in a later stage a cleft appears in the substance of it, and this cavity increases as the follicle grows (Fig. 14-18). At the end of its ovarian development the ovum is surrounded by a relatively enormous structure, the graafian follicle, in which one may distinguish the following parts (Fig. 14-19): the follicle, which is covered by a capsule of connective tissue, or theca folliculi. The outer part of this (theca externa) is dense fibrous tissue and the inner (theca interna) is looser and more vascular, containing cells and abundant cytoplasm, the form and arrangement of which suggest glandular rather than fiber-forming function. Internal to the theca are the follicular cells, the derivatives of the cells of the primary follicle. These form a coating approximately fifteen cells deep around the whole follicle, and the entire layer is now known as the stratum, or membrana, granulosum. At one point there is a mound of follicular cells that bulges into the cavity of the follicle. This is the cumulus oophorus, at the center of which is the ovum. The rest of the follicular cavity is filled with a fluid, the liquor folliculi. This is sometimes seen in sections as a pinkish granular coagulum. The cells of the cumulus that immediately surround the ovum are columnar in form (zona radiata).

The ovum and its follicle are now ready for the extrusion of the egg from the ovary (ovulation). The entire structure has moved out of the periphery of the cortex and lies so near the surface as to produce an elevation. At the end of intra-ovarian development the follicle ruptures, and the ovum is washed into the oviduct by the liquor folliculi. The number of ova discharged at one time and the interval between ovulations varies in different animals. In the human ovary there is usually one ovum discharged, from one ovary or the other, at intervals of 4 weeks.

It has been supposed that in human ovaries the first step of this development of follicles, namely, the separation of ova from the germinal epithelium, has been completed during embryonic life. If that is so, the time required for the maturation of a follicle would vary from 13 to 45 years, according to whether they rupture at the first or the last ovulation of sexual life. It has been shown that in the mouse, cells may be found detaching themselves from the germinal epithelium at any time between puberty and menopause, and it seems probable that the process occurs in this way in other mammals also.

At ovulation the majority of the follicular cells remain in the ovary, and the follicle undergoes changes leading to the formation of the corpus luteum. The first of these is the formation of a clot of blood, coming from the vessels of the theca interna that ruptured at ovulation. The next change involves the alteration of the character of the follicular cells and the cells of the theca interna. In the mature graafian follicle the former are rather small elements, with relatively little cytoplasm. They now enlarge and begin to invade and resorb the blood clot. Ultimately, they fill the center of the follicle with large, pale cells (Figs. 14-16 and 14-20). Each cell has an abundant amount of cytoplasm in which may be seen granules and fat droplets. The theca cells also enlarge and invade the mass at its periphery, along with connective tissue elements and blood vessels. The structure has, in a fresh specimen, a yellow color and is called the corpus luteum. The length of life of the corpus luteum and the size to which it grows depend upon the fate of the ovum that was discharged from the follicle.

If the ovum is fertilized and becomes implanted in the uterine wall, the corpus luteum continues to grow and is called a "true" corpus luteum (of pregnancy). If the ovum is not fertilized, the corpus luteum begins to degenerate about 14 days after ovulation. Such corpora lutea are "false" and are soon replaced by scar tissue (corpus albicans). These relations will be discussed more fully later.

ATRETIC FOLLICLES

In the preceding paragraphs we have discussed the normal development of an ovum and its follicle. It often happens, however, that follicles which have developed to the graafian stage degenerate instead of going on to ovulation. The first step in atresia is the death of the ovum itself, which is followed by the degeneration of the follicular cells; the result is a mass of detritus left at the center of the follicle. The cells of the theca interna undergo a hypertrophy similar, at first, to that occurring in

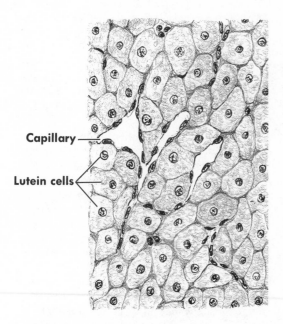

Capillary

Lutein cells

Fig. 14-20
Part of corpus luteum.

corpus luteum formation. Hypertrophy continues, moreover, resulting in the characteristic atretic follicle composed of a ring of enlarged theca cells surrounding it (Fig. 14-17). These cells have at this stage some resemblance to the cells of the corpus luteum but are smaller, less eosinophilic, and not conspicuously vacuolated.

The theca cells gradually come to fill the space left by the degenerating ovum and follicular cells, thus forming a solid mass. In this condition they may remain in the stroma of the ovary for some time. Such masses or strands of theca cells have been called the interstitial cells of the ovary, and they were originally supposed to have a function comparable to that assigned to the interstitial cells of the testis. However, experimental work has not offered any proof that they secrete the hormone responsible for the maintenance of secondary sexual characteristics.

It has now been established that the ovaries elaborate two hormones, estrogen and progesterone. Estrogen is formed mainly by the growing follicles. This hormone is concerned with the growth and development of the female reproductive tract and also the mammary glands. Progesterone, derived from the corpus luteum, is responsible for the secretion of the uterine

glands and also conditions the uterine mucosa for the reception of the fertilized ovum. The formation of these hormones is cyclical in nature and corresponds to changes that occur in the reproductive tract and uterine mucosa. These latter events are activated to a large extent by the gonadotropins secreted by the anterior pituitary gland.

• • •

To sum up, one may find in the ovary, in addition to the connective tissue stroma, the following elements:
1. Germinal epithelium
2. Interstitial cells
3. Primary follicles
4. Growing follicles
5. Graafian follicles
6. Blood clots
7. Corpora lutea
8. Scars
9. Atretic follicles

FALLOPIAN TUBE (OVIDUCT)

The ova, when they are extruded from the ovary, pass into the open end of the oviduct. The relation of the ovary to its duct differs from that of the testis to the ductus deferens. In the latter case the lumina of the convoluted tubules are continuous with that of the duct, and there is no possibility of the spermatozoa escaping from the system into the body cavity. The ova, on the contrary, come out to the surface of the ovary, and the latter is not completely enclosed in the lumen of the oviduct. The end of the oviduct is funnel shaped, with a convoluted, ciliated mucosa. It sweeps over the surface of the ovary, the beat of its cilia pulling the ova into its lumen. Occasionally, however, an egg cell falls out of the open end of the tube, resulting, if it is a fertilized egg, in an abdominal, or ectopic, pregnancy.

Sections of the oviduct vary somewhat in appearance according to the region from which they are cut. At the funnel-shaped end of the tube the folding of the mucosa attains its greatest development, and the lumen is reduced to a narrow channel between the fimbriae (Fig. 14-21). Further down the tube the height of the fimbriae is reduced and the lumen enlarged. The mucosa consists of a ciliated columnar epithelium, resting on a tunica propria. It is said that special preparations show some cells of the epithelium to be nonciliated and glandular.

Columnar epithelium

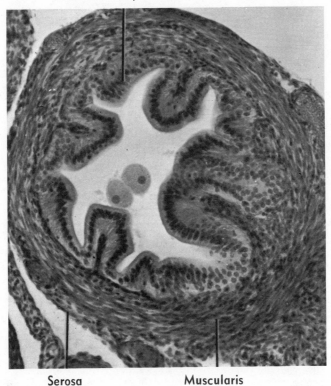

Serosa   Muscularis

Fig. 14-21
Section of fallopian tube of mouse, showing two fertilized eggs in lumen. (×200.) (Specimen courtesy Dr. Henry Browing, Houston, Tex.)

There is no muscularis mucosae, so that the tunica propria blends with the submucosa, and the two layers are sometimes called one. The muscularis has two layers, an inner circular and an outer longitudinal, the two being indistinctly separated.

UTERUS (Figs. 14-22 and 14-23)

The human uterus is a pear-shaped muscular organ with two parts, a body and a neck, or cervix. At its upper, broader end it receives the oviducts; its lower end opens into the vagina.

Its wall consists of three layers: the endometrium, which corresponds to the mucosa and submucosa; the myometrium, or muscularis; and the perimetrium, or serous membrane. The myometrium is a very thick layer of interwoven bundles of smooth muscle, forming three-fourths of the uterine wall. At the lower end, or cervix, of the uterus the fibers are arranged in three fairly distinct layers; the mid-

dle layer is circular, and the outer and inner layers are longitudinal.

Endometrium

The endometrium is lined by columnar epithelium and contains numerous tubular glands that open at the surface. The mucosa undergoes a number of cyclic variations that are related to changes occurring during the ovulatory and menstrual cycle. While the changes that occur in the endometrium are not abrupt, structural differences occur that have resulted in the classification of four morphologically distinct stages: the proliferative, also known as the estrogenic stage; the progravid, or secretory, stage; the premenstrual stage; and, finally, the menstrual stage.

Proliferative stage. The phase of the cycle begins at the termination of the menstrual phase and continues until the thirteenth or fourteenth day of the cycle. It is characterized by the rapid

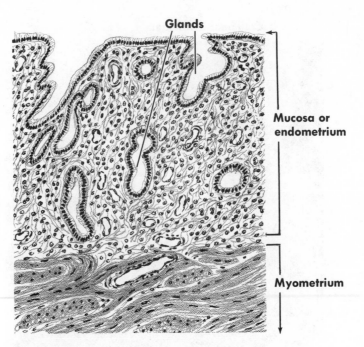

Fig. 14-22
Mucosa and part of muscularis of human uterus.

regeneration of the endometrial wall and a replacement of epithelial cells to cover the surface of the mucosa. Also, the gland cells increase in number, and the glands themselves increase in length. Vascularity of the tissue becomes more pronounced, and indications of edema are also evident.

Secretory (progravid) stage. The secretory stage is characterized by a marked increase in the hypertrophy of the endometrium, which is the result of proliferation of the glandular tissue and a marked increase in edema and vascularity of the mucosa. The secretory stage begins on the thirteenth or fourteenth day of the cycle and continues until the twenty-sixth or twenty-seventh day.

Premenstrual stage. In the premenstrual part of the cycle changes occur in the vascular components that result in a loss of the superficial portion of the mucosa. During this time fragmentation of the glands and the extrusion of blood and tissue debris into the lumen of the uterus occur. The premenstrual stage is confined to 1 or 2 days and is said to terminate at the first external signs of bleeding.

Menstrual stage. The menstrual stage usually occupies 3 to 5 days of the cycle and is characterized by a considerable amount of endometrial destruction, which consists essentially in the sloughing off of the upper three-fourths of the endometrium. It involves the destruction of the epithelium and connective tissue and the rupture of blood vessels.

Pregnancy. During pregnancy the structure of the endometrium undergoes marked hypertrophy to provide for the nutrition of the embryo. For a full description of the placenta the student should consult a textbook of embryology. We shall consider, here, only so much as will explain the place of pregnancy in the female sexual cycle. The changes that take place in the secretory stage are preparations for the implantation of a fertilized ovum.

The probable relations between the uterine cycle and the changes that take place in the ovary (ovulation and the formation of corpora lutea) are as follows: The cycle described is one in which there is no coitus and consequently no fertilization of the ovum. Ovulation probably occurs about the middle of the latter part of the interval between menstrual periods (16 to 20 days after the beginning of the last menstrual flow). The unfertilized ovum travels slowly down the fallopian tube, reaching the uterus in from 8 to 12 days. In the meantime the ruptured follicle is being transformed into

Epithelium

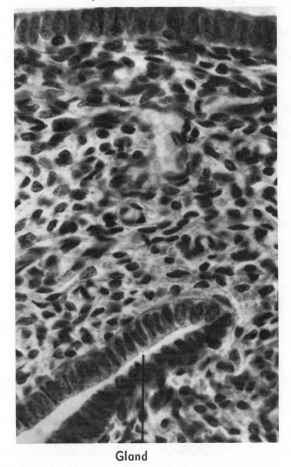

Gland

Fig. 14-23
Section of endometrial wall of human uterus. (×640.) (From Bevelander, G.: Essentials of histology, ed. 6, St. Louis, 1970, The C. V. Mosby Co.)

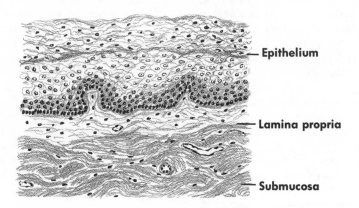

Epithelium

Lamina propria

Submucosa

Fig. 14-24
Human vagina. Epithelium shows a layer of cornification about midway between its base and its surface.

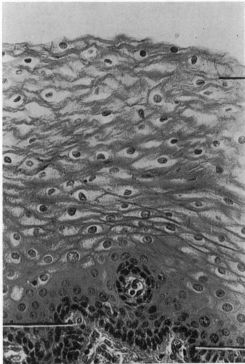

Partly keratinized cells

Papilla

Basal layer

Fig. 14-25
Stratified squamous epithelium of human vagina. (From Bevelander, G.: Essentials of histology, ed. 6, St. Louis, 1970, The C. V. Mosby Co.)

a corpus luteum, and the endometrium is undergoing the progravid hyperplasia. The ovum reaches the uterus when the latter is ready to receive a fertilized egg. But in the cycle under consideration the ovum is dead, and the endometrium enters the menstrual period, during which a part of its mucosa is sloughed off. The ovum also is expelled with the menstrual flow, and the corpus luteum begins to degenerate. If the ovum has been fertilized, it reaches the uterus, as before, when the latter is in the progravid condition. The endometrium provides a suitable place for the embedding of the ovum, which remains in the uterus for the 9 months of the gestation period. If pregnancy occurs, the corpus luteum does not undergo involution but grows larger and persists throughout pregnancy.

The foregoing account is supported by a considerable body of evidence, although it is not definitely proved to be accurate. It appears quite certain that the regulating mechanism of the cycle is in the ovary, not in the uterus, and that it is of endocrine nature.

VAGINA (Figs. 14-24 and 14-25)

The wall of the vagina includes a mucosa, submucosa, and muscularis. As in the oviduct and uterus, the mucosa and the submucosa are blended. The epithelium is of the stratified squamous variety; the muscularis is of interlacing fibers of smooth muscle that form somewhat indefinite circular (inner) and longitudinal coats.

The epithelium of the human vagina undergoes changes during the menstrual cycle, although these are less marked than those of the uterine mucosa. During the premenstrual period a zone of keratinized cells is formed in the middle layers of the epithelium. At the menstrual period the cells above this zone are sloughed off, and the keratinized cells are thus brought to the surface. In some mammals the changes are more marked, so that vaginal smears furnish an indication of the stage of the estrus cycle of the animal from which they are made.

MAMMARY GLAND

The mammary gland is a compound alveolar gland that develops from the lower layers of

Excretory duct   Adipose tissue

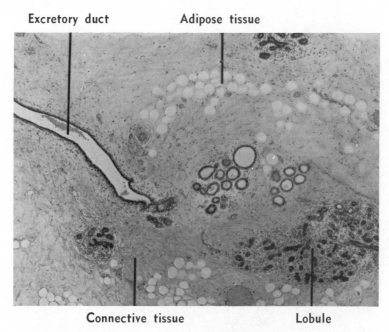

Connective tissue   Lobule

Fig. 14-26
Section of inactive human mammary gland, showing lobules made up chiefly of ducts. (×40.) (From Bevelander, G.: Essentials of histology, ed. 6, St. Louis, 1970, The C. V. Mosby Co.)

Duct

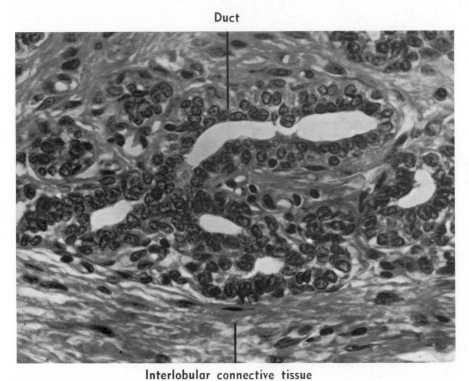

Interlobular connective tissue

Fig. 14-27
Lobule of resting (inactive) mammary gland of cat. (×160.) (From Bevelander, G.: Essentials of histology, ed. 6, St. Louis, 1970, The C. V. Mosby Co.)

Lobule

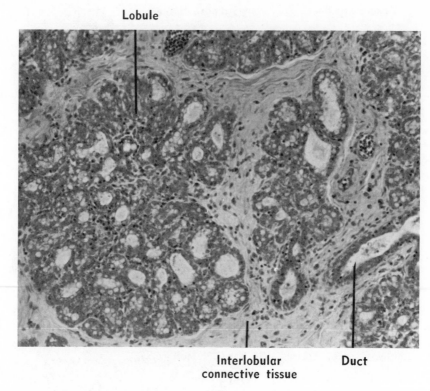

Interlobular
connective tissue   Duct

Fig. 14-28
Section of active (secreting) human mammary gland. (×160.) (From Bevelander, G.: Essentials of histology, ed. 6, St. Louis, 1970, The C. V. Mosby Co.)

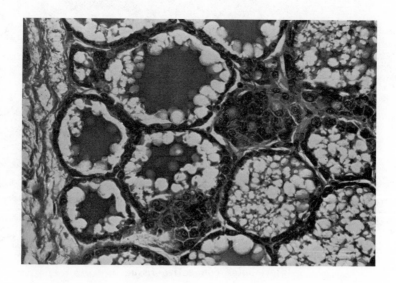

Fig. 14-29
Lactating cat mammary gland, showing follicles and secretion. (From Bevelander, G.: Essentials of histology, ed. 6, St. Louis, 1970, The C. V. Mosby Co.)

the epidermis. It consists of fifteen to twenty lobes separated by broad bands of dense connective tissue. The lobes are divided into lobules by connective tissue septa, from which strands extend into secreting units. The intralobular connective tissue is fine areolar. The alveoli of each lobule open into small intralobular ducts, which unite to form interlobular ducts, and these in turn lead to the main excretory (lactiferous) ducts. The inactive and active phases of the gland are marked by a difference in appearance.

Resting gland

A section of the mammary gland during a period of inactivity hardly resembles a gland at all on first inspection (Fig. 14-26). The secreting tissue is represented by scattered ducts, around the terminal portions of which one may see a few collapsed or very small follicles and a few solid cords of epithelial cells (Fig. 14-27). Such groups of intralobular epithelial tissue lie in a thin investment of loose connective tissue, and this is surrounded by a dense mass of collagenous fibers. The connective tissue occupies by far the greater proportion of the section. Examined under high magnification the ducts are seen to be lined with two or three layers of cuboidal cells, while such follicles as may be found are composed of simple cuboidal epithelium.

Active gland

During pregnancy the epithelial portions of the mammary gland undergo a pronounced hypertrophy, so that by the fifth month of the period of gestation the organ presents a histological picture very different from that of the resting gland (Fig. 14-28). Alveoli have developed from the cords of tissue that were to be seen before. The small areas of intralobular connective tissue have expanded, and the lobules appear as relatively large areas filled with alveoli and ducts. The interlobular connective tissue is correspondingly reduced in amount.

During the later part of the gestation period the development of alveoli and ducts continues, so that at childbirth they occupy the greater part of the section. They are lined with an epithelium that varies from tall columnar, in actively secreting units, to low cuboidal, in those that have been drained of milk (Fig. 14-29). The cells in active alveoli are filled with fat droplets, which distend them at the free surface and give an irregular outline to the lumen. The ducts leading from the alveoli are lined with low columnar cells, which are replaced by pseudostratified epithelium in the excretory ducts. Near the nipple the epithelium changes to stratified squamous, which is continuous with the skin.

Hormonal control of secretion

The mammary glands are under the control or influence of several hormones. Although the glands undergo some development in the preadolescent state, this process is accentuated during adolescence and is under the influence of two ovarian hormones, estrogen and progesterone, the secretions of which are in turn regulated by hormones derived from the anterior pituitary gland. During gestation, production of female hormones is at a high level and the gland attains a presecretory state of development. At term, lactation occurs. This process is maintained by the action of prolactin derived from the anterior pituitary and probably secretions derived from other glands, such as the adrenal gland, as well.

The mammary gland remains in the active condition for a variable period after childbirth and then returns to the resting stage. After the menopause it undergoes involution in which the alveoli and parts of the ducts degenerate and their places are taken by connective tissue.

Blood vessels, lymphatics, and nerves

Blood is brought to the mammary gland by the intercostal, internal mammary, and thoracic branches of the axillary artery. The terminal branches of these vessels lie among the alveoli. Lymph vessels, which are numerous, drain chiefly toward the axilla. Nerves come from both cerebrospinal and sympathetic systems to supply the epithelial tissue and the blood vessels.

15
ENDOCRINE ORGANS

Endocrine glands may be defined as collections of epithelial cells that are not provided with ducts but deliver their secretion (hormone) into the bloodstream. However, there are not many organs that clearly fit this definition. The absence of ducts is easily determined, but the presence of secretion is more difficult to prove. Two methods of experimentation are used in this field: operative removal of the gland in question and injection of substance extracted from it. The first of these is not always practicable. To the second method there may be objections on the ground that extracts from organs do not necessarily represent the secretion elaborated by them. The use of the two methods may be illustrated by the work on the thyroid, which has yielded fairly clear-cut results. If this gland is removed from a laboratory animal, there follows a marked retardation of the metabolic rate, but this becomes normal again when thyroid extract is administered. The extract also raises the metabolic rate of normal (unoperated) animals. Clinical and postmortem evidence also supports the belief that the thyroid contains a substance that influences, directly or indirectly, the rate of metabolism of the body. This effect is not produced by extracts of other glands. Moreover, the thyroid is a ductless organ composed of secreting epithelial cells, so that its morphology supports the conclusion, derived from experimental and clinical work, that it secretes a hormone.

Unfortunately, results are not so clear-cut in the cases of some other organs. In some instances the results of physiological experiments are contradictory; in others they are unsupported by morphological evidences of secretion. One may arrange in the following way the organs that have been believed to have an endocrine function.

Thyroid, parathyroid, hypophysis, adrenal, islands of Langerhans

The thyroid, parathyroid, hypophysis, adrenal, and islands of Langerhans are composed of cells that have the appearance of glandular tissue. Clinical and experimental evidence is preponderantly in favor of the view that each secretes a specific substance which influences some phase of the metabolic activity of the body.

Gonads

There is ample experimental evidence that the testis and ovary produce hormones which control in part the development and maintenance of secondary sexual characteristics and that the ovarian secretion influences the estrus cycle. It is believed that the first of these functions is regulated by the interstitial cells of the two organs, but this point is not definitely proved. Similarly, doubt exists as to the respective roles of the graafian follicles and the corpus luteum in the regulation of estrus. The difficulty in establishing the connecting link between physiological and morphological evidence is obvious; it is impossible to extripate completely the interstitial cells while leaving the other tissues of the gonads intact.

Thymus, pineal

Evidence of the endocrine function of the thymus and pineal glands is weak. The results of physiological experimentation are contradictory, and there is little in the morphology of the organs to suggest that they are secretory in function. They are placed in the endocrine group chiefly because their function is not known. This is true also of various other groups of cells in the body.

Other organs

A fourth group may be made of organs from which, at various times, investigators have claimed that they have isolated hormones. For instance, a substance called secretin has been extracted from the wall of the duodenum, and it has been shown that this substance stimulates the alveoli of the pancreas. There are, however, no cells in this region to which the elaboration of the substance can be assigned; in other words, we have a "secretion" without a gland to form it.

Liver

The liver is sometimes grouped with the endocrine organs. The preceding grouping of organs indicates a part, at least, of the confusion existing in this field. The complications of the physiological side of the science are great because all members of the endocrine group are closely interrelated, and disturbance of one may be expected to affect some or all of the others. Fortunately, the histology is less complicated than the physiology. We shall now discuss the thyroid, parathyroid, hypophysis, and adrenal. The islands of Langerhans and the gonads, also in good standing as endocrines, have already been described. (See Pancreas, Testis, Ovary.)

THYROID GLAND

The thyroid gland (Fig. 15-1) consists of two lobes and a connecting isthmus. It lies in the neck in contact with the upper part of the trachea and the lower end of the pharynx. The thyroid is enclosed in a connective tissue sheath derived from the cervical fasciae.

Trabeculae arising from this facial sheath penetrate the gland, subdividing it into lobules, and provide a pathway for the vascular and nerve supply of the gland. The connective tissue that makes up the stroma of the gland is largely reticular in nature and is extremely rich in nerve and vascular plexuses.

The structural unit of the thyroid is the follicle, which consists of a layer of simple epithelium enclosing a cavity (follicular cavity) containing a colloid secretion. The colloid elaborated by the cells is usually rich in iodine and contains the thyroid hormone. The shapes of the follicles, their contents, and the character of their epithelium vary with the functional condition of the gland. In the hypoactive condition the follicles are round or oval with regular outlines. They are lined with low cuboidal epithelium, which stains deeply with eosin and has indistinct cell walls. The lumen of each follicle is filled with colloid, which appears as a structureless red mass in hematoxylin and eosin preparations. In the hyperactive state, on the other hand, the follicles may have a folded, irregular shape. In this condition they are lined with tall columnar cells, the cytoplasm of which stains lightly. The colloid is pale in color during the active phase of glandular activity, and many follicles may be found that contain little or none of this substance. The two conditions described represent the extremes. A normal thyroid may contain some follicles of each sort, but the majority will be in a condition intermediate between the two. The secretion of the thyroid gland is a compound rich in iodine. It is probable that the colloid represents stored secretion. The hormone is carried away from the gland through the capillaries in the connective tissue surrounding the follicles.

In addition to the principal cells of the thyroid already mentioned, there are other cells, often larger and laden with mitochondria, known as the *parafollicular cells*. They are said to elaborate *thyrocalcitonin*.

The cells of the thyroid secrete a colloid material that contains thyroglobulin and several enzymes. Thyroglobulin is a glycoprotein rich in iodinated amino acids. The secretory process is complex and not fully understood. It consists of synthesis, storage, and release of the hormone into the capillaries surrounding the follicles. The primary function of the thyroid is to regulate metabolism. It is also concerned with the growth, development, and differentiation of the organism. Hyperfunction results in increased bodily metabolism; conversely, hypofunction results in decreased metabolism. The number and variety of functions affected by the thyroid are extensive and diverse. Hypothyroidism frequently results in the enlargement of the gland, a condition referred to as goiter. Other functions regulated by the thyroid, which has intricate interrelationships with other endocrine glands, affect carbohydrate metabolism, heart rate, bodily growth, mental activity, and tooth eruption. It has also been shown that the thyrotropic hormone (TSH) elaborated by the anterior pituitary stimulates release of thyroxine. Removal of the thyroid results in the hypertrophy of the beta cells in the anterior lobe of the pituitary.

Recently, the existence of another hormone affecting calcium homeostasis has been postu-

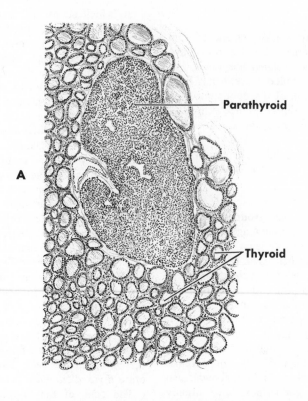

Parathyroid

Thyroid

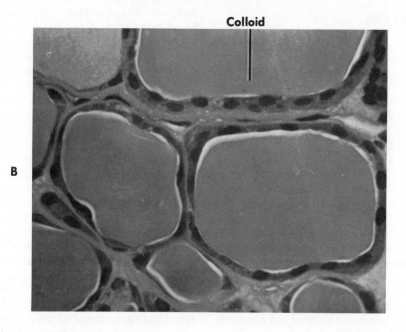

Colloid

Fig. 15-1

A, Parathyroid gland and part of thyroid of monkey, low magnification. B, Follicles of human thyroid, showing epithelium of different heights and colloid secretions in follicles. (×640.) (B from Bevelander, G.: Essentials of histology, ed. 6, St. Louis, 1970, The C. V. Mosby Co.)

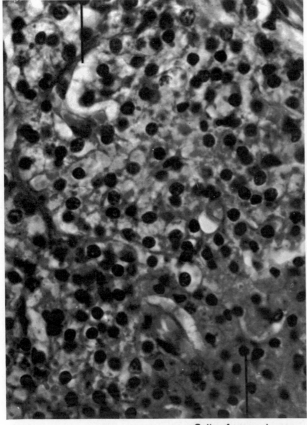

Fig. 15-2
Parathyroid, human. (×640.)

Cells of parenchyma

lated. This new hormone was referred to as *calcitonin* and was believed to originate in the parathyroids; however, more recent evidence indicates that it is produced by parafollicular cells of the thyroid, so the term *thyrocalcitonin* has been suggested for this principle. The action of this hormone is believed to be hypocalcemic, thereby preventing plasma calcium from rising above normal levels.

PARATHYROID GLANDS

The parathyroid glands (Fig. 15-2) are paired and in man are usually four in number. The glands are surrounded by a framework of reticular tissue, which divides the gland into poorly defined lobules. The lobules are subdivided into sheets or cords by fine extensions of the trabeculae. The connective tissue of the gland contains blood vessels, nerves, lymphatics, and adipose tissue. The cells of the gland are enclosed by a network of reticular fibers in which is found a dense network of capillaries.

The parenchyma of the parathyroid is made up of two kinds of cells in the adult human, chief cells and oxyphil cells, the former being most numerous. The chief cells are polyhedral in shape and exhibit a round, centrally located nucleus and well-defined cell membranes. Chief cells are of two kinds, light and dark. The light cell is most numerous, is slightly larger, and exhibits a clear cytoplasm; both kinds contain glycogen and secretory granules. Evidence appears to indicate that the light cells may be an inactive form of the dark cells.

Oxyphil cells are larger than chief cells, are fewer in number, and exhibit small, dense nuclei and acidophilic cytoplasm. They occur either singly or in groups and do not make their appearance until the fourth or fifth year. The cytoplasm is densely packed with mitochondria. With advancing age, their number increases. Thus far, these cells have been observed only in humans, monkeys, and cattle.

The plasma levels of calcium in the normal

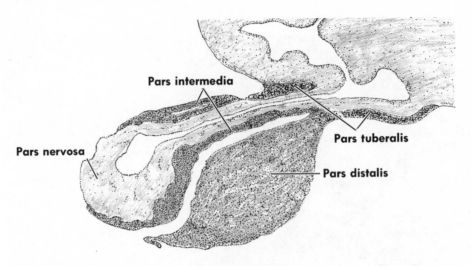

Fig. 15-3

Hypophysis of cat, midsagittal section, under low magnification to show topography.

mammal are remarkably stable, usually in the in the vicinity of 10 mg./100 ml. The presence and normal function of the parathyroids prevent the plasma calcium from dropping to levels that would be incompatible with the animal's survival. Removal of the parathyroids results in a decrease of plasma calcium, with resultant tetany and death in most mammals. The administration of parathyroid hormone will raise the serum calcium and result in bone resorption. Parathyroid hormone exerts a direct effect on the process of bone resorption, which is highly complex and poorly understood. It is believed that the resorption is caused by osteoclasts, which in turn release calcium into the body fluids. Parathyroid hormone has been purified and is known to be a peptide of low molecular weight (6,000 to 8,000). Commercial preparations have not been used extensively, since vitamin D and its related compounds are effective in treating hypoparathyroidism.

HYPOPHYSIS

The hypophysis or pituitary gland consists of two lobes, each of which is again subdivided (Fig. 15-3). These parts, unlike the lobes of a secretory gland such as the parotid, are composed of tissues that differ from each other in function and (partially) in origin. The gland is actually two organs intimately associated. One part of it, the glandular or *adenohypophysis*, develops from the roof of the oral cavity of the embryo; the other part, the *neurohypophysis*, develops as an outgrowth of the floor of the brain. The hypophysis is located in a fossa of the sphenoid bone, the *sella turcica*, and is invested by an extension of the dura mater. The buccal portion loses its connection with the oral cavity and becomes a solid mass of cells. In some animals the nervous portion retains a cavity in its center.

The adenohypophysis is divided by a lumen in two unequal parts. The *pars distalis* lies anterior to the lumen, and the *pars tuberalis,* an extension of the pars distalis, envelops the neural stalk. The third component, the *pars intermedia,* consists of a thin cellular portion located posterior to the lumen. The anterior lobe refers to the pars distalis and the pars tuberalis; the posterior lobe refers to the pars intermedia and the pars nervosa (the infundibular stalk and median eminence).

The pars distalis of the anterior pituitary gland is composed of glandular cells, which are arranged in irregular clumps and cords that are in intimate relation to vascular sinusoids. The anterior lobe is enveloped in a dense connective tissue capsule. Internally, fine reticular fibers arising from the capsule surround the cords of the parenchymal cells and serve to support them and the vascular elements.

The glandular cells are classified as *chromophilic* or *chromophobic* on the basis of their affinity or lack of affinity for routine dyes. The

Connective tissue capsule   Basophil

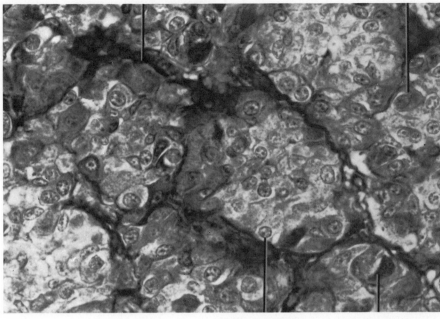

Chromophobe   Eosinophil

Fig. 15-4
Section of anterior pituitary gland of monkey, showing several follicles. (Mallory-azan; ×640.) (From Bevelander, G.: Essentials of histology, ed. 6, St. Louis, 1970, The C. V. Mosby Co.)

chromophilic cells are classified as *acidophilic* or *basophilic* according to the staining reactions of their specific granules.

Chromophil cells

The acidophils are round or ovoid and measure from 15 to 19μ in diameter. They possess a prominent Golgi apparatus, numerous rod-shaped mitochondria, and refractile granules that are recognizable with the light microscope. The acidophils are believed to secrete the *growth hormone* (somatropin) and *prolactin* (mammotropin).

In some species two types of acidophils may be differentiated. Those cells whose granules exhibit an affinity for orange G are known as *alpha* acidophils, and those whose granules stain intensely with azocarmine are known as *epsilon* acidophils. Studies with the electron microscope have confirmed the presence of these two kinds of acidophils. In the alpha type the granules are small (approximately 300 mμ) and closely packed. In the epsilon type the granules are approximately 900 mμ in diameter and appear to be scattered throughout the cytoplasm.

The basophils are oval or angular, are slightly larger than the acidophils, and possess a nucleus that resembles that of the acidophils. The Golgi apparatus is somewhat removed from the nucleus and granules are smaller in most species examined and are PAS positive. *Thyrotropic* and *interstitial cell–stimulating hormones* are believed to be elaborated by these cells.

The granules of the basophils are less numerous and smaller than in the eosinophils. In some mammals two types of basophils have been recognized. In one type, the beta basophil, the granules have an affinity for aldehyde fuchsin; in the other type, the delta basophil, the granules do not react to this stain.

Chromophobe cells

The chromophobes are relatively smaller than the chromophils. The organelles are similar to those observed in the latter, but they are usually devoid of granules. It was formerly believed that these cells were "reserve" cells capable of differentiating into various kinds of chromophils. More recent evidence indicates that these cells are diverse in nature and that a degree of cytological differentiation does exist; they are, however, the antecedent of only one kind of chromophil.

Hormones produced by the pars distalis

The pars distalis is known to produce six hormones, which consist of proteins or polypeptides.

Somatotrophic hormone (STH). One of the earliest hormones to be recognized was the growth, or somatotrophic, hormone (STH), which stimulates body growth, particularly that of the epiphyses of long bones. Hypophysectomy in growing animals results in a cessation of growth, which can be overcome by the administration of the hormone. Underproduction of the hormone results in dwarfism, overproduction in gigantism. If overproduction occurs when the epiphyseal plate has calcified, a thickening of the bones of the face, skull, hands, and feet occurs. This condition is known as *acromegaly.*

Thyrotropic hormone (TSH). The thyroid-stimulating hormone maintains the integrity of the thyroid epithelium and is responsible for stimulating thyroid secretion. Hypophysectomy results in the atrophy of the thyroid, which in turn may be restored by administration of the hormone.

Adrenocorticotrophic hormone (ACTH). The adrenocorticotrophic hormone controls the growth and secretion of the adrenal cortex. Hypophysectomy results in atrophy of the cortex, which can be alleviated by administration of ACTH.

Follicle-stimulating hormone (FSH). The follicle-stimulating hormone stimulates growth of the follicles in the ovary and spermatogenesis in the seminiferous tubules of the testis. Atrophy of the gonads following hypophysectomy can be partially alleviated and the gonads restored to their normal state by the administration of FSH, but complete restoration also requires some luteinizing hormone.

Luteinizing hormone (LH); interstitial cell–stimulating hormone (ICSH). After stimulation by FSH the luteinizing hormone contributes to the maturation of the ovarian follicle and also to ovulation. In the male, ICSH stimulates the interstitial cells of Leydig in the testes to produce testosterone, responsible for the maintenance of the secondary sexual characteristics. This latter effect is augmented by appropriate administration of FSH.

Prolactin (lactogenic hormone) (LTH). Prolactin initiates secretion of milk after hypertrophy of the mammary gland in response to stimulation of ovarian hormones during pregnancy. It also has been shown in the rat that LTH initiates and maintains the secretion of progesterone; hence the synonym, luteotropic hormone.

Pars tuberalis

The pars tuberalis consists of a thin band of cells enveloping the infundibular stalk. The main cells are cuboidal or polyhedral; the cytoplasm is faintly basophilic and contains small granules. The cells arranged in cords or clusters are in intimate association with a rich supply of blood vessels. Occasional small, colloid-laden vesicles occur among the cells. In addition, there are undifferentiated cells and also small acidophils and basophils. The function of the pars tuberalis is not known.

Pars intermedia

In man the pars intermedia is rudimentary. It occupies a position adjacent to the residual lumen and is composed of cells and scattered follicles containing colloid. The cells are basophilic and blend with those of the pars distalis. The cells lining the colloid vesicles are frequently ciliated. The only known function of this part of the gland is the secretion of *melanin-stimulating hormone.*

Neurohypophysis

The neurohypophysis is composed of the infundibular process—the infundibulum and the median eminence of the tuber cinereum. The infundibulum and median eminence of the tuber cinereum have in common the same type of cell, nerve, and blood supply and elaborate similar active substances. The cells of the neurohypophysis are small, have numerous processes, and are known as *pituicytes.* Unlike neuroglia, which they resemble, their cytoplasm contains fat and pigment granules. The nuclei of the pituicytes are round, and the cytoplasmic processes often extend to capillary walls or the septa of the gland.

The nerve cells in the supra-optic and paraventricular nuclei of the hypothalamus elaborate secretory products, which are transmitted by nerve fibers and are stored in the neural lobe and in nerve fiber terminations known as *Herring bodies.*

Two active fractions have been isolated from

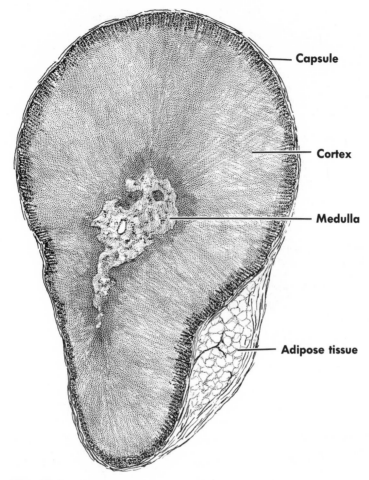

Capsule

Cortex

Medulla

Adipose tissue

Fig. 15-5
Section through adrenal gland of rabbit, showing the relation of its parts.

the neurohypophysis. They have been identified as polypeptides. One of these, *oxytocin,* stimulates uterine contraction during late pregnancy and also activates the myoepithelial cells of the mammary gland resulting in the flow of milk. The second fraction, *vasopressin,* is an antidiuretic (ADH) hormone. It also has the ability to raise blood pressure.

ADRENAL GLAND

The adrenal (suprarenal) gland is like the hypophysis in that it is in reality two glands having different functions and arising from different sources. One of these is the cortex, which is derived from mesodermal tissue. The other is the medulla of the organ, which comes from the same group of cells as those that form the sympathetic ganglia (Fig. 15-5).

The entire gland is surrounded by a capsule of connective tissue. From the capsule delicate connective tissue fibers pass into the cortex at the hilus. They continue into the stroma of the gland as reticular fibers supporting the arterioles and capillaries of the cortex and the sinusoidal vessels of the medulla. The capsule also gives rise to cells that replace the cells of the cortex.

Cortex

The cortex is composed of cords of cells, between which lie capillaries in a fine network of reticular tissue. Three zones are distinguishable, though they are not sharply delimited one from another. They are the zona glomerulosa, zona fasciculata, and zona reticularis.

In the zona glomerulosa the cells are pale and

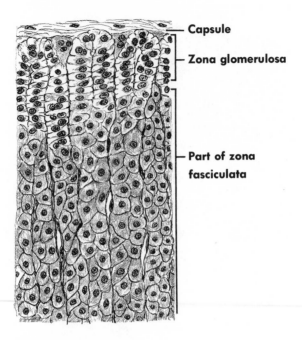

Capsule

Zona glomerulosa

Part of zona fasciculata

Fig. 15-6
Outer portion of cortex of adrenal gland of rabbit.

columnar (Fig. 15-6); they are arranged in oval groups separated from each other by fine vascular connective tissue. The nuclei stain intensely, and the cytoplasm is faintly basophilic.

The zona fasciculata is the widest zone of the cortex and is composed of polygonal cells, in the cytoplasm of which fat (lipoid) droplets are present; cells in the zone are arranged in cords that radiate from the center of the gland; the cords are usually two cells in width, being cuboidal and often binucleate. In the outer portion of the fasciculata the cells contain droplets of cholesterol and fatty acids. In the usual preparations these areas appear as vacuoles, giving the cell a spongy appearance. They are sometimes called spongiocytes.

In the zona reticularis, the innermost zone of the cortex, the cords of cells, rather than running in a radial direction, break up into a network, in the spaces of which the capillaries are to be found; the cells of the reticular zone are somewhat smaller and darker than those of the fascicular zone (Fig. 15-7). Many cells have picnotic nuclei and contain pigment granules.

Medulla

The medulla consists of irregularly arranged groups of cells that have a granular cytoplasm

and polygonal outlines (Fig. 15-7). With hematoxylin and eosin, their color is faintly purple. They react strongly to chromium salts and are therefore called chromaffin cells. Even without this specific stain they are readily distinguished from the cortical cells by their basophilic reaction, their larger size, and their arrangement. Among the cords is a network of capillaries such as is characteristic of endocrine organs.

Functions of the adrenal gland

The cortex is essential to life, and destruction or removal of the cortex results in Addison's disease, which is fatal. It regulates electrolyte balance and maintains carbohydrate balance, effecting glycogen stores in the liver and muscles; glycogen in turn is associated with normal fat and protein metabolism. Another important function of the cortex is the maintenance of connective tissue throughout the body. Connective tissue diseases are often dramatically arrested by the administration of cortisone, an active steroid principle present in the cortex. Deficiency of the hormone is believed to affect adversely other functions such as blood pressure, sexual libido, and vascular permeability. The activity of the adrenal cortex is controlled in part by the adrenocorticotrophic hormone

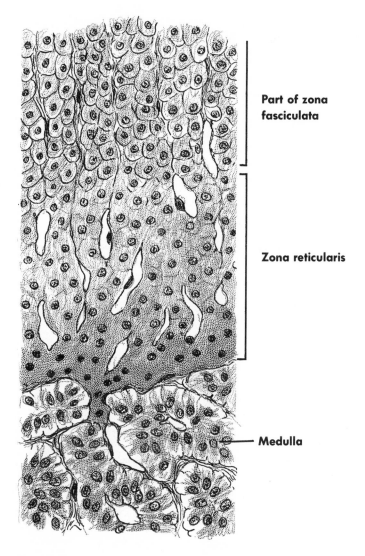

Fig. 15-7
Inner portion of cortex and part of medulla of adrenal gland of rabbit.

(ACTH) derived from the adenohypophysis whose effect is chiefly on the cells of the zona fasciculata.

Unlike the cortex the medulla is not essential to life. It elaborates two substances, *epinephrine* and *norepinephrine,* which are catecholamines located in the chromaffin granules of the cells. Epinephrine increases oxygen consumption and the mobilization of glucose from glycogen stored in the liver. It also causes contraction of smooth muscle, increases cardiac output, and is active in situations of stress or emergency. Epinephrine will also stimulate the secretions of ACTH

by the adenohypophysis under experimental conditions. Norepinephrine, believed to be a precursor of epinephrine, serves as a transmitting agent of the heart and blood vessels.

PINEAL BODY

The pineal body, also known as the *epiphysis cerebri,* is a small, flattened, conical body attached to the roof of the third ventricle by a slender stalk. It is divided into lobules by connective tissue septa derived from the capsule in which it is enclosed. When the pineal body is stained with hematoxylin and eosin, it appears to consist of cords of epithelial cells, which are irregular in shape and have a large nucleus and pale-staining cytoplasm. These are the most numerous cells that occur in this organ and are known as *pinealocytes.* When stained with silver, they are shown to have long radiating processes that terminate in the supporting connective tissue in bulbous processes. Also present are neuroglial cells (interstitial cells), which are believed to serve as supporting elements. At the sixth or seventh year in the human being the pineal body attains its maximum development and from this time on it undergoes retrogressive changes. The human pineal body often contains concretions, *acervuli* (brain sand), which are extracellular in location and are composed of a mineralized organic matrix having a lamellate appearance.

The function of the pineal gland is not well understood. The pineal in man has been shown to contain *serotonin* and *melatonin.* It is believed to exert a neuroendocrine function and to participate in hormonelike mediation. The details of these processes still await clarification.

16
INTEGUMENT

The skin consists of an epidermal and a dermal layer (corium) and rests upon the subdermal connective tissue. The epidermis is a stratified squamous epithelium, modified in some portions of the body by the addition of a thick cuticular layer and in others by the development of the hair and nails. The corium is a layer of dense connective tissue, in which are located the various glands of the skin and the hair follicles. The subdermal, or subcutaneous, tissue is also fibrous, but it is more loosely arranged than the corium and generally contains adipose tissue.

HAIRLESS SKIN (Figs. 16-1 and 16-2)

No hair grows on the palms of the hands or the soles of the feet. They are covered with thick skin, which consists of the following parts.

Epidermis

Stratum corneum. The outer layer of the corneum makes up about three-fourths of its thickness. It consists of cornified nonnucleated cells, the outer layers of which are detached from the surface in ragged patches (desquamation). The inner layers of the stratum corneum are compact, and here the outlines of individual cells are easily visible.

Stratum lucidum. Beneath the stratum corneum is the stratum lucidum, which consists of several rows of flattened nonnucleated cells. They form a hyaline, highly refractile band, which appears homogenous and stains deeply with eosin.

Stratum germinativum. The remainder of the epidermis constitutes the stratum germinativum and has many of the characteristics of the lower layers of stratified squamous epithelium. There are no very flat cells, such as one sees at the surface of the esophageal lining, since in the skin the surface cells have undergone cornification and form the stratum corneum. The cells nearest the stratum lucidum are spindle shaped, with their long axes parallel to the surface of the skin. There are from two to five layers of cells in which the cytoplasm is full of granules that stain deeply with hematoxylin. These layers make up the stratum granulosum, which is prominent because of its color. On closer examination it may be seen that the stratum granulosum differs from other epithelia in the arrangement of its cells. Instead of being closely applied to each other, they are separated by narrow spaces so that each is surrounded by a light line (in section). This is demonstrable in ordinary preparations. In exceptionally good preparations and under high magnification it may be seen that the polygonal cells below the stratum granulosum are also separated by clefts and that the spaces are traversed by minute cytoplasmic bridges, uniting each cell to its neighbors. The name *prickle cells* is sometimes given to the polygonal cells and those of the stratum granulosum because of these protoplasmic strands.

The basal cells of the stratum germinativum are modified columnar cells with deeply staining cytoplasm and indistinct cell boundaries. The boundary between the epidermis and the corium is irregular because of the great number of papillae formed by the corium. Granules of pigment (melanin) are present in the stratum germinativum of the skin. In the white race, melanin occurs in the basal cells only, except in deeply pigmented areas like the nipples and the circumanal tissue. In dark-skinned races it extends further into the germinativum. Some investigators believe that the epithelial cells elaborate melanin; others believe that it is formed and passed on to the epithelium by certain cells of the corium called melanoblasts. The

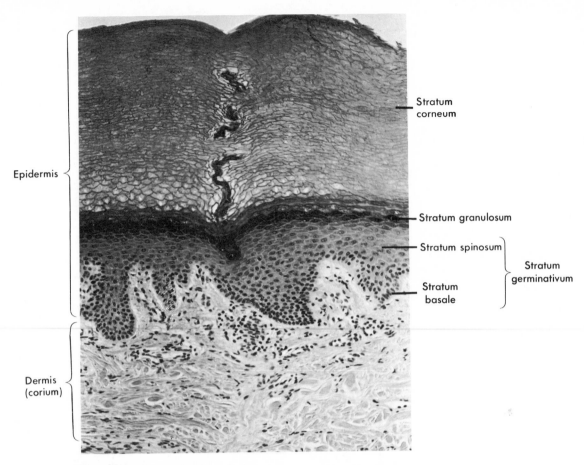

Epidermis

Stratum corneum

Stratum granulosum

Stratum spinosum

Stratum basale

Stratum germinativum

Dermis (corium)

Fig. 16-1
Section of thick skin of human, showing duct of sweat gland in epidermis. (×160.)

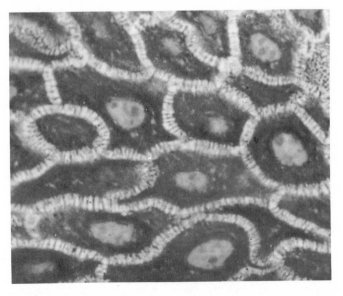

Fig. 16-2
Photomicrograph of part of the stratum spinosum of human gingival epithelium, showing intercellular bridges. (×1,200.)

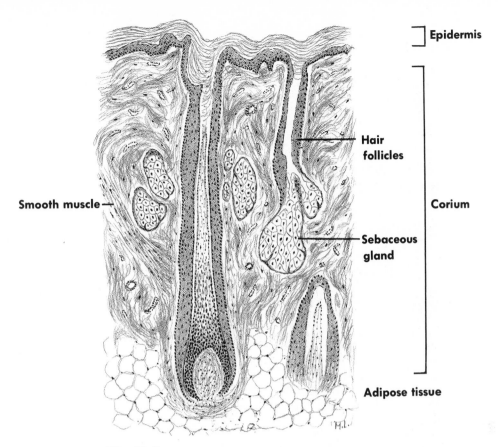

Fig. 16-3
Human scalp.

melanoblasts lie directly beneath the epithelium and send projections into it between the cells.

Corium

The corium, or dermis, is a compact layer of connective tissue containing numerous collagenous and elastic fibers. In it are the sweat glands, which will be described later. Some of the papillae that the corium sends into the epidermis contain capillary loops; others contain nerve endings.

HAIRY SKIN (Fig. 16-3)

In the skin of the greater part of the body the stratum germinativum of the epidermis extends into the corium to form hair follicles. These are most extensively developed in the scalp, which may be used as an example of hairy skin. In this locality, protection is afforded by the hair, and the cornified layer is much thinner than it is on the hands and feet. In some cases it is reduced to less than half the thickness of the germinative layer; the stratum lucidum is much reduced or entirely lacking, and there are few granular cells.

A hair follicle has two layers. The outer layer is a poorly defined connective tissue sheath; the inner layer is a continuation of the germinative layer of the epidermis. At the base of the follicle the connective tissue forms a papilla, which projects into the epithelium, and at this point also the epithelium is continuous with the hair shaft. This part of the follicle is enlarged to form the bulb.

A sebaceous gland and a strand of smooth muscle are associated with the hair follicle. The axis of the latter is never exactly perpendicular to the surface of the scalp, and the muscle and gland lie in the wider angle of the two that the follicle makes with the surface.

The hair itself is epithelial and under high magnification may be seen to consist of the following layers:

1. A cuticula of transparent overlapping scales.

2. A cortex of flattened cornified cells containing pigment.

3. A medulla of cuboidal cells, usually in two rows.

The follicle is composed of two sheaths, the

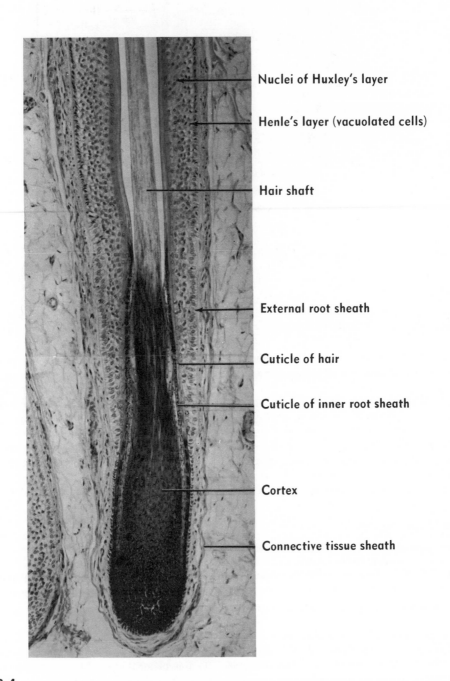

Nuclei of Huxley's layer

Henle's layer (vacuolated cells)

Hair shaft

External root sheath

Cuticle of hair

Cuticle of inner root sheath

Cortex

Connective tissue sheath

Fig. 16-4
Parasagittal section of human hair. (×160.) (From Bevelander, G.: Essentials of histology, ed. 6, St. Louis, 1970, The C. V. Mosby Co.)

outer of which is connective tissue, the inner, epithelium. The former is divided into three layers:

1. On the outside there is a layer of loose connective tissue containing blood vessels. The fibers of this sheath, some of which are elastic, run longitudinally.

2. The middle layer consists of white fibrous tissue in which the fibers are circularly arranged.

3. The innermost layer is hyaline but may contain white fibers longitudinally disposed (membrana vitrea).

The epithelial sheath consists of two parts, outer and inner as follows:

1. The outer epithelial sheath is an impocketing of the skin that grows thinner as it nears the bulb of the hair.

2. The inner epithelial sheath is still further subdivided as follows:

(a) Henle's layer, located outside Huxley's layer, is composed of flattened or cuboidal cells with a clear cytoplasm. The cytoplasm contains longitudinal fibrils, and nuclei are present only in those cells lying deep in the follicle.

(b) Huxley's layer lies outside the root sheath and is composed of several rows of elongated cells containing eleidin. Near the surface the nuclei of these cells are lacking or rudimentary.

Next to the hair there is a cuticle of nonnucleated cornified cells, the cuticula of the sheath.

GLANDS OF THE SKIN

The glands of the skin are of two kinds, the sweat glands and the sebaceous glands.

Sweat glands

Sweat glands are distributed over most of the surface of the body. They are simple tubular glands with convoluted secreting portions. The latter may lie in the subcutaneous tissue or in the deeper portion of the cortium, and they are lined with cuboidal or columnar epithelium. The cytoplasm contains secretory granules or droplets.

The ducts of the sweat glands are lined with a double layer of stratified cuboidal cells resting upon a thin basement membrane. The inner layer exhibits a homogeneous dark-staining cytoplasm, and the surface of the cells is refractile. In the epidermis the cellular constituents disappear, and the duct consists of a noncellular channel in the epidermis.

In some regions of the body, such as the axilla, the mammary areolae, and the circumanal region, the sweat glands are much larger than those located in the palms and other areas. These glands are of the apocrine type, producing thicker secretions than the sweat formed by the smaller (merocrine) glands. Also included in this group of larger glands are the wax-secreting *ceruminous* glands, located in the external auditory canal and the margin of the eyelid. The secretion of the glands is carried to the lower border of the epidermis, where it passes into a coiled channel through the tissues to emerge on the surface by way of a minute pore.

Sebaceous glands

Sebaceous glands are almost always associated with hair follicles, opening through ducts into the spaces between the follicles and the hair shafts. Structurally, they are different from any other glands we have described hitherto. Their secreting portions are not composed of a single layer of cells grouped around a lumen but are rounded masses of cells. At the periphery of each mass the cells are cuboidal; in the center they are polygonal. The central cells are filled with vacuoles, so that their appearance is somewhat like that of developing adipose tissue cells. The secretion of the sebaceous glands is accompanied by the breaking down of the central cells, and their remains are poured out with the oily accumulation into the hair follicle. The cells thus destroyed are replaced from the peripheral layer.

NAILS (Fig. 16-5)

The nails are modifications of the epidermis, They include the following parts.

1. The body with its free edge is composed of several layers of clear, flattened cells that differ from the stratum corneum of the skin in that they are harder and also possess shrunken nuclei. The proximal part of the nail body lying under the fold of skin is called the root.

2. The nail wall is the fold around the proximal and lateral borders of the nail, marked off from the latter by the nail groove. The wall consists of skin that has all the layers of other parts of the skin except, sometimes, the stratum lucidum. The stratum corneum of the wall at the proximal part of the fold extends out over the body of the nail (eponychium).

3. The nail bed is the skin under the body of the nail. It lacks the stratum corneum and

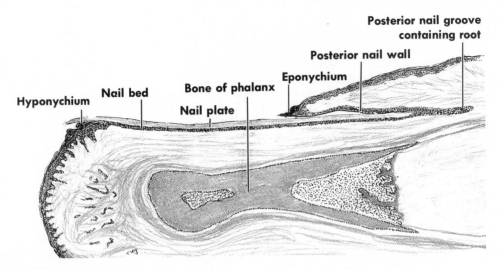

Hyponychium   **Nail bed**   **Bone of phalanx**   **Posterior nail wall**   **Posterior nail groove containing root**

Nail plate   **Eponychium**

Fig. 16-5
Finger of newborn infant.

stratum lucidum, consisting of the stratum germinativum only. Under the proximal part of the nail, in the region called the lunula, the germinativum thickens. It is from this region, the matrix, that growth of the nail takes place, the superficial cells of the matrix being transformed into nail cells. The corium of the nail bed has its connective tissue fibers arranged in two groups: (a) a group running in the long axis of the nail and (b) a group running vertically to the periosteum of the underlying bone. The dermal papillae of the nail bed form ridges that run in the long axis of the nail.

17
ORAL CAVITY

LIPS

The lips are muscular organs covered on the outside by skin and on the inside by the mucous membrane of the mouth. The muscles of the lips are striated and consist of the orbicularis oris and the mimetic. The lip is usually sectioned vertically in preparation for microscopic study and, when so cut, presents the cross sections of the orbicularis oris as a sort of core, with a relatively small number of strands of the mimetic muscle cut longitudinally (Fig. 17-1).

The skin covering the outside of the lip is like that of the greater part of the body. It consists of stratified squamous epithelium that is cornified at the surface and rests upon a layer of connective tissue. In the latter are sweat glands, sebaceous glands, and the bases of hair follicles. In the region transitional between skin and oral mucosa, hair follicles and glands disappear, and the epithelium is somewhat modified. Its basal layer follows a very irregular course, so that there are tall projections of the underlying connective tissue extending toward the surface of the lip. These cells are not pigmented but are well supplied with blood vessels, giving this part of the lip a brighter color than that of the surrounding skin.

On the oral surface the epithelium changes again. The height of the connective tissue papillae gradually diminishes, as does the cornification of the surface, and at the base of the lip, on the inside, the mucous membrane is like that lining other soft parts of the oral cavity. In this region there are seromucous glands lying in the connective tissue between the epithelium and the muscle.

LINING OF THE ORAL CAVITY

The epithelium lining the oral cavity is of the stratified squamous variety. It rests on a tunica propria of reticular or fine areolar tissue, which blends, in most parts of the cavity, with a submucosal layer of areolar tissue. Beneath the submucosa lie tissues that vary in different parts of the mouth. In the cheeks and lips, for example, the mucosa and submucosa lie against muscle, making a soft and somewhat elastic wall of the oral cavity. In the hard palate and the gingivae, on the other hand, the layers in question lie directly against bone. Modifications of the mucous membrane are correlated with these differences in the tissue it covers.

Lips and cheeks (Fig. 17-2)

The inner surface of the lip is a good example of conditions in parts of the mouth that are bounded by muscle. The epithelium is not cornified. It has a surface layer of flattened cells that slough off in patches. Connective tissue papillae are low; the tunica propria blends without demarcation with the submucosa. The latter is fairly thick and in some regions contains glands, the ducts of which penetrate the mucosa and open into the oral cavity.

Gingivae and hard palate

In places where the mucosa and submucosa lie over bony tissue, as in the gingivae and hard palate, modifications of arrangement are to be observed. In the gingival region the connective tissue papillae of the tunica propria are long and slender and close together. The submucosa blends with the periosteum of the underlying bone, and in the region immediately surrounding each tooth, fibers are present that are specialized as part of the apparatus by which the tooth is held in its socket. There are no glands in this portion of the oral mucosa.

In the hard palate the papillae of the tunica

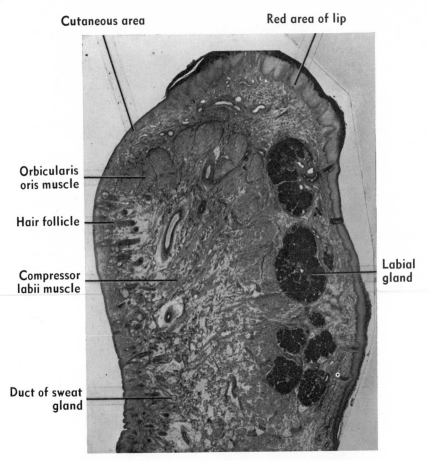

Cutaneous area   Red area of lip

Orbicularis oris muscle

Hair follicle

Compressor labii muscle

Labial gland

Duct of sweat gland

Fig. 17-1

Parasagittal section of human lip in newborn infant. (×14.) (Section courtesy Dr. Sol Bernick, Los Angeles, Calif.)

propria are well developed, and there is a layer of elastic fibers that forms a line of demarcation between the mucosa and submucosa. The latter coat blends here, as in the gingivae, with the periosteum of the underlying bone. There are mucous glands in the submucosa of the posterior palatal region; numerous fat cells occur in the corresponding layer of the anterior palatal region.

TONGUE

The tongue is primarily a muscular organ. It is covered with a mucous membrane consisting of stratified squamous epithelium, parts of which are modified to conform to its function as an organ of mastication and of taste.

The striated muscles of the tongue are in three main groups: longitudinal, transverse, and sagittal fibers, arranged in interlacing groups and embedded in areolar and adipose tissue.

The mucosa covering the dorsal surface of the tongue is modified to form a great number of elevations, or papillae. It should be noted that these papillae are different from the projections of connective tissue of the epithelium that have been mentioned in descriptions of other parts of the oral mucosae. The papilla of the tongue is an elevation of both connective tissue and epithelium. Within each of them there may also be projections of the tunica propria into the epithelium, which are termed *secondary papillae*. The distribution and characteristic forms of the papillae of the tongue are as follows.

Filiform papillae

Filiform papillae are the most numerous of the papillae and are distributed over the entire dorsal surface of the tongue. Each consists of a conical elevation of the tunica propria and

198

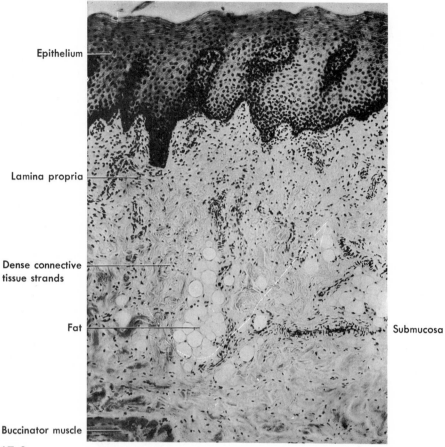

Epithelium

Lamina propria

Dense connective
tissue strands

Fat

Submucosa

Buccinator muscle

Fig. 17-2
Section through mucous membrane of cheek. Note the strands of dense connective tissue attaching the mucous membrane to the buccinator muscle. (From Sicher, H., editor: Orban's oral histology and embryology, ed. 6, St. Louis, 1966, The C. V. Mosby Co.)

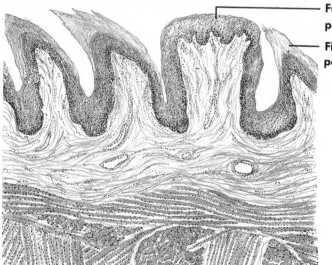

Fungiform papilla

Filiform papilla

Fig. 17-3
Dorsal surface of tongue of dog.

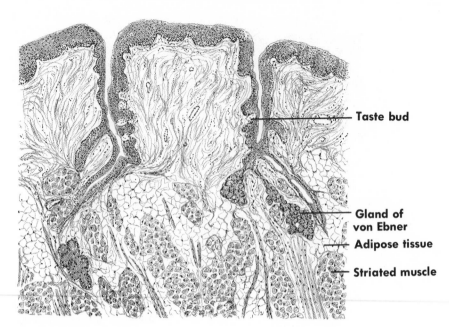

Fig. 17-4
Circumvallate papilla.

Labels: Taste bud, Gland of von Ebner, Adipose tissue, Striated muscle

stratified squamous epithelium. The whole papilla is inclined in an anteroposterior direction. Its surface epithelium is cornified, the cornification extending in strands, which gives this type of papilla its name (threadlike) (Fig. 17-3). They may have one or more secondary papillae.

Fungiform papillae

Fungiform papillae are distributed unevenly among the filiform papillae on the dorsal surface of the tongue, being most numerous near the margin of the organ but never so numerous as the filiform variety. They are club shaped, with flattened free surfaces and a diameter somewhat greater than that of the basal portion of a filiform papilla. The epithelium covering them shows little, if any, cornification and is relatively thin. This, combined with the fact that they have a rich blood supply, gives them a red color in the living state. Their secondary papillae are low (Fig. 17-3). Taste buds are sometimes visible on the free surfaces of fungiform papillae but are small and not always noticeable.

Foliate papillae

Foliate papillae are well developed on the tongues of certain rodents but are rudimentary in man. When fully developed, they have some features in common with fungiform papillae, being club shaped with flat tops. The types are readily distinguishable, however, by the following facts: The foliate papillae occur in groups along the lateral margins of the tongue and are not intermingled with filiform papillae; they have numerous prominent taste buds set close together along their sides; and finally, they are characterized by the presence of the secondary connective tissue papillae that occupy approximately three-fourths of the depth of the primary papilla. Lingual glands occur in the same part of the tongue as do the foliate papillae (Fig. 17-5).

Vallate (circumvallate)

Vallate (circumvallate) papillae are the largest papillae of the tongue and the least numerous. There are only from twenty to thirty of them, arranged along the sulcus terminalis, and they are so large as to be macroscopically visible. Each projects a short distance above the surface of the tongue but is, as the name implies, surrounded by a deep groove (Fig. 17-4). Their secondary papillae are short and are usually limited to the upper surface. The outstanding characteristic, aside from their size and positions, is as follows: The walls of the grooves surrounding them are beset with large taste buds, and the grooves serve as the point of exit for the ducts of conspicuous serous glands that are

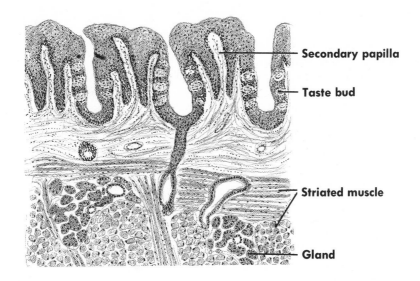

Fig. 17-5
Foliate papillae.

Stratified squamous epithelium

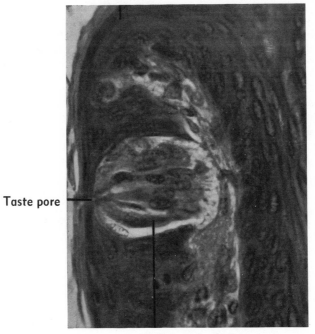

Cell in taste bud

Fig. 17-6
Taste bud. (×640.) (From Bevelander, G.: Essentials of histology, ed. 6, St. Louis, 1970, The C. V. Mosby Co.)

present in this part of the tongue (Ebner's glands).

The taste buds are composed of two kinds of cells: the specialized taste cells and the supporting cells. In ordinary sections the two kinds may be distinguished by their nuclei, those of the taste cells being dark and spindle shaped and those of the supporting cells pale and round or oval shaped (Fig. 17-6). The taste bud as a whole is a flask-shaped structure lying in the epithelium and opening onto the surface through a minute circular pore. In specimens treated with silver nitrate, nerve fibers may be traced into the center of the buds.

• • •

The ventral surface of the tongue is covered by mucous membrane not unlike that lining the lip and cheeks. In all parts of the organ the interlacing bands of striated muscle are a characteristic feature. In regions where glands occur, their secreting portions lie in the connective tissue that forms a stroma around the muscles, producing an arrangement of glandular and muscular tissue not often seen in other organs. It may be said that the tongue has no submucosa, this layer being replaced by a mixture of connective tissue, muscle, and glands.

GLANDS OF THE ORAL CAVITY

Saliva, the fluid in the oral cavity, is secreted principally by three large glands, the parotid, the submaxillary, and the sublingual, which lie outside the lining of the cavity and communicate with it by means of large ducts. Contributions to the saliva are made also by numerous smaller glands that are situated in the submucosa of some parts of the wall of the oral cavity and among the muscles of the tongue. They are of three kinds—serous, mucous, and seromucous—and are located as follows:

Serous
  Tongue, in region of vallate papillae (Ebner's)
Mucous
  Anterior surface of soft palate (palatine)
  Hard palate, lateral posterior region
  Tongue, borders near foliate papillae (lingual)
  Tongue, root
Seromucous
  Tongue, anterior portion (anterior lingual)
  Lips (labial)
Posterior to the sulcus terminalis there are

no papillae on the dorsal surface of the tongue. It is covered by stratified squamous epithelium like that lining the remainder of the cavity at this point. The tunica propria is reticular tissue and contains condensations of lymphoid tissue and the palatine and lingual tonsils described in Chapter 8. There are mucous glands in the submucosa of the fauces.

PHARYNX

The oral cavity opens, through the fauces, into the pharynx, a region in which the respiratory and digestive systems are only partly separated by the soft palate. The respiratory part, or nasopharynx, has a lining characteristic of the respiratory tract, namely, an epithelium of the pseudo-stratified variety and a tunica propria, which is separated from the submucosa by an elastic membrane. The oropharynx, or digestive part, is intermediate in composition, as it is in position between the oral cavity and the esophagus. It is lined with stratified squamous epithelium and has a tunica propria containing many elastic fibers, some of which form a fairly definite membrane at the border of the mucosa. The submucosa may be of considerable extent and contain the secreting portions of mucous glands. In some parts of the pharynx, however, the elastic membrane of the mucosa rests immediately over the muscular layer, and the glands are pushed down among the strands of muscle, as they are in the tongue. Such arrangements have given rise to the statement that the pharynx has no submucosa. It is obvious, however, that in a transitional region like the pharynx different conditions obtain in different parts. Sections of the lower part of the pharynx are in fact difficult to distinguish from sections of the upper part of the esophagus.

The muscular layer of the pharyngeal wall consists of bundles of striated muscle obliquely set to form a constrictor arrangement. The bundles interlace and do not form regular layers.

NASAL MUCOSA

The epithelium of the respiratory part of the nasal cavity consists of the pseudo-stratified, ciliated, columnar type. Many goblet cells are present as in the case of the trachea. The underlying tunica propria, which is separated from the epithelium by a basement membrane, contains many mixed glands that open to the surface of the epithelium. In addition to the loose connective tissue one may observe aggregations of lymphoid tissue and many unmyelinated nerve fibers.

Overlying the superior meatus and the dorsal anterior region of the nasal cavity the epithelium contains many nerve cell bodies, lacks goblet cells, and is modified to form an olfactory organ. Since the processes of the cells are difficult to follow, the epithelium frequently is classified as stratified columnar. The surface cells appear to be columnar. The mucosa is supplied with special glands known as Bowman's glands, which probably produce the secretion frequently noted over the surface of this organ.

INDEX TO PART ONE

Meissner's plexus, 117, 125
Melatonin, 190
Membranes, serous, 33
Mesangium, 155–156
Microglia, 72
Microtubules, 11
Mitochondria, 9–11
Monocytes, 76
Motor neuron, 59–62
Mucosa of digestive tract, 109–117, 119–122, 124
Multicellular glands, 107–108
Muscle, 51–58
    cardiac, 56–57
    circulation and innervation of, 58
    diagnostic features of, 58
    skeletal, 52–56
    smooth, 51–52
    striated, 52–56
Muscularis of digestive tract, 109–111, 114, 117, 120–122, 124
Myelin sheath, 63, 65
Myocardium, 88–89
Myometrium, 173

N

Nails, 195–196
Nasal mucosa, 202–203
Nasal passages, 142–144
Nasopharynx, 144
Nephron, 153–155
Nerve cell bodies, 59
Nerve cells, 59–62
    of dorsal root ganglia, 61
    in spinal cord, 61
Nerve endings, 68–70
    motor, 68–69
    sensory, 70
Nerve fibers, 59, 62–65
    myelinated, 63–64
    in sheath of Schwann, 63, 64
Nerves, 65–67
Nervous tissue, 59–72
Neurofibrils, 59
Neuroglia, 70–72
Neurohypophysis, 184, 186–187
Neurons, 59–62
Neuroplasm, 59
Neutrophilic leukocytes, 74, 76
Nissl bodies, 59
Nodes of Ranvier, 63, 65
Norepinephrine, 187
Nucleic acids, 4–5
Nucleoloneme, 12
Nucleolus, 12
Nucleus, 12

O

Oligodendroglia, 71–72
Oral cavity, 109, 197–203
    glands of, 202
    lining of, 197–198
Osteoblasts, 38, 40
Osteoid bone, 40
Ovary, 169–171, 180
Oviduct, 172–173

Ovulation, 171
Oxytocin, 187

P

Palate, hard, 197–198
Palatine tonsils, 98–99
Pancreas, 132–133
    blood and nerve supply of, 133
Paneth cells, 117, 120
Papillae
    filiform, 198–200
    foliate, 200
    fungiform, 200
    vallate, 200–202
Papillary ducts of kidney, 157–158
Parafollicular cells, 181
Parathyroid glands, 180, 183–184
    hormonal control of calcium by, 184
Parotid, 126–129
Pars distalis, 184–186
Pars intermedia, 184, 186
Pars tuberalis, 184, 186
Pedicles, 155
Penis, 166–168
Perikaryon, 59–62
Perimetrium, 173
Perineurium, 65
Periosteum, 47
Peyer's patches, 117, 120
Pharyngeal tonsil, 99
Pharynx, 202
Pigment granules, 12, 14
Pineal body, 180, 189–190
Pinealocytes, 190
Pituicytes, 186
Pituitary gland, 180, 184–187
Plasma, blood, 77
Plasma calcium, hormonal control of, by parathyroids, 184
Plasma cells in connective tissue, 30–31
Plasma membrane, 6–8
Podocytes, 155
Polymorphonuclear leukocytes, 74
Portal canal, 138
"Prickle" cells of epithelium, 24
Procallus, 50
Proerythroblasts, 79
Progesterone, 172, 179
Prolactin, 185, 186
Promyelocytes, 78–79
Prostate, 166
Protoplasm, 3–4
Proximal convoluted tubules of kidney, 156
Purkinje fibers, 89

R

Rectal columns of Morgagni, 122
Rectum, 121–122
Reflex mechanism, 67–68
Reproductive system
    female, 168–179
    male, 161–168
Respiratory tract, 142–150
    lower parts of, 144–150
        alveolar ducts in, 148–150

Part two

DENTAL HISTOLOGY AND EMBRYOLOGY

1

DEVELOPMENT OF THE FACE

In a study of the development of the face and associated structures it is necessary to consider briefly the origin and development of certain organ systems and masses of tissue that are directly involved at one time or another in this process. When considered in terms of chronological development, it is evident that single systems or parts of systems do not arise independently of one another, yet for the sake of simplicity of description we shall at times describe the development of isolated structures.

As early as the third or fourth week of development in the human embryo, the digestive tract is already present as a hollow tube that, until this time, has been closed at both the caudal and cephalic ends by a plate of ectodermal tissue, the buccopharyngeal membrane. In this, the 3-week stage of development, the cephalic plate has already ruptured. This rupture results in establishing a communication between the pharyngeal part of the alimentary tract and the large cavity that lies just below the forebrain, known as the stomodeum. The relation of these structures is shown diagrammatically in Fig. 1-1, A. With the stomodeum established the first important step in the development of the face is completed. The stomedeum is later involved in the formation of those structures that we recognize as the oral and nasal cavities in the adult.

Examination of the head of the embryo in the third or fourth week, such as the one shown in Fig. 1-1, B, demonstrates two paired structures, the maxillary and mandibular processes. At this time they form the lateral walls of the primitive oral cavity.

As indicated, these processes derived from the first branchial arches play an extremely important part in the formation of the face. Ac-

cordingly, we shall consider the role that they play in this particular development. Fig. 1-1, C, a lateral view of the head of a 3-week embryo, shows not only the relation of the two processes to the oral cavity but also the line of union between them, which is later recognized as the angle of the mouth. In a slightly later stage of development a median unpaired structure, the frontal process, makes its appearance as shown in Fig. 1-1, E and F. In the sixth week of development two additional paired structures arise. They appear first on the lateral surfaces of the head as two small ectodermal plaques, which are known as the nasal, or olfactory, processes. About 1 week later an inverted U-shaped elevation of tissue surrounds each olfactory plaque, the limbs of which are known respectively as the lateral and medial olfactory processes. These structures, in conjunction with the maxillary processes, take part in the formation of the nose and maxillary arch, or upper jaw. By the end of the seventh week the olfactory plaques hollow out into pits, and thus the primitive external nares are established. The pits deepen and are separated from the mouth cavity by a membrane that soon ruptures and then gives rise to an internal orifice, the primitive choana.

The nasolacrimal groove separating the maxillary and lateral nasal processes closes over superficially, while the deep part remains as the nasolacrimal duct.

By the time the nasal processes have reached the stage of development just described, certain changes have also occurred in the maxillary and mandibular processes. Considering first the development of the maxillary region of the face, one should note that while in the 3-week embryo (Fig. 1-1, B and C) the maxillary processes are

3

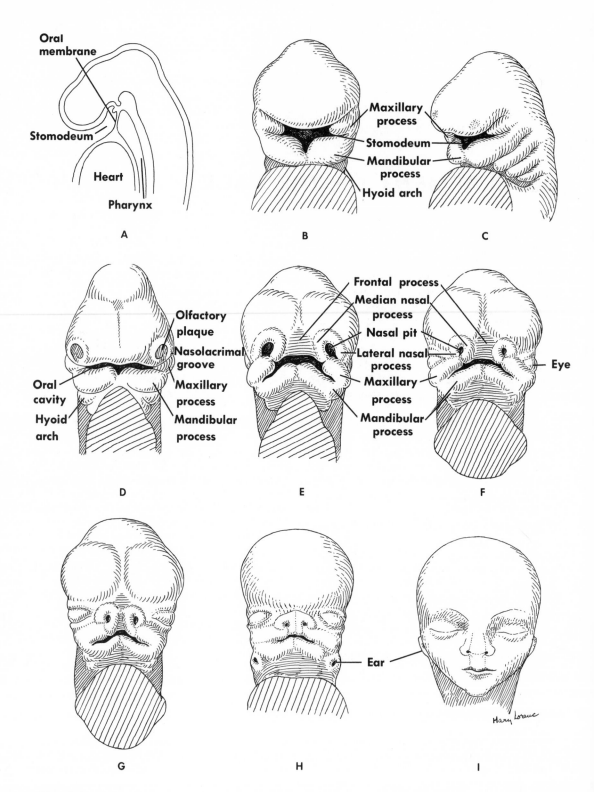

Fig. 1-1

Stages in development of face and jaw from approximately 6 weeks to term.

relatively small structures located on the lateral surface of the face, in the 6-week embryo (Fig. 1-1, *E*) they have increased in size and have grown toward the midline of the face.

In this growth the medial migration of the maxillary processes impinge upon the medial nasal processes and crowd them toward the midline. Thus, by 10 weeks these two pairs of structures form a complete maxillary arch with the component parts aligned from side to side as follows: maxillary process—medial nasal process—medial nasal process—maxillary process. During the time in which the maxillary arch develops a caudal migration of the frontal process and a medial migration of the two lateral nasal processes also occur, the former giving rise to the bridge, the latter to the alae of the nose. An additional feature in the development of the nose is the establishment of the primitive nasal septum. This occurs when the two medial walls of the medial nasal processes meet in the midline of the face and fuse. The net result of the rearrangement of the nasal processes is the formation of two primitive nasal cavities located just under the primitive forebrain.

The mandible in the meantime has also developed to a considerable extent. The mandible is derived from the paired mandibular processes that previously arose as bifurcating limbs of the first branchial arch. These processes eventually migrate from their lateral position to a point in the midline where fusion occurs. This is illustrated in Fig. 1-1, *B* to *E*.

The embryonic mandible is supported by a semirigid crescentic bar of cartilage known as Meckel's cartilage. The position of this cartilage is shown in Figs. 2-2 and 2-3. Almost as soon as membranous bone appears in the human mandible (8 weeks), resorption of the tissue comprising Meckel's cartilage begins. In the mandible proper the cartilage is replaced by fibrous tissue. It should be recalled, however, that Meckel's cartilage itself is not the tissue that calcifies. In the proximal region Meckel's cartilage gives rise to the sphenomandibular ligament, the malleus, and incus.

2

DEVELOPMENT OF THE TONGUE AND PALATE

While the changes described in Chapter 1 have been taking place on the external part of the face, some important developments have also occurred internally.

TONGUE

The tongue is essentially a pharyngeal derivative; secondarily, it grows forward into the oral cavity. In terms of developmental components the tongue is derived from (1) a mucous membrane and (2) skeletal muscle that invades the sac and completely fills it.

The mucous membrane of the tongue arises from two regions: The body or apical part that bears papillae arises anteriorly to the second branchial arches; the root is derived chiefly from the second arch and also to a lesser extent from the third and fourth arches. In the later stages of development the root is distinguishable from the body by the presence of a well-defined, V-shaped groove, the sulcus terminalis.

The anlagen of the mucous membrane coverings of the tongue can be recognized in embryos of the fifth week. They consist of a median swelling, the tuberculum impar, located on the floor of the pharynx between the first pair of pouches and a pair of larger lateral swellings, located on the mandibular arches. The future root can be observed as a ventral elevation at the juncture of the median union of the second branchial arches. This is known as the copula. Between the tuberculum impar and the copula a depression known as the thyroid diverticulum occurs.

Later development of the tongue consists of a rapid proliferation of the lateral swellings (located on the medial surface of the mandibular arches), which fuse with the tuberculum impar and eventually meet at the midline almost completely overshadowing the tuberculum. The copula in the meantime enlarges to form the root of the tongue. Eventually, the third and fourth arches also contribute to the formation of the tongue. The 5th and 7th nerves, derived from the first and second branchial arches, supply the mucosa of the body of the tongue; the glossopharyngeal (9th) and the vagus (10th), derived from the third and fourth arches, supply the root.

By the seventh week the tongue becomes fairly well separated from the mandible and is elevated from the floor of the mouth by the infiltration of striated muscle internally. The 12th nerve supplies these muscles. It is assumed, therefore, that this muscle tissue has undergone a cranial migration from the postbranchial myotomes.

PALATE

During the sixth week, three anlagen of the palate also appear. One of these is a median structure that takes its origin from the medial nasal process; the others, two lateral anlagen, are derived from the maxillary tissue. They are known as the medial and lateral palatal processes, respectively. The medial nasal process does not actually become incorporated into the anterior part of the hard palate but, as previously described, retains its relation with the maxilla as the premaxillary part of this bony structure.

A comparison of two important stages in the early development of the palate is shown in Figs. 2-1 to 2-3. Fig. 2-2 shows the relative size, shape, and relations of the combined nasal and oral cavities. (This is known as the open

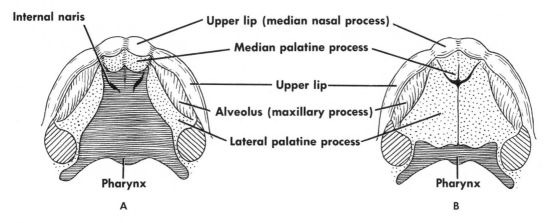

Fig. 2-1
A, Palatal view of developing maxilla and anlagen, which give rise to palate. B, Palatal view of fully formed hard palate.

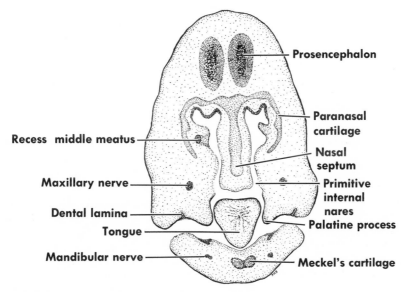

Fig. 2-2
Coronal section through 20-mm. pig embryo head (open palate stage).

palate stage.) This cavity is roughly H shaped, the upper half of the H representing the future nasal cavity, the lower half representing the oral cavity. Each arm of the nasal part, as seen in section, is enclosed by incomplete rings, the nasal cartilages. They are remnants of the walls of the olfactory pockets. In the medial migration of these latter structures the two medial walls fuse to form the primitive septum of the nose; the lateral walls remain as the outer margins

of the growing cavity. Reference to Fig. 2-2 shows, in addition, the relation of the nasal cavities to the primitive forebrain vesicles.

In the lower, or oral, part of the cavity the position of the tongue at this stage of development is largely responsible for the shape of this orifice. As shown in Fig. 2-2, it projects above the mandibular tissue to such an extent that its superior surface lies just below the nasal septum. One should also note the position of the

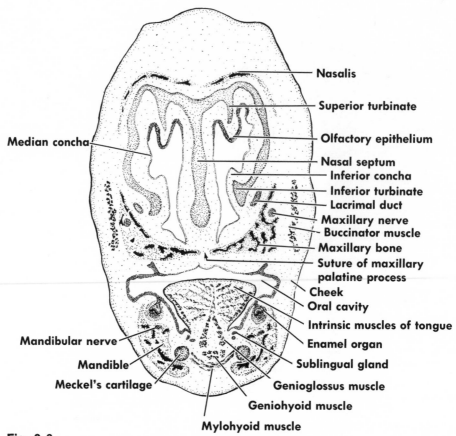

Fig. 2-3

Coronal section through 37-mm. pig embryo head (closed palate stage).

lateral palatal flaps, disposed vertically, which appear in a frontal section as paired folds approximating either side of the base of the tongue.

The development of the palate from this, the open palate stage, to the closed palate stage consists in the main of two important changes. First, the tongue drops to an inferior position in the oral cavity, and second, the two lateral palatal flaps grow in a medial and superior direction because of the unequal rate of growth of the lower part of the palatal flap. This growth continues until the two lateral palatal processes meet in the midline and begin to fuse in the nineteenth week. This fusion first occurs in the anterior region and proceeds posteriorly. In the extreme anterior region the median palatal process, a derivative of the median nasal process, lies between the lateral palatine processes, and in this area the two lateral shelves fuse with it instead of with each other (Fig. 2-1, *B*).

At the time that fusion occurs, ossification

of the anterior part of the palate also begins. This eventually results in the formation of the hard palate. Posteriorly, the palate continues as a shelf of soft tissue to its apex, the uvula. The unfused backward prolongations of the palatine folds on the lateral walls of the pharynx give rise to the palatine arches, which separate the oral cavity from the pharynx. Reference to Fig. 2-3 shows the relations of the former oral region, which is now completely separated into a superior (nasal) cavity and an inferior (oral) cavity. This delimitation is effected by the fusion of the hard palate, which serves as the roof of the oral cavities and floor of the nasal cavities.

In connection with the formation of the hard palate and the resulting separation of the primitive oral cavity it should be noted that the separation occurs in the anterior part of the oral cavity. Posteriorly, these two cavities remain in communication as the nasopharynx. It seems

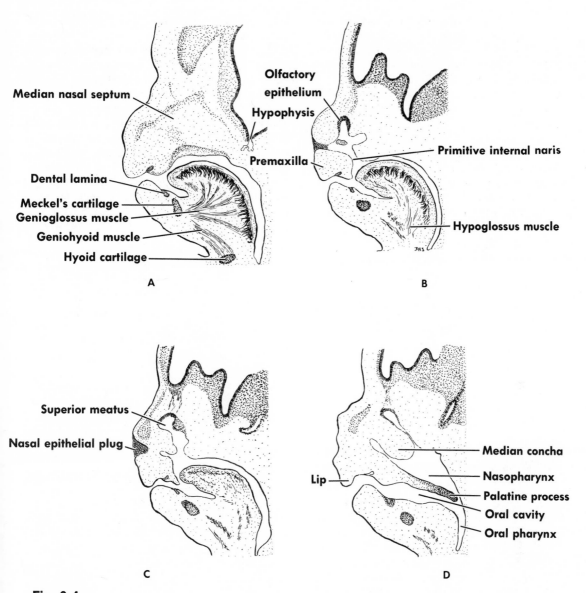

Fig. 2-4.

A, Midsaggital section through jaws of embryo. **B** to **D,** Representative sagittal sections progressively lateral to that shown in **A. D,** Palatine process lateral to tongue (which no longer appears at this level). Reveals *prospective* separation of nasal and oral cavities with only pharyngeal communication.

appropriate to point out in this connection that when frontal sections of the embryonic head are examined it is important to orient oneself in regard to the level from which the section is taken, so that the structures that appear in the preparation will be correctly interpreted. If, for example, an open palate stage of the embryonic face is cut coronally so that the plane of section passes posteriorly to the region in which the lateral palatal flaps have not yet

fused in the midline, the maxilla itself will appear in the position in which one would expect to find the palatal flaps. Sections farther anterior in the same series will correct this misleading impression and show more clearly the actual relations between the palate and the maxilla.

If one compares the structure of the nasal cavity shown in Fig. 2-2 with that shown in Fig 2-3, one can readily ascertain that the most striking difference between the two is the enclosure of the nasal cavity inferiorly by the palate. The shape and relations of the nasal cartilages are for all purposes similar to those shown in Fig. 2-3, the open palate stage. The nasal septum meanwhile continues to grow inferiorly until it meets the cephalic surface of the palate, eventually dividing the nasal cavity into right and left chambers.

It is important to remember that the cartilaginous plates that form the framework of the primitive nose comprise the central core around which the soft parts of the face are subsequently laid down.

Anomalies in the development of the palate and upper lips sometimes occur. Failure of the lateral palatine processes to unite in the normal midline position gives rise to a malformation known as cleft palate, or uranoschisis. There are many variations of this condition; clefts in the soft palate usually occupy a midline position, while those involving the hard palate are either unilateral or bilateral and lie to one side of the midline. Cleft palate is frequently associated with imperfect fusion of the lip. This condition is known as harelip. This abnormal development has been produced experimentally by interfering with metabolic events during embryogenesis.

3
EARLY DEVELOPMENT OF THE TEETH

The teeth are derived from two distinct embryonic tissues: (1) ectoderm, which gives rise to the enamel organ and subsequently the enamel (crown) of the tooth; (2) mesenchyme, the precursor of all the other parts of the tooth and associated supporting structures.

In a study of the development and structure of the teeth it is necessary to have available a series of sections of the jaw taken at appropriate intervals in the process of development. The following description that deals with the histogenesis of the teeth is based on the study of a number of stages of the developing mammalian tooth, which has been chosen to illustrate the most important phases of tooth development.

EARLY DEVELOPMENT

The dental anlagen are differentiated in the human embryo at about the sixth week. At first these structures consist of a continuous ridge of tissue, one for each jaw, which appear as solid proliferations of the oral epithelium extending into the underlying mesenchyme. These laminae are to be found in a position that is approximately at right angles to the surface epithelium. They extend around the arch of each jaw and are known as the dental laminae. For orientation of these structures in regard to other parts of the jaw, see Fig. 3-1, a midsaggital section through the head of an 8-week embryo.

Almost as soon as the dental lamina is differentiated, one can observe that it is made up of two separate parts. One part consists of a vertical labial ingrowth, which marks off the future lip and vestibule; this is known as the labial lamina. The second part continues as a lingual prolongation of epithelium that eventually gives rise to the enamel organs. The latter structure is known as the dental lamina. Sectional views of the early development of these structures are shown in Figs. 2-4, 3-1, 3-2, and 3-3.

The tooth buds arise as outgrowths of the dental laminae. Ten of these buds normally arise in each jaw at the sites corresponding to the location of the future deciduous teeth (Fig. 3-3).

In the developing jaw one may now distinguish between the dental lamina, which is a continuous proliferation of tissue, and the ten separate tooth buds. These buds appear first as solid structures; later they become hollowed out because of growth and differentiation and by an invasion of the underlying mesenchyme. In this latter form they serve more or less as a mold in which the crown of the developing tooth is fashioned.

We shall now direct our attention to the development occurring in the buds. For the sake of clarity we wish to repeat that the dental lamina is as a whole U shaped, foreshadowing the shape of the dental arch. This relation is clearly shown by the examination of serial sections of these structures, in which one sees the alternation of buds and regions devoid of buds in which only sections of the lamina itself are apparent. When isolated sections are examined, one may sometimes see on one side of the jaw a developing bud consisting of a solid core of cells (Fig. 3-3); on the other side one may see part of the lamina that lies between the two buds. It is thus obvious that it is extremely important to orient oneself in regard to the sections that are available for study.

ENAMEL ORGAN

After the appearance of the labial laminae, differentiation in addition to growth plays an extremely important role in the development of the tooth. This is clearly illustrated by the section of the tooth represented in Figs. 3-4 and 3-5. The changes that lead to the stage of development illustrated by Fig. 3-4 are as follows: (1) The epithelial bud becomes somewhat removed from the oral epithelium but is still attached to it by a narrow strand of cells, the dental lamina. (2) The mesenchyme at the base of the epithelial bud undergoes a rapid proliferation. In this process a condensation of mesenchymal cells, collectively known as the mesenchymal knot (dental papilla), causes a depression in the distal wall of the epithelial bud, which is now called the early enamel organ. Accompanying these changes in the external configuration of the tooth germ, certain changes occur in the arrangement of the tissues therein.

As the mesenchymal cells that lie at the base of the tooth bud proliferate, a concomitant division of tooth bud cells results in partial envelopment of the mesenchyme (Fig. 3-4). The derivatives of the basal cell layer are the inner enamel epithelium and outer enamel epithelium, while the derivatives of the spiny cell layer form a loose network of cells invested in a metachromatic ground substance to form the

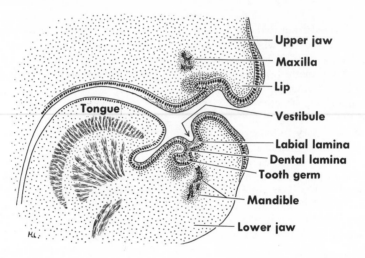

Fig. 3-1
Sagittal section through jaws of human embryo of approximately 8 weeks. Note relation of the vestibule, lips, dental lamina, and tooth germ.

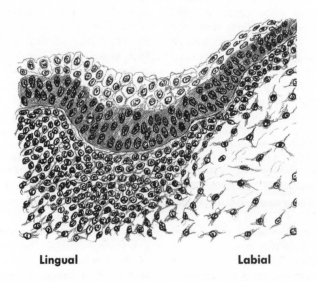

Lingual   Labial

Fig. 3-2
Coronal section through dental anlage, showing first indication of its division into labial and lingual proliferation.

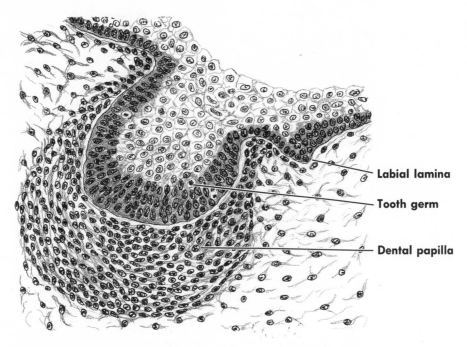

Fig. 3-3
Coronal section, showing relation of early tooth germ (bud) and labial lamina.

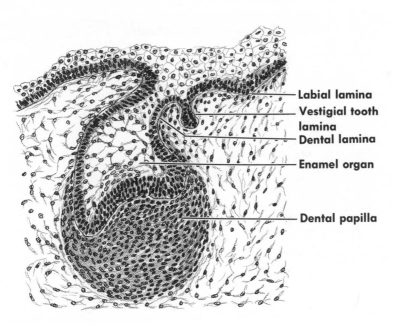

Fig. 3-4
Coronal section through early enamel organ.

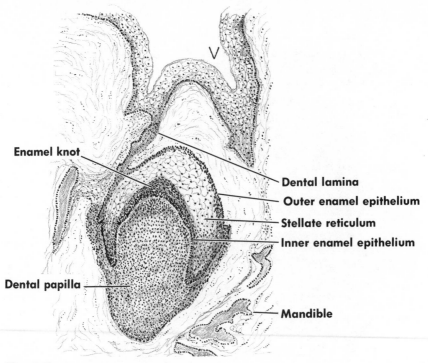

Enamel knot

Dental lamina

Outer enamel epithelium

Stellate reticulum

Inner enamel epithelium

Dental papilla

Mandible

Fig. 3-5
Intermediate stage in development of human enamel organ. **V,** Vestibule.

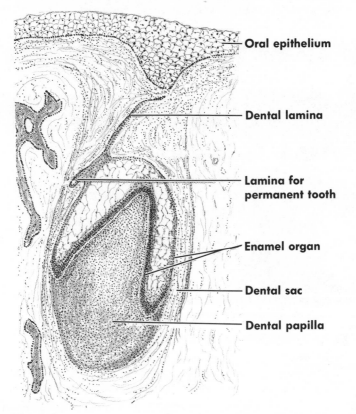

Oral epithelium

Dental lamina

Lamina for permanent tooth

Enamel organ

Dental sac

Dental papilla

Fig. 3-6
Late enamel organ.

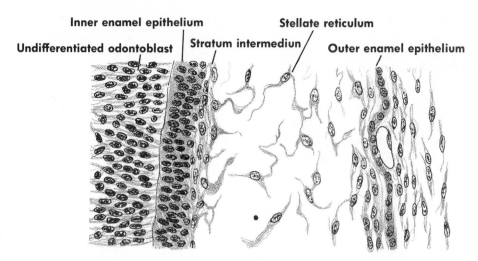

Inner enamel epithelium   Stellate reticulum

Undifferentiated odontoblast   Stratum intermediun   Outer enamel epithelium

Fig. 3-7

High magnification of lower parallel lines in Fig. 4-3.

third tissue of the early enamel organ known as the stellate reticulum. In the intermediate stages (Fig. 3-5) and late enamel organ stage (Fig. 3-6) most of the cell division seems to take place in the region of junction between the inner and outer enamel epithelia and in further development of the tooth in that region known as the cervical loop. Division in the latter region results in the addition of cells to the stellate reticulum as well as to the inner and outer epithelia. The overall effect is broadening and lengthening of the enamel organ, thus enclosing more of the rapidly proliferating dental papilla.

In the early enamel organ and intermediate stages (Fig. 3-5) some enamel organs show an additional proliferation of the inner enamel epithelium, known as the enamel knot. The significance of this tissue, which soon disappears, is not well known.

In the early development of some teeth (for example, the deciduous canines and first molars) an additional lamina, the vestigial tooth germ lamina, makes its appearance (Fig. 3-4) but soon disappears. The vestigial lamina, which does not appear in the development of the deciduous incisors, is said to be a remnant of a primitive prelacteal dentition.

In the latter stages of enamel organ development, proliferation of cells in the cervical region increases the length of the enamel organ so that it assumes the shape of a bell or inverted goblet. The dental lamina is reduced in size, and a structure not hitherto observed appears as a

small projection on the lingual aspect of the enamel organ. This is the anlage for the permanent, or succedaneous, tooth. At this stage (Fig. 3-6) the whole enamel organ and dental papilla are enclosed in a saclike structure known as the dental follicle, or dental sac. It is derived from the mesenchyme and consists of two general layers: an inner vascularized layer containing a few reticular fibers and an outer, more fibrous layer containing many reticular fibers and primitive cells. A fourth layer, known as the stratum intermedium, appears in the enamel organ adjacent to the inner enamel epithelium, and this layer is characteristic of the late enamel organ stage.

One can differentiate the following tissues in the enamel organ proper from without inward: (1) outer enamel epithelium, (2) stellate reticulum, (3) stratum intermedium, and (4) inner enamel epithelium located at the periphery of the embryonic pulp chamber and separated from the latter by a basement membrane (Fig. 3-7). These tissues constitute the enamel organ proper. During subsequent development of the tooth each of these components undergoes several changes in shape, arrangement, function, and ultimate fate. These changes will be discussed in connection with the formation of the tooth.

The formation of cusps in multicusped teeth involves the formation of an enamel organ whose inner enamel epithelium is folded to outline the origins of the future cusps and sulci.

SUMMARY OF EARLY DEVELOPMENT

The dental anlage, which consists of a band of tissue in each jaw, appears at approximately the sixth week. Soon thereafter one can observe that this anlage (the dental lamina) is made up of a labial downgrowth and a lingual proliferation. The former gives rise to the lip and vestibule, the latter to the enamel organs.

The tooth germs arise as outgrowths of the dental laminae. They become invaginated by underlying mesenchyme, remaining meanwhile suspended by the dental lamina. Invagination of the tooth germ continues; accompanying this change, differentiation of the elements of the growing enamel organ eventually gives rise to four distinct cell layers, which will subsequently be intimately involved in the elaboration of enamel. The dental lamina at this stage of development begins to atrophy.

4
DEVELOPMENT OF DENTIN

Dentin is laid down in the developing deciduous tooth in the fifth to the sixth month of intrauterine life, just previous to the appearance of the embryonic enamel. The development of this tissue, like that of membranous bone, consists in establishing a fibrous matrix in a fluid ground substance, which subsequently becomes impregnated with a hard calcifying substance. Dentin is first differentiated on the tip of the crown, then it gradually envelops the entire pulp cavity.

Studies aided by the use of the electron microscope show that prior to the initial formation of dentin the incompletely differentiated odontoblasts and ameloblasts abut each other at their distal surfaces. These cell surfaces are separated by a minute space bounded by the distal cell membrane of the odontoblast and the ameloblast, respectively. This region represents the future dentinoenamel junction (Fig. 4-1). Shortly before dentinogenesis occurs the differentiating odontoblasts exhibit a prominent basal nucleus, numerous mitochondria, an extensive rough endoplasmic reticulum, scattered ribosomes, and a Golgi apparatus, all located in a supranuclear region. The presence of these organelles are indicative of protein synthesis as an important function of the cell.

Subsequent events leading to the elaboration of dentin consist of the formation of a specialized zone at the terminal surface of the cell that is known as predentin. The predentin area arises as the result of (1) the formation of a terminal protoplasmic extension of the cell, Tomes' dentinal process (Fig. 4-2), (2) the retreat of the odontoblast pulpward, (3) the proliferation and appearance of reticular (Korff's) fibers (Figs. 4-2 and 4-3), and also (4) the elaboration and transport of tissue fluid and ground substance components to this area.

The preceding events give rise to an arrangement in which the odontoblast has retreated from its original position, maintaining contact, however, with the dentinoenamel junction by means of the protoplasmic extension known as Tomes' dentinal process (Figs. 4-4 to 4-6). When the relations and events described have taken place, mineralization occurs in the area described as predentin (Fig. 4-8).

Mineralization occurs as a gradual and incremental process. The triggering of mineral deposition results in the accumulation of minute amounts of hydroxyapatite in increments that appear as isolated collections of immature crystals in the cuspal area. The crystals appear in isolated patches of ground substance and in and on the collagen fibers (Figs. 4-7 and 4-8).

After the initial zone of predentin has been established, increase in the amount (that is, additional increments) consists of the elaboration of an additional zone of predentin and a corresponding pulpward shift of the odontoblasts. While the second zone of predentin is being formed the initial or peripheral zone undergoes partial mineralization (Fig. 4-6). This process is repeated several times until eventually the entire matrix becomes uniformly mineralized except for the space occupied by Tomes' dentinal process (the dentinal tubule), which does not mineralize.

Tomes' dentinal processes as previously mentioned are vital protoplasmic extensions of the odontoblasts. In mature dentin they extend from the region of the pulp to the periphery of the dentin, occupying spaces in this tissue known as the dentinal tubules. Structurally, the processes are relatively homogeneous except for the temporary presence of microtubules. During dentin formation they exhibit dense granules that appear to be incorporated

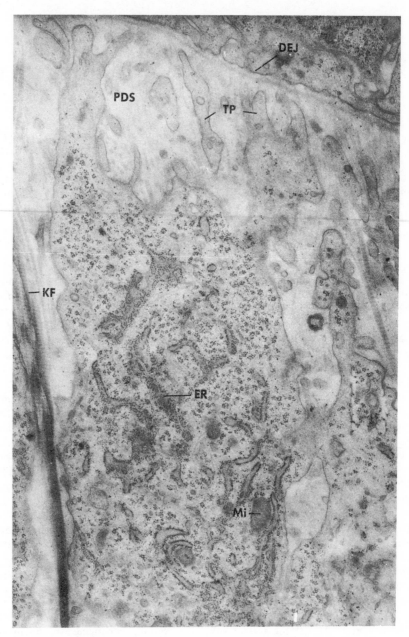

Fig. 4-1
Electron micrograph of odontoblast prior to mineralization of dentin. **ER**, Endoplasmic reticulum; **DEJ**, dentino-enamel junction; **Kf**, Korff's fibers; **Mi**, mitochondrion; **PDS**, predentin space; **TP**, Tomes' dentinal process. (From Bevelander, G., and Nakahara, H.: The formation and mineralization of dentin, Anat. Rec. **156**(3):303, 1966.)

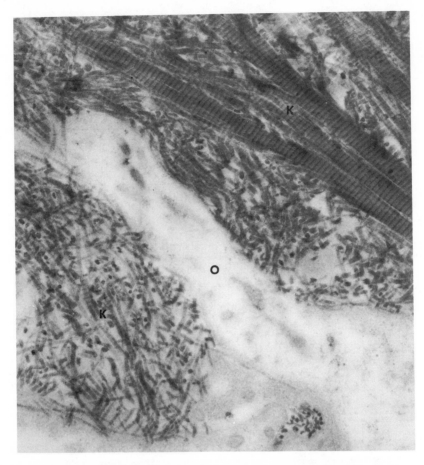

Fig. 4-2
Electron micrograph showing region of predentin. **K,** Korff's fibers of two different diameters; **O,** odontoblast process. (From Bevelander, G., and Nakahara, H.: The formation and mineralization of dentin, Anat. Rec. **156** (3):303, 1966.)

into the matrix. These granules are probably derived from the Golgi apparatus and accordingly contribute a mucoprotein component to the matrix.

In summary, dentinogenesis consists of the differentiation of the odontoblast into a cell disposed to elaborate protein that is conveyed to a zone known as predentin. The structural protein consists of reticular or collagen fibers derived at least in part from the pulp. Other proteins (nonstructural) mucopolysaccharides are probably derived from the Golgi apparatus and the endoplasmic reticulum. Predentin formation at first preceeds and then accompanies mineralization. This latter process results in the eventual mineralization of the entire matrix except for the space occupied by Tomes' dentinal process.

The odontoblasts are derived from mesodermal cells in the pulp and during their development and active functional span lie in a ground substance containing glycogen, mucopolysaccharides, and acid polysaccharides. When the odontoblasts attain their functional state and calcification of dentin occurs, these cells contain appreciable amounts of alkaline phosphatase, mucopolysaccharides, and nucleic acids.

One concept regarding the role of polysaccharides in calcifying tissues is that these substances become depolymerized and thereby offer reactive molecules that readily combine with calcium. It has been suggested that the presence of mucopolysaccharides in cells also rich in alkaline phosphatase provide a milieu favorable for enzymatic activity.

In a study of stained sections of the develop-

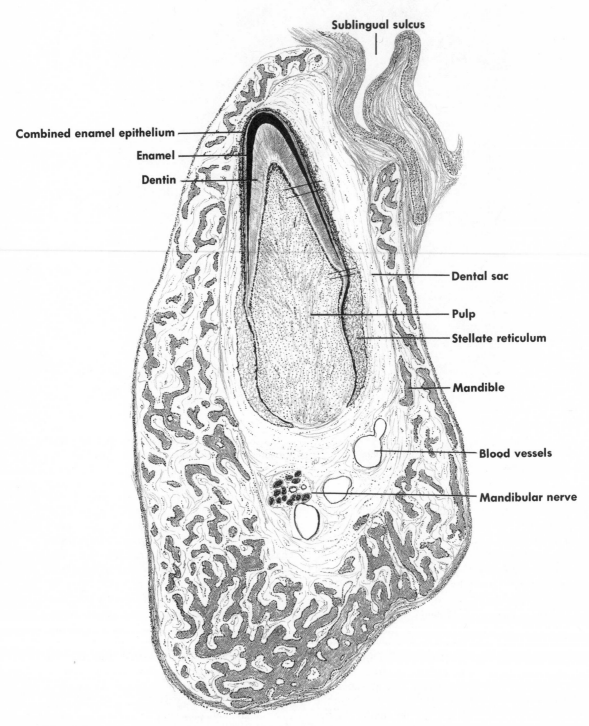

Sublingual sulcus

Combined enamel epithelium —

Enamel —

Dentin —

— **Dental sac**

— **Pulp**

— **Stellate reticulum**

— **Mandible**

— **Blood vessels**

— **Mandibular nerve**

Fig. 4-3
Coronal section of developing jaw with anterior tooth, showing early dentin and enamel formation.

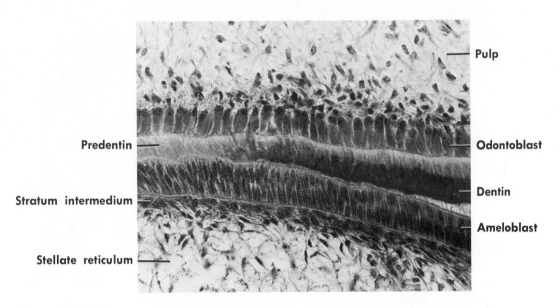

Fig. 4-4
Section of developing tooth, showing development of dentin.

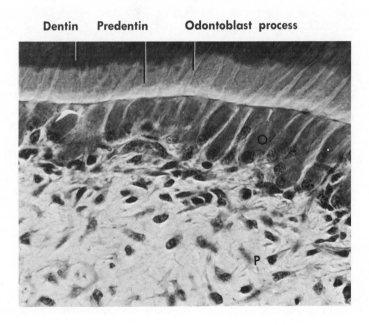

Fig. 4-5
Section of developing tooth, showing dentin and predentin. (×640.) **O**, Odontoblast; **P**, pulp.

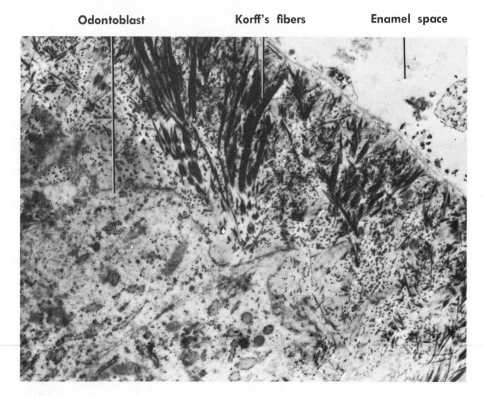

Odontoblast　　　**Korff's fibers**　　　**Enamel space**

Fig. 4-6
Electron micrograph of developing dentin. (×8,800.)

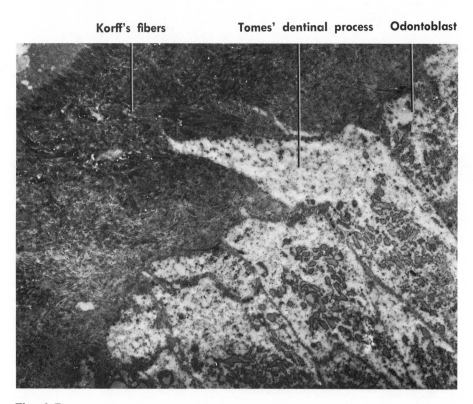

Korff's fibers　　　**Tomes' dentinal process**　　　**Odontoblast**

Fig. 4-7
Electron micrograph of developing dentin. (×4,000.)

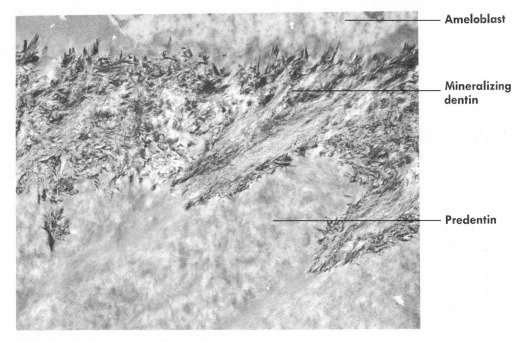

Ameloblast

Mineralizing dentin

Predentin

Fig. 4-8

Electron micrograph showing early stage of mineralization of dentin. (From Bevelander, G., and Nakahara, H.: Formation and mineralization of dentin, Anat. Rec. **156** (3):303, 1966.)

ing tooth examined at the optical level one can observe that the calcified substance of dentin appears first as exceedingly fine droplets that stain intensely with hematoxylin. These droplets later coalesce and form calcoglobules. Various stages in the calcification of dentin are illustrated in Figs. 4-4 to 4-7.

The growth of dentin is incremental; that is, it increases by the gradual rhythmic deposition of one layer upon another. The growth of dentin is divided into two steps: The first consists of the deposition of a given incremental organic layer (predentin) that occurs in advance of its calcification. The second step consists of calcification of the initial increment. The difference in the time relations of these two stages is indicated by the width of the predentin. Under normal conditions the rate of organic apposition and the rate of calcification are relatively constant.

5

DEVELOPMENT OF ENAMEL

Shortly after dentin has been deposited on the tip of the developing crown, enamel formation begins. Examination of the inner enamel epithelium of the calcifying tooth shows in the cervical region that the epithelia is of a low, more or less cuboidal form whereas at the tip of the crown these cells are of the tall columnar variety. During the maturation of these cells a shift in the position of the nucleus and other cellular constituents occurs, which results in the nucleus being located in the surface of the cell that lies adjacent to the stratum intermedium. The reversal in polarity of these cells is probably correlated with the fact that the enamel is produced at the dentinal surface (Figs. 5-3 and 5-4).

Although a number of details of enamel formation are still somewhat obscure and controversial, it is generally believed that the ameloblasts play approximately the same role in the formation of enamel that the odontoblasts play in the formation of dentin.

The first step in enamel formation consists of the elaboration of Tomes' enamel process and the ground substance in which it lies. Mineralization leading to the formation of the rods first occurs on the surfaces of the distal part of Tomes' process (Figs. 5-1 and 5-5). Crystal formation continues and Tomes' process is gradually infiltrated with crystals. As the distal part of the process mineralizes the ameloblasts retreat and continue to elaborate Tomes' process as well as ground substance. Crystal initiation and growth continues, eventually giving rise to an elongated structure that is roughly cylindrical in shape, the enamel rod (Fig. 5-7).

In addition to the rods, enamel exhibits mineralized material, the interrod (interprismatic) substance, similar in all respects to the rod in composition. It surrounds each rod, and mineralization occurs in the organic ground substance (Fig. 5-2).

The end result of the process of amelogenesis is the formation of enamel composed of elongated rods and the interrod substance. Although enamel consists of approximately 90% mineral, there is a considerable amount of organic substance in this tissue in the form of eukeratin. In addition, each rod is enclosed in a rod sheath.

Before enamel is deposited the stellate reticulum begins to disappear, first at the tip and gradually from the entire crown of the tooth (Fig. 4-3). The disappearance of the reticulum brings the other remaining epithelial layers of the enamel organ together in a layer known as the combined (united) epithelium. The ameloblasts retain their morphological characteristics until the crown erupts. During this phase of tooth development the ameloblasts elaborate a horny pellicle-like layer, or cuticle, which is firmly attached to the outer enamel surface. This cuticle is extremely resistant to acids and is known as Nasmyth's membrane. The function of this enamel cuticle is questionable. Some authorities believe that it may be a protective covering for the crown, particularly in the region of the pits and fissures.

In the apical part of the tooth the enamel epithelium persists in part until after eruption. It appears as a loop or duplicature that turns inward toward the midline of the root. This portion of the remaining inner and outer enamel epithelium is known as Hertwig's sheath (Fig. 5-6). It acts as a limiting membrane to aid in the shaping of the root and to give rise to additional odontoblasts to produce the dentin of the root.

Developing enamel is incompletely calcified and contains relatively large amounts of organic material and water. Therefore, after decalcification incidental to preparing a section of the

Text continued on p. 31.

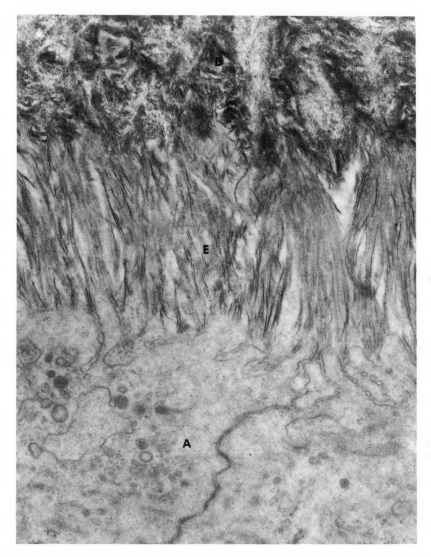

Fig. 5-1
Electron micrograph of early stage of mineralization of enamel and dentin. **A**, Ameloblast; **E**, enamel; **D**, dentin. (From Bevelander, G.: Atlas of oral histology and embryology, Philadelphia, 1967, Lea and Febiger.)

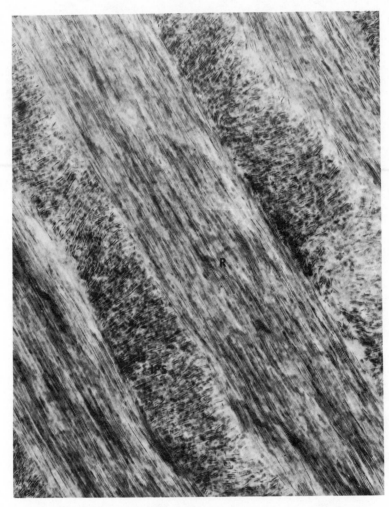

Fig. 5-2
Electron micrograph of partially mineralized enamel. **R,** Rod; **IPS,** interprismatic substance. (From Bevelander, G.: Atlas of oral histology and embryology, Philadelphia, 1967, Lea and Febiger.)

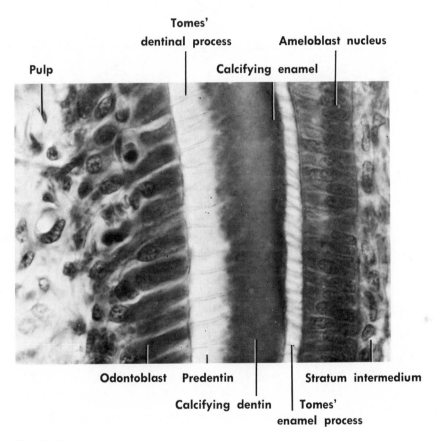

**Tomes'
dentinal process**

Ameloblast nucleus

Calcifying enamel

Pulp

Odontoblast   **Predentin**   **Stratum intermedium**

Calcifying dentin   **Tomes'
enamel process**

Fig. 5-3
Section of developing incisor, showing formation of enamel and dentin. (×640.)

27

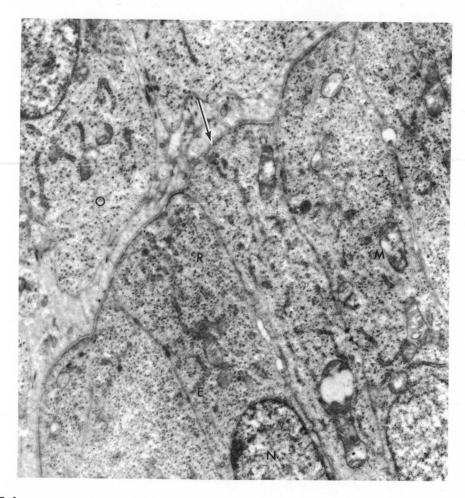

Fig. 5-4

Electron micrograph of young ameloblasts. (×8,000.) **E,** Endoplasmic reticulum; **M,** mitochondrion; **N,** nucleus of ameloblast; **O,** odontoblast; **R,** ribosomes. Arrow indicates dentinoenamel junction.

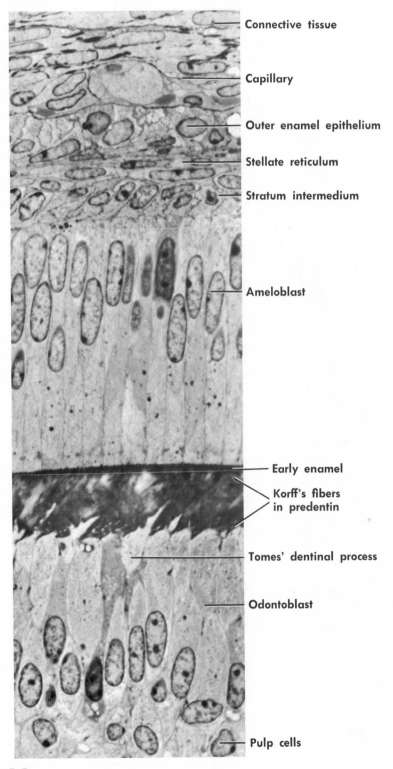

Connective tissue

Capillary

Outer enamel epithelium

Stellate reticulum

Stratum intermedium

Ameloblast

Early enamel

Korff's fibers
in predentin

Tomes' dentinal process

Odontoblast

Pulp cells

Fig. 5-5
Section of incisor of 4-day-old rat, showing all components of developing tooth. (×1,600.)

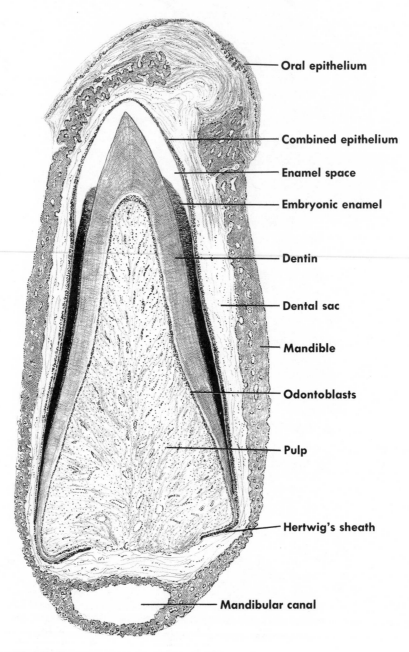

Oral epithelium

Combined epithelium

Enamel space

Embryonic enamel

Dentin

Dental sac

Mandible

Odontoblasts

Pulp

Hertwig's sheath

Mandibular canal

Fig. 5-6
Late stage of developing unerupted tooth in mandible.

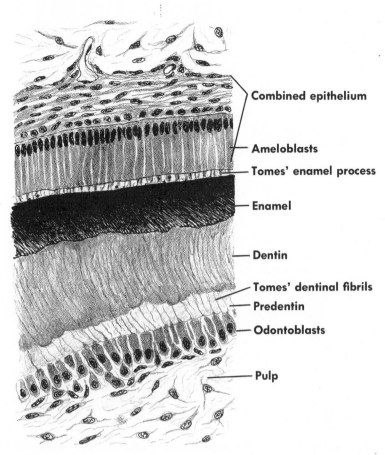

Fig. 5-7

Drawing of calcifying tooth, showing increments of dentin and enamel.

tooth a stainable residue is left. In contrast with mature enamel, on the other hand, the organic material has been almost entirely replaced by calcified matrix.

The role of the ameloblast is similar to the role of the odontoblast, but there are also some differences that have been observed. Ameloblasts are ectodermal in origin and secrete the protein matrix (keratin) upon which the mineral salts are deposited. They are in physiological contact with the constituents of the enamel organ, which contain, as does the embryonic pulp, polysaccharides of several varieties. The ameloblasts acquire alkaline phosphatase, nucleic acids, and mucopolysaccharides as they become functional. The ameloblasts are in physiological continuity with enamel during the period enamel is elaborated. When the tooth erupts, the ameloblasts are lost. From this time on enamel is physiologically a relatively inert tissue. This latter feature is in marked contrast to the vital characteristics exhibited by mature dentin.

6
MATURE DENTIN

MORPHOLOGY

Mature dentin makes up the bulk of the calcified tooth (Figs. 6-1 and 6-2). It is composed of an organic part that consists of collagenous fibers, Tomes' dentinal fibrils, a cementing substance, and polysaccharides. The inorganic part of dentin is present in the form of hydroxyapatite. Dentin is laid down in a rhythmic fashion, and one may often observe striations in dentin indicative of this process called the lines of Owen.

The outstanding morphological characteristic of dentin is the system of dentinal tubules, which extend through the matrix from the free surface of the odontoblasts to the dentinocemental or dentinoenamel junction. The dentinal tubules are not straight but are frequently S shaped. The tubules are widest at the pulpal surface (2 to 3μ) and taper to about 1μ at their termination. In the peripheral region the tubules branch dichotomously into two to four branches (Fig. 6-2). Each tubule also has many branches known as tubiculi (Fig. 6-3). These tubiculi afford an extensive system of communication between adjacent dentinal tubules.

The dentinal tubules are potential spaces that contain Tomes' dentinal process. In the living state there is no unoccupied region of the tubule except for a minute capillary space that allows for the circulation of a tissue fluid. When observed in transverse section (Figs. 6-7 and 6-8), the dentinal tubules are approximately circular in outline. The ends of the coronal tubules sometimes penetrate the enamel, carrying with them part of the dentinal matrix (Fig. 6-5). These extensions are known as enamel spindles.

Variations in the structure of dentin are quite numerous, as the following examples show. On the periphery of the root one can observe an imperfectly calcified zone of dentin, which in ground sections of the tooth has a granular appearance (Fig. 6-11). This zone is known as Tomes' granular layer. Aside from the fact that this zone appears consistently in the roots of all teeth, nothing further can be said regarding it with any degree of certainty.

In both deciduous and permanent teeth a zone of dentin is laid down adjacent to the pulp cavity that appears somewhat different from the more peripherally located dentin. This tissue is known as circumpulpal secondary dentin. It is formed during the latter part of tooth formation and is present in all mature teeth. There are several varieties of secondary dentin; the types that occur most frequently are of the regular and irregular variety.

Secondary dentin may form as a result of irritation or stimulation. One can observe in the tooth shown in Fig. 6-12 that the pulp cavity is gradually filling in directly under the abraded surface. This condition is quite common. The formation of caries or the preparation incident to placing restorative materials in the teeth may also stimulate the formation of secondary dentin, as shown in Fig. 6-13. This tissue, not to be confused with the usual circumpulpal variety, is more properly known as adventitious or reparative secondary dentin.

Some changes that are of a regressive or protective nature also produce differences in the appearance and structure of dentin. These variations result from differences in the degree of calcification. In Fig. 6-14, for example, the apical one-third of the root appears more transparent than the coronal dentin. In other parts of the tooth, as shown in Fig. 6-14, another variation, known as sclerosed dentin, is shown. In this condition the tubules are usually replaced

Text continued on p. 40.

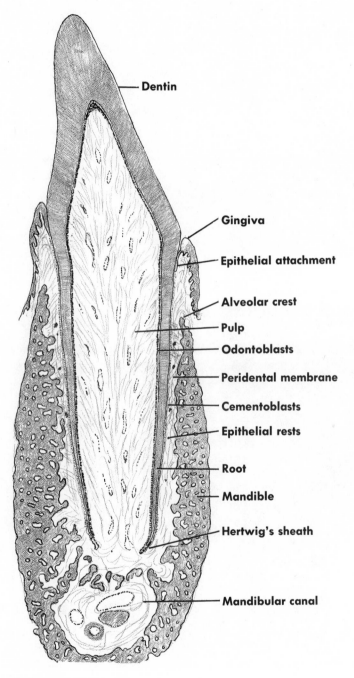

— Dentin

Gingiva

Epithelial attachment

Alveolar crest

Pulp

Odontoblasts

Peridental membrane

Cementoblasts

Epithelial rests

Root

Mandible

Hertwig's sheath

Mandibular canal

Fig. 6-1
Erupted young deciduous tooth in mandible.

33

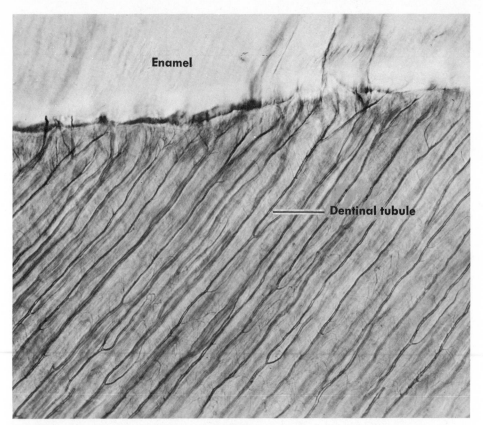

Fig. 6-2

Longitudinal ground section of dentin.

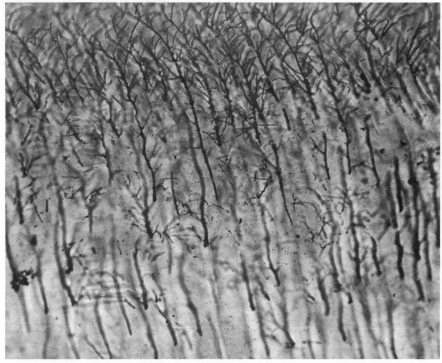

Fig. 6-3

Longitudinal section of decalcified dentin stained with silver. Note numerous tubiculi that branch from dentinal tubules.

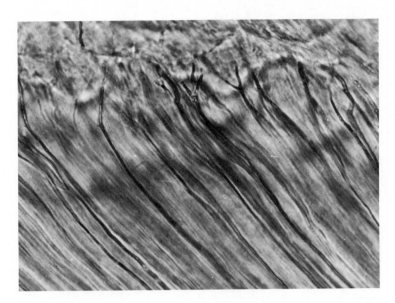

Fig. 6-4
Ground longitudinal section of dentin, showing tubules and matrix.

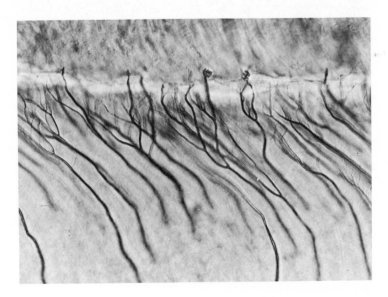

Fig. 6-5
Section of dentin, showing arrangement of tubules in region of dentinoenamel junction. Extensions of tubules into enamel are known as enamel spindles.

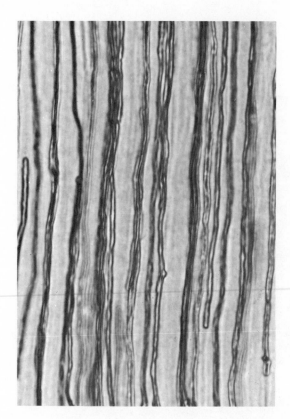

Fig. 6-6
Longitudinal ground section of dentin, showing dentinal tubules and intervening matrix.

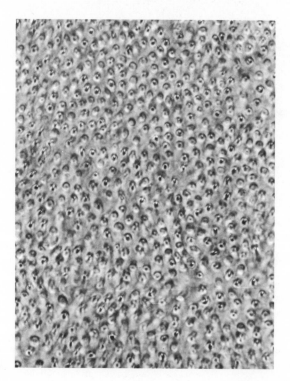

Fig. 6-7
Transverse ground section of dentin, showing tubules and matrix.

Peritubular dentin   **Matrix**   **Dentinal tubule**

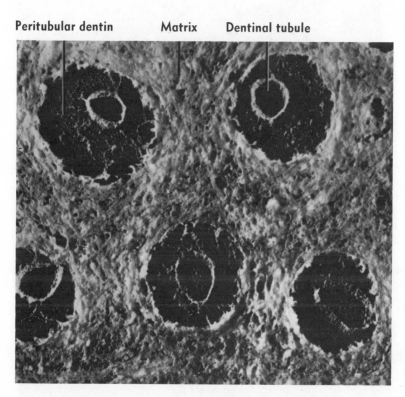

Fig. 6-8
Electron micrograph of demineralized transverse section of dentin. (×5,000.) (Courtesy Dr. David Scott, Cleveland, Ohio.)

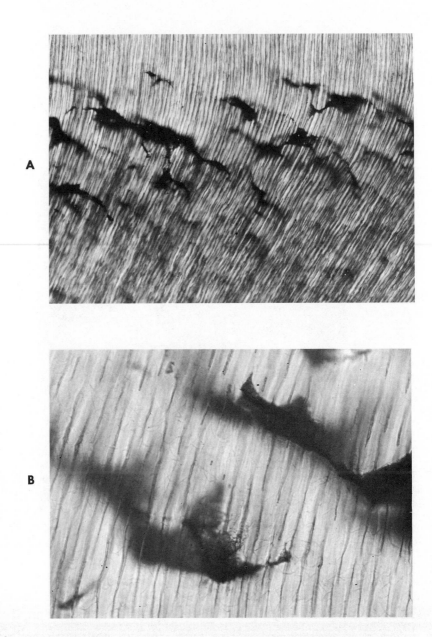

Fig. 6-9
A, Coronal dentin; dark crescentic areas are interglobular dentin. **B,** Interglobular dentin; note tubules traverse these areas.

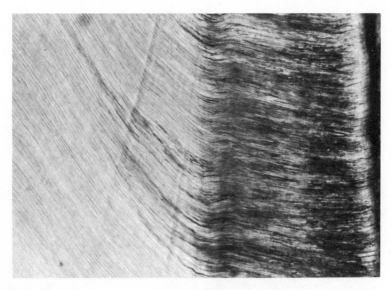

Fig. 6-10
Ground section of root dentin, showing primary (light) and secondary (dark) dentin.

Dentin   Tomes' granular layer   Cementum

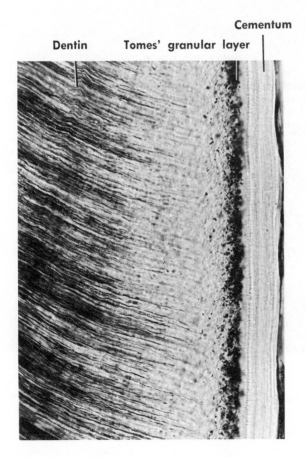

Fig. 6-11
Ground section of root of tooth,
showing Tomes' granular layer.

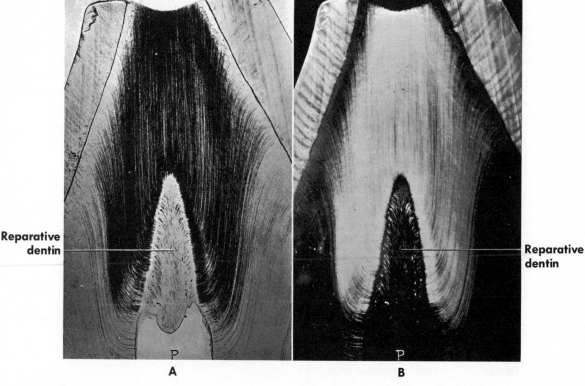

Reparative dentin

Reparative dentin

A B

Fig. 6-12

Dead tracts in dentin of vital tooth resulting from attrition and exposure of a group of dentinal tubules. Corresponding to dead tract is reparative dentin formation. **P,** Pulp. Dead tracts appear dark in transmitted light, **A,** and white in reflected light, **B.** (From Bevelander, G.: Dentin. In Sicher, H.: Orban's oral histology and embryology, ed. 6, St. Louis, 1966, The C. V. Mosby Co.)

by calcified tissue. Imbrication lines, or lines of Owen, may also be observed. They appear as bands or lines of varying width and density.

More extensive irregularities, which consist of areas completely devoid of mineral salts, are known as interglobular dentin (Fig. 6-9). Interglobular zones are especially prominent in dentin that develops under conditions such as deficiency or imperfectly balanced calcium-phosphorus levels, rickets, avitaminosis, and hypoparathyroidism or hyperparathyroidism. In short, any condition that impairs the normal mineral metabolism will be reflected in the structure of the developing dentin.

SENSITIVITY

Dentin is sensitive to various stimuli. It reacts to tactile, thermal, and chemical stimulation. Sensitivity, however, is not uniform in all teeth.

The teeth of some individuals are more sensitive than those of others. Different areas in the same tooth may also vary as to the degree of sensitivity at different times.

The mechanism by means of which a sensation is transmitted through dentin to the pulp is not clearly understood in spite of the many studies that have been made. Whatever the method may be, the presence of nerve fibers cannot be demonstrated in dentin; nerve endings, however, have been observed in the predentin.

CHEMICAL COMPOSITION

Dentin is made up of approximately 70% inorganic and 30% organic material. In comparing these ratios with those of bone, cementum, and enamel it is apparent that the chemical composition of dentin, bone, and cementum

40

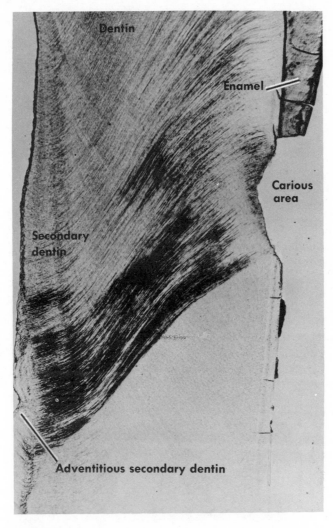

Fig. 6-13
Longitudinal section of anterior tooth.

is very similar. Enamel, however, has a much higher mineral content. The inorganic component of dentin consists chiefly of calcium triphosphate (hydroxyapatite) plus small amounts of sodium and magnesium and other calcium salts. The organic component of dentin, exclusive of Tomes' dentinal fibrils, is chiefly collagen and a ground substance.

AGE CHANGES

Certain changes in dentin relate to the age of the individual. Some of these have already been described in connection with the formation of sclerotic and secondary dentin.

Dentin may, and usually does, continue to form after the eruption of the tooth. This fact is of special importance in connection with the formation of the apex of the root, which is not fully formed until several years after eruption of the tooth.

As long as the pulp tissue remains intact, slow appositional growth may continue. As a consequence the pulp chamber may be and usually is gradually reduced in size.

VITALITY

Vitality used in connection with a tissue, cell, or organ usually refers to one or more charac-

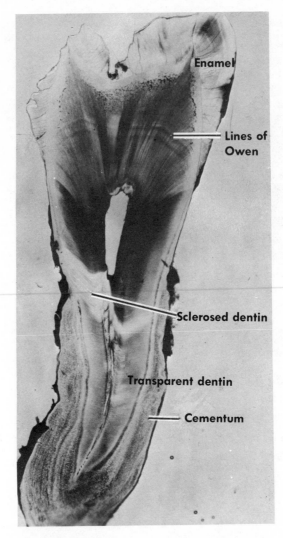

Fig. 6-14
Mesiodistal section of adult premolar.

teristics, such as respiration, anabolism, catabolism, excretion, or irritability. The intensity or degree of the vital processes that occur in living tissues varies considerably at different times or in different physiological states.

Normal dentin exhibits certain characteristics, already described. Dentin is in communication with the pulp by means of Tomes' dentinal fibrils. It undergoes changes in the relative degree of calcification, and it also exhibits the property of irritability. In addition, there is a gradual maturation of the reticular fibers, which become collagenous. From the examples cited one may assume that dentin is a vital tissue. It should be recalled, however, that dentin, like other tissues in the body, frequently undergoes regressive changes. As a result of this the vitality of the tissue may be considerably altered.

7
MATURE ENAMEL

MORPHOLOGY

The morphological unit of structure of enamel is known as the enamel rod or prism. The enamel rods are continuous structures that originate at the dentinoenamel junction and terminate at the free enamel surface. These rods measure from 0.002 to about 0.005 millimeter in diameter. Examination of ground sections of enamel under high magnification shows that the rods are frequently interrupted by numerous cross striations, as shown in Fig. 7-1. In transverse section, the human enamel rods are roughly polygonal in shape. One or more of the surfaces may be convex or concave. The highly calcified rods are separated by a minute interprismatic space, which in mature enamel is also calcified. The rod is covered by a membrane, the enamel rod sheath (Figs. 7-2 and 7-3).

Direction of the rods

The direction of the enamel rods varies in different teeth, but in general, the rods are arranged as follows: At the tip of the cusp they are arranged radially; from the tip of the cusp to the cementoenamel junction they deviate from the radial arrangement, gradually assuming more of an acute angle in reference to the dentinal tubules as the cementoenamel junction is approached. In teeth with pits or fissures the rods incline toward the base of these structures (Fig. 7-10).

Striae of Retzius

In longitudinal ground sections of enamel that are observed at low magnification one may observe a number of brown lines that represent the contour (growth) lines of the enamel. They are known as the striae of Retzius. Their origin is at the dentinoenamel junction, and they extend in an arc to the free surface of the enamel.

In transverse sections of the enamel, such as that shown in Fig. 7-5, these striae have a concentric arrangement. These structures terminate at the surface of the enamel in slight indentations of the surface that are known as perikymata (Fig. 7-4).

Lines of Schreger

The so-called lines of Schreger appear in the enamel of some teeth as the result of the wavey direction of the enamel rods. When sections of the enamel are examined under reflected light, these areas appear as alternating light and dark bands (Fig. 7-6, parazones and diazones).

Gnarled enamel

A further variation in the direction of the rods also frequently appears in sections of enamel. This consists of an intertwining of the rods, giving rise to what is known as gnarled enamel. This configuration of the rods is apparently an adaptation that increases the strength of the enamel.

Organic constituents of enamel

(1) The rods and interprismatic areas, although calcified, contain organic substance (keratin); (2) enamel is covered by a hornified cuticle; (3) in ground transverse sections of enamel one can usually observe (a) projections of the dentinal tubules, the enamel spindles (Fig. 7-7), (b) fan-shaped structures that originate at the dentinoenamel junction, known as tufts (Fig. 7-7), and (c) lamellae (Fig. 7-8), which are poorly calcified areas in the enamel and extend from the dentinoenamel junction to the surface of the enamel. These latter are easily confused with fractures.

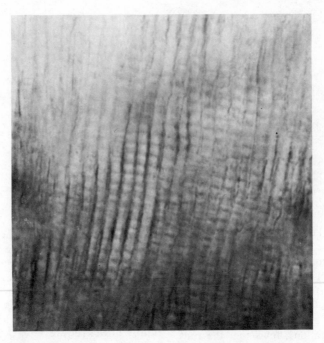

Fig. 7-1
Ground section of enamel, showing enamel rods and cross striations.

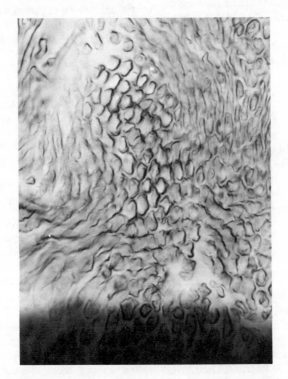

Fig. 7-2
Ground section of enamel, showing rods cut transversely.

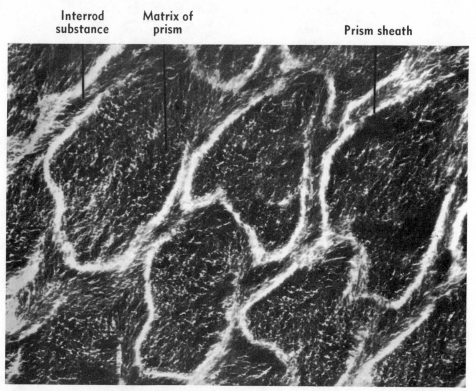

Interrod substance   Matrix of prism   Prism sheath

Fig. 7-3
Electron micrograph of cross section of demineralized enamel. (×10,000.) (Courtesy Dr. David Scott, Cleveland, Ohio.)

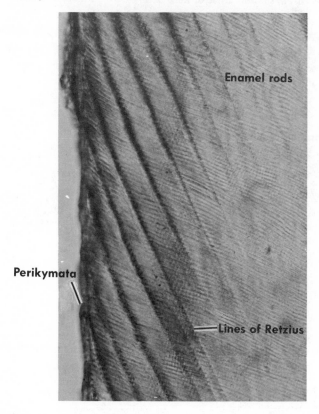

Enamel rods

Perikymata

Lines of Retzius

Fig. 7-4
Longitudinal section of periphery of enamel.

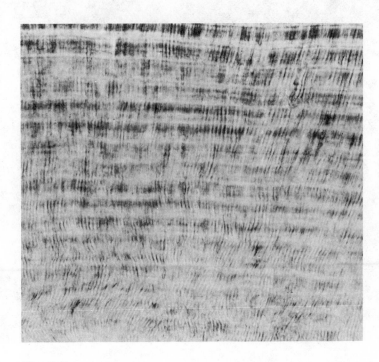

Fig. 7-5
Ground transverse section of crown, showing striae of Retzius.

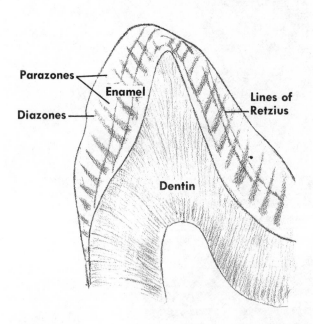

Fig. 7-6
Drawing of crown of tooth, showing lines of Schreger.

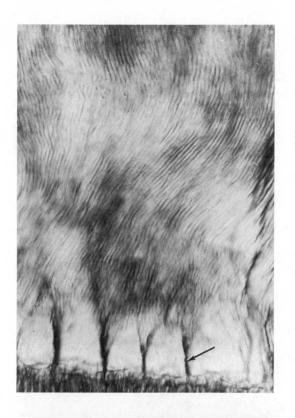

Fig. 7-7
Ground section of tooth, showing enamel tufts (arrow).

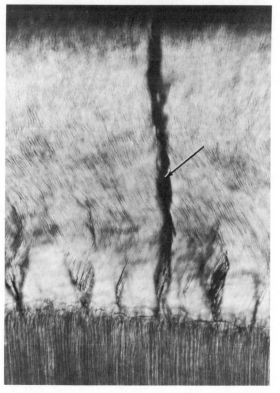

Fig. 7-8
Ground section of tooth, showing enamel lamella (arrow).

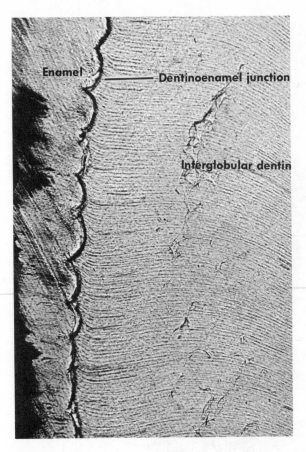

Fig. 7-9
Longitudinal section through crown of tooth.

Dentinoenamel junction

The dentinoenamel surface marks the peripheral plane of the coronal dentin. It is from this region that the enamel rods take origin. This margin, known as the dentinoenamel junction, is sometimes smooth and even (Fig. 7-9), sometimes irregular. The irregularities usually consist of a number of scallop-shaped depressions (Fig. 7-9).

Pits and fissures

The pits and fissures are narrow grooves or channels that appear as depressions in the surface of the enamel (Fig. 7-10). They represent the lines of fusion between the calcification centers of the tooth. These regions of the crown are usually the last to develop enamel, and in these areas the development is frequently arrested. This gives rise to an area in the crown in which the enamel is relatively much thinner than in other parts of the crown. This, together with other factors, makes the region of the pits and fissures a site at which enamel caries frequently occur.

Enamel hypoplasia

Hypoplastic enamel is caused by a disturbance in the process of enamel formation that occurs before the eruption of the tooth. It manifests itself in the erupted tooth in several ways, commonly as an imperfection in external form, in deficient calcification, or in the partial absence of the tissue (Fig. 7-11).

Chemical composition

Enamel is the hardest tissue in the body. In the mature tooth it is made up of approximately 98% inorganic and 2% organic material. The

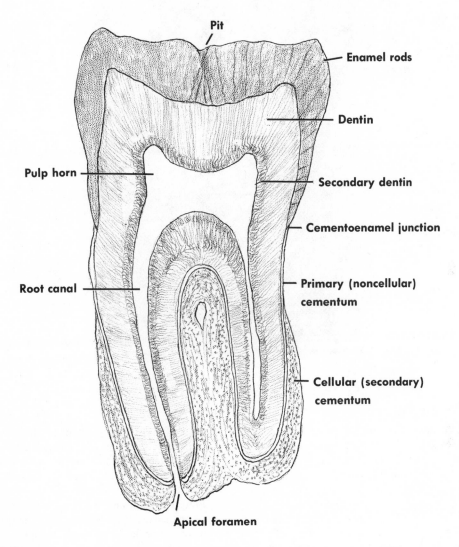

Pit

Enamel rods

Dentin

Pulp horn

Secondary dentin

Cementoenamel junction

Root canal

Primary (noncellular) cementum

Cellular (secondary) cementum

Apical foramen

Fig. 7-10
Drawing of ground section of molar to show relationship of calcified tissues. Note direction of enamel rods.

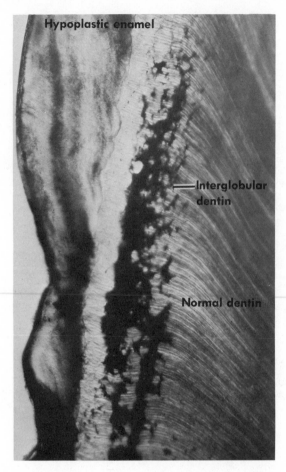

Fig. 7-11

Longitudinal section through crown of tooth, showing enamel hypoplasia.

inorganic salts of enamel are present in the form of hydroxyapatite. The main organic constituent of enamel is keratin. There is also a small amount of moisture in enamel.

Vitality

The fact that the enamel of the erupted tooth does not have any direct connection with vital tissues, such as blood vessels and nerves, has led to the assumption that this tissue is nonvital.

Recent studies that investigate the exchange of mineral components of enamel have shown that in the erupted tooth small amounts of minerals (phosphorus and sodium) may be taken up by the enamel.

Fluoride solutions may displace phosphate from the surface layers to produce an insoluble calcium fluoride. This and related problems still await further study.

8
CEMENTUM

Cementum is formed when the root is fairly well developed. The cells responsible for the elaboration of this tissue are derived from mesenchyme in the dental sac. At the appropriate time the mesenchymal cells differentiate to form relatively large round or oval cells exhibiting prominent cell processes (Figs. 8-1 and 8-2). These cells are known as cementoblasts. At the beginning of cementogenesis they occupy a position adjacent to the root surface and are arranged in a row consisting of one or more cells in thickness. The cytoplasm contains a prominent nucleus, an extensive rough endoplasmic reticulum, a prominent Golgi system, and numerous mitochondria. These cells are similar to osteoblasts, and the formation and structure of cementum is similar to bone. The cells or their processes lie in close contact to the root surface separated by a zone of ground substance. The collagen fibers making up the peridental ligament are derived from the activity of the fibroblasts in the peridental space and terminate at the surface of the root and alveolus, respectively. The cementoblasts elaborate ground substance and reticular or collagenous fibers. Mineralization occurs on and around these fibers, giving rise to mineralized cementum enclosing or anchoring the peridental fibers within the cementum (Figs. 8-3 and 8-4).

The deposition of cementum is incremental, which results in the formation of several layers, or increments. The end product of this process is one in which a thin layer of calcified tissue is deposited on and firmly attached to the entire root surface. Embedded in the cementum are the collagenous fibers of the peridental ligament. The opposite ends of these fibers are embedded in the alveolar bone and are typical Sharpey's fibers. This complement of fibers is responsible for supporting the tooth in the socket.

Histologically, cementum is divided into two types: cell-free (primary) and cellular (secondary). Primary cementum is usually distributed quite uniformly on the entire surface of the root. Secondary cementum is usually confined to the apical one-third of the root (Figs. 8-4 and 8-5).

In ground sections of the tooth, primary cementum appears as a hyaline structureless substance. Secondary cementum, which is deposited later than primary cementum, is similar in appearance to bone. In secondary cementum the cementoblasts become trapped in the calcifying tissue, and as in bone, the cells come to lie within spaces known as lacunae.

The coronal termination of cementum at the cementoenamel junction is somewhat variable. It may extend precisely to the termination of enamel, it may fail to extend to the enamel, or it may extend beyond the cervical termination of the enamel.

Certain conditions may affect the cementum or cause it to react in a somewhat unusual manner. A condition known as hypercementosis may occur. In this condition an unusually large amount of cementum is deposited upon the root of the tooth. Sometimes the amount of cementum that is laid down may be so extensive that a calcified union between the tooth and the alveolus may exist. This condition is known as ankylosis. Occasionally, small isolated islands of cementum are deposited in the peridental space. These structures are known as cementicles.

In addition to the important mechanical function performed by cementum in anchoring the fibers to the root of the tooth, there is another process in which it may take part. Frequently,

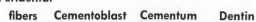

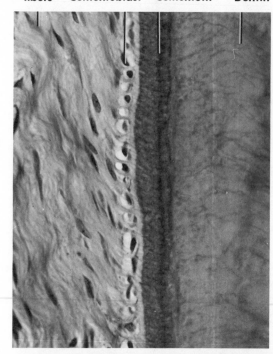

Fig. 8-1
Section of root, showing cementoblasts
and cementum.

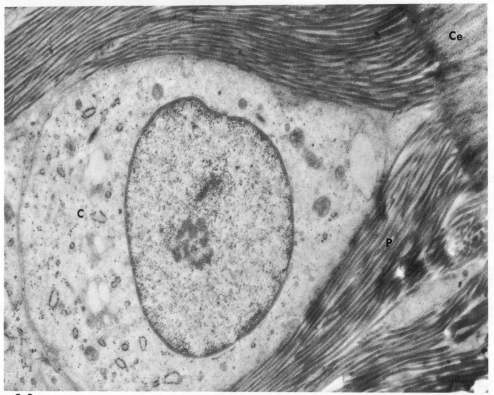

Fig. 8-2
Electron micrograph showing cementoblast, **C,** close to cementum, **Ce,** surrounded by principal fibers, **P,** that are inserted into cementum. (From Bevelander, G., and Nakahara, H.: The fine structure of the peridental ligament, Anat. Rec. **162**(3):313, 1968.)

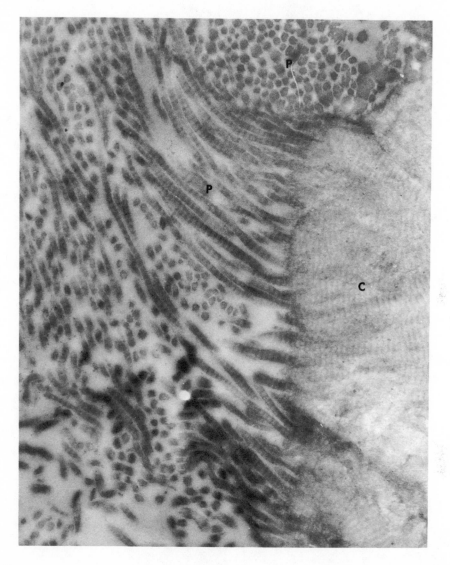

Fig. 8-3
Electron micrograph showing arrangement and insertion of principal fibers into cementum. P, Principal fibers; C, cementum. (From Bevelander, G., and Nakahara, H.: The fine structure of the peridental ligament, Anat. Rec. **162**(3):313, 1968.)

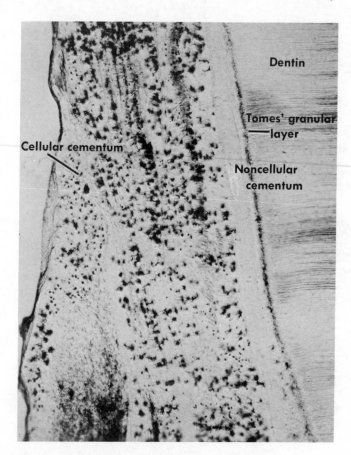

Fig. 8-4
Longitudinal section of peripheral part of root.

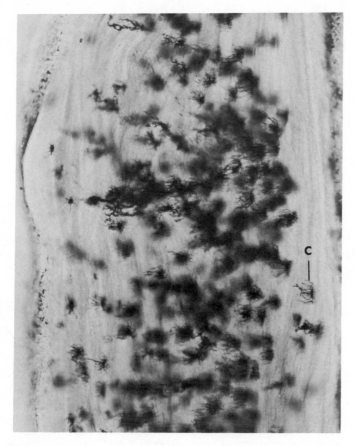

Fig. 8-5
Ground section of cementum showing several cementocytes, C.

the root undergoes resorption; that is, both cementum and dentin are destroyed. In this condition new cementum may replace the lost tissue of the root and effect a functional repair. This situation is also frequently brought about in cases in which a fracture of the root takes place.

Cementum is similar in chemical composition to bone and dentin. It contains about 70% inorganic mineral salts and approximately 30% organic matter and moisture.

9
THE PULP

As previously mentioned, the dental pulp consists essentially of connective tissue. The most numerous cell in the pulp, as is true for all connective tissues, is the fibroblast. In addition, other cells, such as macrophages and undifferentiated mesenchymal cells, are present in varying numbers at different times during the life of the pulp (Fig. 9-1). The pulp cells are located in a tissue fluid ground substance containing reticular and collagen fibers (Fig. 9-2).

Specialization of certain cells on the periphery of the pulp cavity gives rise to cylindrical cells that have already been recognized as the odontoblasts. Just below the odontoblasts one may observe a region known as the subodontoblastic zone. In the pulp of young teeth this zone is made up of a few cells that appear to be in a partially developed state. In older teeth this area is sometimes completely devoid of cells. In this latter condition this area is known as the cell-poor zone of Weil. The significance of these differences in the histological appearance of this region is not well understood.

The blood supply of the pulp enters the tooth through the apical foramen and is accompanied by an adequate lymphatic drainage. The arteries have narrow lumina and usually some smooth muscle fibers in the walls. The veins, which may be more numerous, are characterized by exceedingly thin walls and relatively wide lumina. In young teeth the vascularity of the pulp is very extensive (Fig. 9-3). In the older tooth, however, the vascular elements are gradually lost or replaced with other tissue. The vessels of the pulp in the region of the odontoblasts terminate in loops. In many instances these vessels can be observed in intimate contact with the odontoblasts.

The nerve supply of the pulp consists of both myelinated and nonmyelinated fibers. The latter accompany the vessels as they pass through the pulp (Fig. 9-4). Most myelinated fibers terminate in the region just below the odontoblasts as the subodontoblastic plexus. The terminal portions of these fibers, when studied by appropriate techniques, appear to be beaded or looped (Fig. 9-5). On the basis of their morphology these nerve endings transmit sensations of pain and touch. Some investigators have described the presence of nerve fibers within the dentinal tubules. We believe that this observation needs more confirmatory evidence before it can be accepted.

AGE CHANGES IN THE PULP

The pulp tissues are subject to a number of changes during the life of the tooth. This variation in the character of the tissue is for the most part of a regressive nature that results from certain conditions that affect the tooth in particular or from certain systemic conditions. The changes in the pulp tissues just referred to are of two general types: (1) a change in the histological make-up of the tissue or (2) a change in the relative amount of the tissue.

Changes in the composition of the pulp tissue

In the embryonic pulp and in the pulp of young teeth the basic connective tissue elements have the arrangement and composition typical for young vital connective tissue, with more cells and less fibers per unit area than occur later in the life of the tooth. In the normal intact tooth with advance in age there is a gradual tendency toward a reduction in the number of cells, especially fibroblasts, and an increase in the number

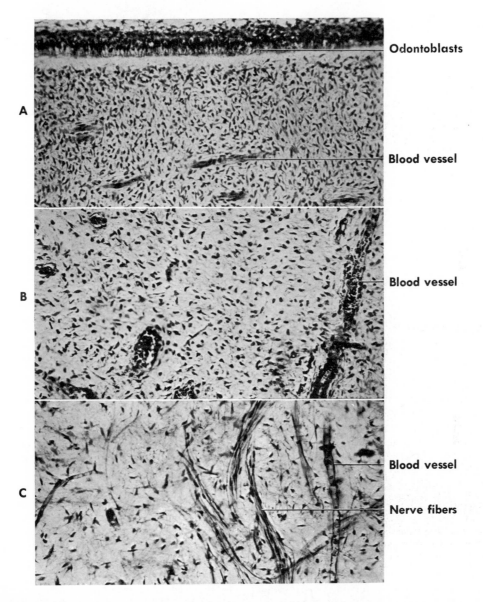

Odontoblasts

Blood vessel

Blood vessel

Blood vessel

Nerve fibers

Fig. 9-1

Age changes of dental pulp. Cellular elements decrease and fibrous intercellular substance increases with advancing age. **A,** Newborn infant. **B,** Nine-month-old infant. **C,** Adult. (From Sicher, H.: Orban's oral histology and embryology, ed. 6, St. Louis, 1966, The C. V. Mosby Co.)

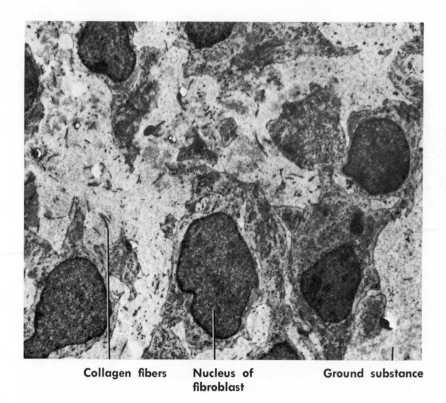

| Collagen fibers | Nucleus of fibroblast | Ground substance |

Fig. 9-2
Electron micrograph of young pulp.

of connective tissue fibers. In addition, changes in the vitality of the cells occur, and various retrogressive or atrophic changes occur in the pulp, such as fatty and hyaline degeneration, reticular atrophy, etc. Other less obvious differences in older pulps also have been observed: These consist of a diminution or loss of enzyme activity and a change in the chemical composition of the ground substance.

The aforementioned changes in the pulp can and do occur in teeth without showing any unfavorable clinical symptoms. It is, however, important to recognize that retrogressive changes in the pulp do occur and, when present, reduce the vitality or resilience of this tissue—a factor of great importance in any projected clinical treatment of the tooth.

Changes in the relative amount of tissue

It will be recalled that one of the important functions of the pulp tissue during early life is elaboration of dentin. This function is retained during the life of the tooth. Dentin formation

is particularly important in the several instances in which secondary dentin is elaborated under areas of attrition, caries, and cavity preparations.

Other kinds of calcification also occur in the pulp. In the pulp horns, concretions arise. In some instances they lie free in the pulp, in others they are attached to and become embedded in dentin. They are known as denticles of the free or attached variety, respectively (Fig. 9-6). In the root canal, calcification also occurs, in this instance a diffuse type consisting of numerous small concretions. Calcification of the type described occurs in a large percentage of all adult teeth. This type of calcification indicates a retrogressive change and is usually accompanied by other retrogressive changes (for example, fibrosis).

Other important facts to recognize concerning the pulp are the following: The pulp tissue is more extensive in the young tooth than in the tooth of the mature individual. The thickness of dentin in the coronal part of the de-

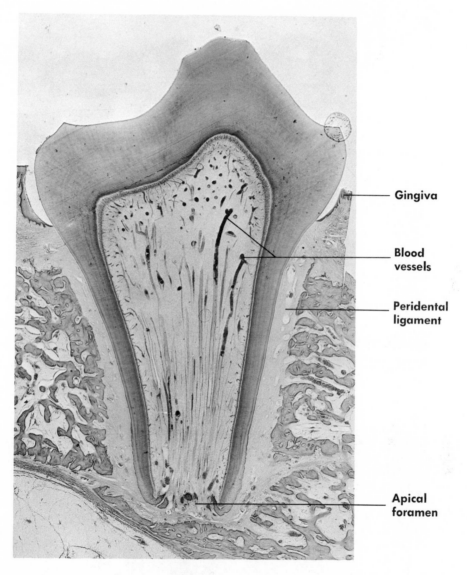

Gingiva

Blood
vessels

Peridental
ligament

Apical
foramen

Fig. 9-3
Longitudinal section of young tooth showing pattern of distribution of blood vessels in pulp. (From Bevelander, G.: Atlas of oral histology and embryology, Philadelphia, 1967, Lea and Febiger.)

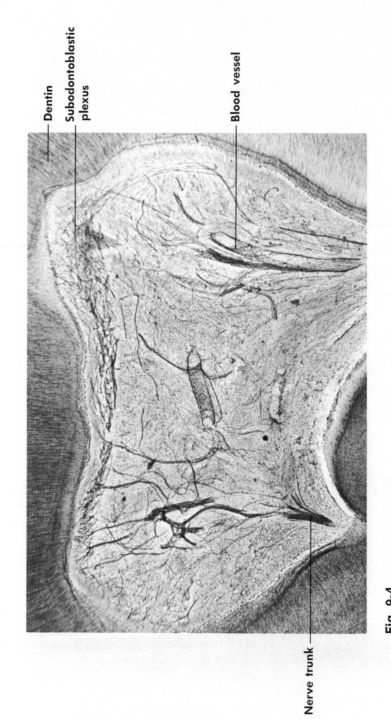

Fig. 9-4
Distribution of nerves in the pulp. (Courtesy Dr. Sol Bernick, Los Angeles, Calif.)

Dentin

Subodontoblastic
plexus

Blood vessel

Nerve trunk

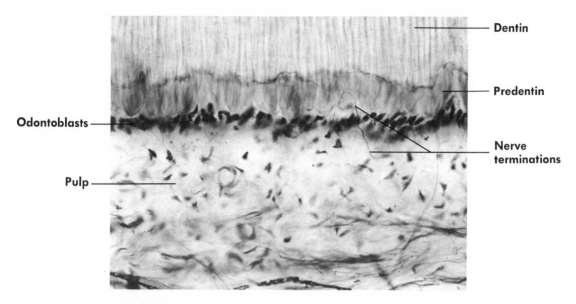

Dentin

Predentin

Odontoblasts

Nerve
terminations

Pulp

Fig. 9-5
Section of periphery of pulp and inner margin of dentin showing nerve terminations. (Courtesy Dr. Sol Bernick, Los Angeles, Calif.)

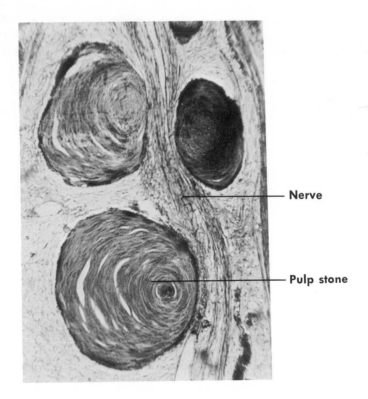

Nerve

Pulp stone

Fig. 9-6
Portion of pulp showing pulp stones. (From Bevelander, G.: Atlas of oral histology and embryology, Philadelphia, 1967, Lea and Febiger.)

ciduous or young permanent tooth is less than in the tooth of the mature individual.

The topography of the pulp is extremely variable. The extent of the pulp horns and especially the high degree of variability in the number and position of root canals and accessory root canals cannot be ascertained with any degree of accuracy except by nonclinical methods such as the corrosion or sectioning techniques.

The dental pulp, as previously described, is derived from mesenchyme and in the mature tooth consists essentially of a mass of connective tissue permeated by vascular elements and nerve fibers. Topographically, the pulp is divided into two areas: (1) the pulp horn or horns occupying the region roughly corresponding to the cusp and (2) the narrow, slender portion occupying the space usually referred to as the root canal (Fig. 10-1). The entire space occupied by the pulp is referred to as the pulp chamber.

10

THE PERIDENTAL LIGAMENT

The *peridental ligament* is a term used to designate several groups of fibers that are responsible for maintaining the tooth in a relatively fixed position in the socket and also for supporting and helping to maintain normal relations of the gingiva (Fig. 10-1). The part of the ligament attached to the alveolus is derived from the dental sac. Before eruption the fibers in the root region are arranged parallel to the long axis of the tooth. During or shortly before eruption the fibers are inserted into the cementum and alveolus, and as the tooth erupts several groups of fibers gradually assume the arrangement observed in the fully erupted or mature tooth.

In the erupted tooth the fibers that make up the ligament are located in various loci and have an arrangement that differs in various parts of the gingiva and root. They are collectively known as the *principal* fibers and consist of stout collagen bundles.

The gingival fibers arise at the cemento-enamel junction and splay out to the various parts of the gingiva, terminating in the lamina propria. A relatively small number of *circular* fibers interlace with the gingival fibers. The *transseptal* group connects the cervical portions of adjacent teeth. The fibers run from the cementum of one tooth, over the alveolar crest to the cementum of an adjacent tooth. They are observed most clearly in mesiodistal sections of teeth. The remainder of the groups of fibers are attached to the cementum and alveolus. The *alveolar crest* fibers (Fig. 10-2) originate in the cervical cementum. Some of these fibers are attached to the alveolar crest, others continue to the alveolar mucosa. The *horizontal fibers* occupy an apical position in reference to the alveolar crest and as their name implies are arranged in an approximately horizontal

position in reference to the surface of the root and the alveolus (Figs. 10-3 and 10-4). The *oblique* fibers (Fig. 10-5), located apically to the horizontal group, comprise the most extensive group of fibers. The *apical* group is located in the region of the apex. They are considered to be radially arranged. There is, however, a great deal of irregularity in the disposition of these fibers. The *interradicular* group, present in multirooted teeth, extends from the surface of the root to the surface of the bone in the region of furcation.

The gingival fibers are primarily concerned with maintaining the gingival tissues in their normal functional relation to the surface of the surface of the tooth and in so doing provide an effective seal between the oral cavity and the peridental space. The transseptal fibers tie the teeth together. This "splint" effect prevents undue mesial and distal excursions of the teeth. The alveolar crest fibers prevent tilting of the cervical part of the tooth and also anchorage of the alveolar mucosa. The horizontal fibers are also arranged to prevent excessive tilting, whereas the oblique fibers are arranged to take up vertical forces. The apical fibers are so arranged to prevent excessive excursion of the root.

The alveolar fibers are embedded in the cementum of the root and the inner surface of the alveolus. They consist of bundles of collagen fibers. These bundles are so arranged that there is a "slackness" which tends to prevent their disruption during mastication and also allows for a slight physiological movement of the teeth.

The stresses to which the teeth are subjected during normal use consist of a composite of forces exerted from several directions. The arrangement of the several groups of alveolar fibers function as a unit in transmitting these

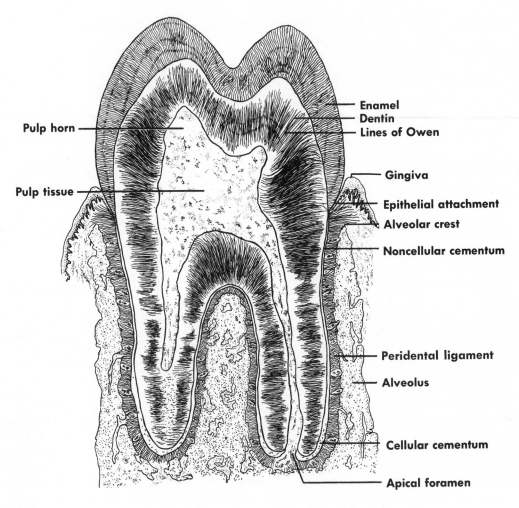

Fig. 10-1
Section of human maxillary molar cut buccolingually to show general relationships of tooth and surrounding tissues.

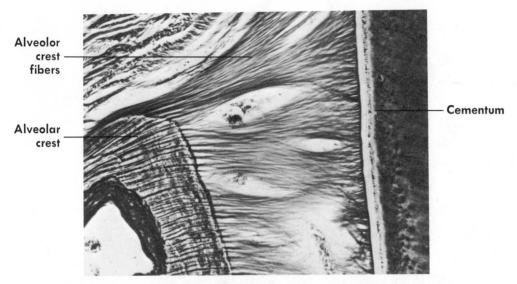

Alveolor crest fibers

Alveolar crest

Cementum

Fig. 10-2
Alveolar crest and alveolar crest fibers. (Courtesy Prof. M. Catloni, Houston, Tex.)

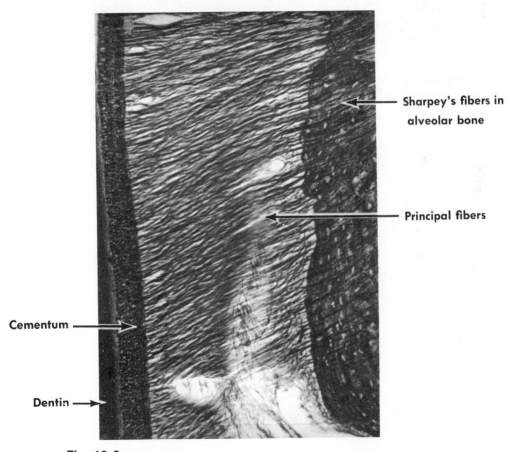

Sharpey's fibers in alveolar bone

Principal fibers

Cementum

Dentin

Fig. 10-3
Illustration showing structure and some of the relationships of peridental ligament.

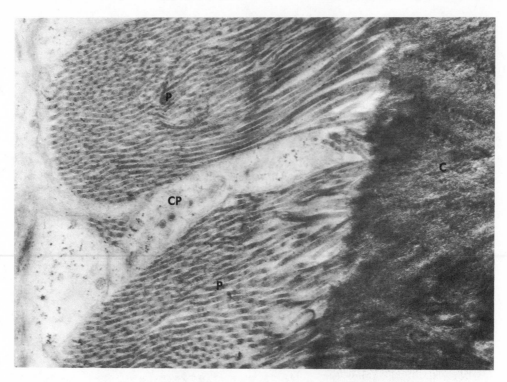

Fig. 10-4
Electron micrograph of portion of peridental space and cementum. **C,** Cementum; **CP,** cementoblast process; **P,** principal fibers. (From Bevelander, G., and Nakahara, H.: The fine structure of the peridental ligament, Anat. Rec. **162**(3):313, 1968.)

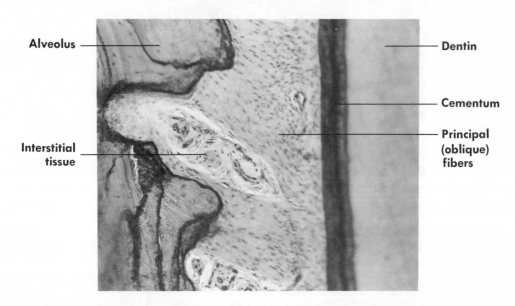

Fig. 10-5
Alveolus and peridental ligament. (From Bevelander, G.: Atlas of oral histology and embryology, Philadelphia, 1967, Lea and Febiger.)

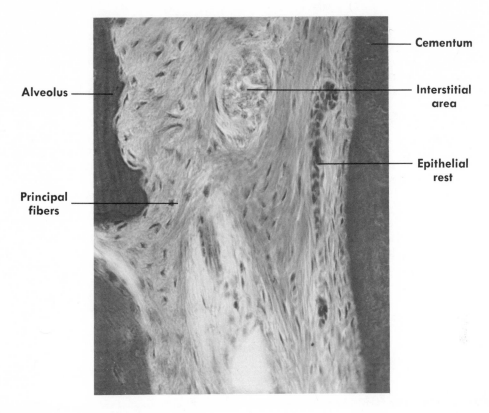

Alveolus

Principal
fibers

Cementum

Interstitial
area

Epithelial
rest

Fig. 10-6
Peridental ligament. (From Bevelander, G.: Atlas of oral histology and embryology, Philadelphia, 1967, Lea and Febiger.)

forces to the various parts of the alveolus. The resulting vector is transmitted to the alveolus as a pull on the bone. This is a fortunate arrangement since this type of force is conducive to the maintenance and growth of bone, whereas the opposite (pressure) effect is conducive to bone resorption.

INTERSTITIAL TISSUE

The *interstitial tissue* consists of islands of loosely arranged connective tissue located between bundles of principal fibers (Fig. 10-5). Within this loose connective tissue are nerves, blood vessels, lymphatics, fibroblasts, histiocytes, and undifferentiated mesenchyme cells.

CELLS IN THE PERIDENTAL SPACE

In addition to fibroblasts, the most numerous cell in the area, the following may also be observed. Osteoblasts occur on the alveolar surface. On the root surface cementoblasts appear as a single or multilayered row of cells. During root resorption osteoclast-like cells are also

present. During the development of the tooth, remnants of enamel epithelium are apparently trapped in the peridental space. These remnants may be observed as rows or nests of cells known as epithelial rests (of Malassez) (Fig. 10-6). They have the potential to give rise to cysts. Another structure, a noncellular calcified concretion known as a cementicle, is also of frequent occurrence

FUNCTIONAL ADAPTATIONS AND RETROGRESSIVE CHANGES

The tooth is subjected to normal stresses during the masticating process, and it has already been pointed out how the structure and arrangement of the supporting apparatus copes with this problem. Following attrition of the cusps the teeth reposition themselves to some degree because of a process known as mesial drift. During this process there is repositioning or rearrangement of the principal fibers. Repositioning of the teeth is frequently brought about by orthodontic treatment. This is possible because of a number of changes that occur when the tooth is subjected to sustained pressure. Two important changes that are involved in this process are alveolar growth of the surface of the alveolus on the area from which pressure is exerted and a resorption on the surface subjected to pressure. A rearrangement and reinsertion of peridental fibers also accompanies this process. Less radical and spectacular changes similar to those just described occur during any slight repositioning of the tooth.

Retrogressive changes result in partial or complete loss of function. Briefly, one of the chief etiological factors resulting in loss of function is the absence of an antagonist. Vitamin deficiencies, such as lack of vitamin C, are known to result in connective tissue disorders in the peridental ligament as well as in other parts of the body. Other nutritional deficiencies may also result in retrogressive changes in the ligament. In connection with epithelial down growth, often associated with gingival recession, loss of fiber attachment occurs on the region of the root covered by the epithelium. The retrogressive changes mentioned may be observed histologically as a decrease in the peridontal space, loss of fiber attachment, decrease in number of fibers and cells, and other atrophic changes. Another important cause of retrogressive changes is neglect or improper mouth hygiene, which usually results in accumulation of calculus, inflammation of the gingiva, and eventually loss of attachment fibers of the ligament.

11

THE ALVEOLUS

Until this juncture our remarks have been confined to the development and structure of the tooth only. The reader is by this time undoubtedly aware that without the presence and function of a group of structures that immediately surround the cervical part of the crown and the root serving to retain the teeth firmly in their anatomical relationship, the teeth would be nonfunctional or lost. Although these structures are intimately related and often blend one with the other, it is useful for the purpose of description to separate them into the *gingiva,* the *peridental membrane,* and the *alveolar processes.*

The alveolar process as such develops in connection with the growth of the jaw and the eruption of the teeth. The alveolar processes are not actually separate entities but are the parts of the maxilla and mandible that are especially designed to accommodate and support the teeth in the socket. In an attempt to understand the gross relationships of the teeth and the mandible and maxilla in which they are located, it will be helpful to recall the structure of these bones. This is best performed by referring to a section of the bones. Examination of a transverse section of the mandible, for example, reveals a simple basic arrangement: an outer and inner plate of compact bone separated internally by a varying amount of cancellous bone. Anteriorly, the labial surface of both jaws is very thin and is composed entirely of compact bone. Posteriorly, this situation varies because of the peculiarities of the configuration of the maxilla and mandible, respectively.

If one now visualizes the sectional view of the mandible and recalls the basic arrangement of the bone, a peripheral compact layer and internal loose or cancellous mass, the following description will help in understanding the relationship the erupted tooth bears to this bone.

If one were to conceive, for *illustrative purposes only,* that the mandible as just described consisted of an elastic-like substance and if one were to take a tooth and insert it into the mandible in its proper anatomical position from the occlusal surface rootward, one might then observe the following: (1) A space would have been created to accommodate the tooth; this would be the socket. (2) Since the periphery of the bone is compact, the insertion of the tooth into the bone would result in pushing this layer of compact bone rootward. This dense layer would then surround the root. This corresponds to the alveolus proper, or *lamina dura.*

The end result of this imaginary process is one that would duplicate the relationship of the tooth, socket, and supporting bone that actually does exist, namely, a tooth in a socket surrounded in the root region by a relatively thin plate of dense bone, the alveolus proper, which in turn is buttressed by radiating trabeculae that terminate in the cortical plate of the mandible (Fig. 11-1).

Histologically the alveolus is made up of compact bone (Fig. 11-2). The surface adjacent to the root is sometimes referred to as bundle bone. It is characterized by lamellae, which are arranged parallel to the long axis of the tooth. The peripheral portion of the alveolus is made up of the usual compact bone arranged in haversian systems.

In some of the areas of the jaw the lamina dura is interrupted by the passage of blood vessels, which give rise to a perforated structure. In this situation the name *cribriform plate* is used to designate this structure.

Between the lamina dura and the external plates of the jaw itself there is a system of

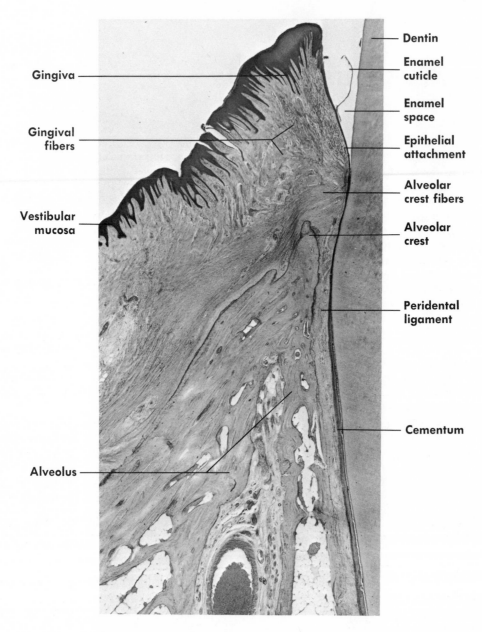

Gingiva

Gingival
fibers

Vestibular
mucosa

Alveolus

Dentin

Enamel
cuticle

Enamel
space

Epithelial
attachment

Alveolar
crest fibers

Alveolar
crest

Peridental
ligament

Cementum

Fig. 11-1
Section showing supporting structures of tooth. (×22.5.)

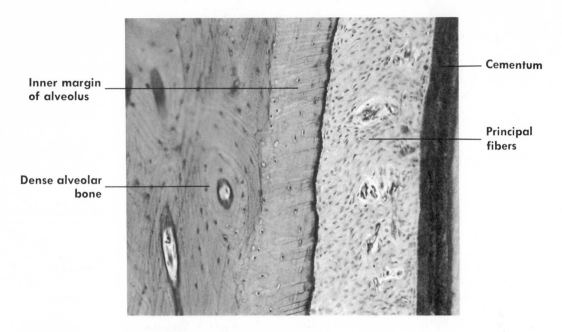

Inner margin
of alveolus

Dense alveolar
bone

Cementum

Principal
fibers

Fig. 11-2
Alveolus and peridental ligament. (From Bevelander, G.: Atlas of oral histology and embryology, Philadelphia, 1967, Lea and Febiger.)

trabeculae of membrane or cancellous bone that is known as the supporting bone. The trabeculae of the supporting bone are arranged so that they are well adapted to take up the mechanical stresses that are transmitted to them by the peridental membrane and the tooth. Between the sockets and the root the trabeculae are arranged, in general, in a horizontal position; at the fundus of the alveoli the trabeculae are arranged in a more nearly vertical direction.

In sectional view the alveolus usually appears tapered at the region of the cementoenamel junction, where it terminates. This is known as the *alveolar crest.*

The alveolus proper is fairly constant throughout the life of the tooth. Various conditions, such as a change in pressure, the presence or absence of an antagonist, or the removal of the tooth from the socket, have an effect upon the amount and character of the supporting bony tissue. In general, the supporting bone responds to the functional conditions to which it is subjected; increase in the load that this tissue must bear results in the addition of supporting trabeculae, and decrease or loss in function is accompanied by a corresponding decrease in the supporting tissue.

It should be apparent from the preceding discussion that bone is a relatively labile tissue. It has the ability to increase when subjected to increased functional demands and to rearrange itself when the direction of stress placed upon it is modified, and a lack of function causes a resorption of this tissue. These changes result from the ability that bone possesses to react to various physiological stimuli. In addition to the foregoing a loss of bone, especially in the region of the alveolar crest, often occurs. This bone loss is known as *alveoloclasia.* The bone loss is accompanied by loss of peridental fibers, which in turn results in loss of tooth support in this area.

12
THE GINGIVA

The gingiva may be defined as the modified portion of the oral epithelium that encloses the cervical part of the tooth and is continuous with the mucosa covering the alveolus. Grossly the gingiva consists of a band of tissue exhibiting a scalloped appearance at the apical or free surface and extends for some distance in a coronal direction between the teeth, giving rise to the interdental papillae. The gingiva normally appears pink in color, whereas the alveolar mucosa arising at the mucogingival junction is a deeper red because of the presence of numerous small blood vessels occurring near the surface.

For purposes of description the gingiva may be divided into the following parts (see Fig. 12-1): The gingiva tapers at the most coronal aspect, and this portion is known as the *gingival crest.* The gingiva is covered with epithelium on its outer surface, and the basal layers are thrown into deep folds or pegs. The inner (tooth) surface of the gingiva is also covered by epithelium, which extends from the gingival crest to the cementoenamel junction. The apical part of the inner epithelium is similar to the surface epithelium, namely, a thick stratified epithelium exhibiting extensive pegs. This part of the inner epithelium forms part of the outer boundary of the space known as the *gingival sulcus.* The inner boundary of the sulcus is the surface of the tooth; the base is the site at which the epithelium is attached to the enamel. The remainder (the rootward part) of the inner epithelium, known as the *epithelial attachment,* is derived from the stratum intermedium.

Returning again to the outer surface of the gingiva one frequently (but not invariably) observes a prominent indentation of the surface known as the *gingival groove.* This groove, when present, appears at the level of the base of the sulcus. The part of the gingiva located coronally in reference to the groove or more accurately to the base of the sulcus is known as the *free gingiva,* so called because it is not attached to the tooth. Continuing rootward from the level of the base of the gingival sulcus the remainder of the gingiva is known as the *attached gingiva,* since it is attached to the surface of the enamel. The epithelium of the alveolar region changes in character at the mucogingival junction, becoming thinner, and no longer exhibits epithelial pegs.

HISTOLOGICAL FEATURES

The gingiva are covered with a rather thick stratified squamous epithelium, the base of which is thrown into deep folds, the *epithelial pegs* (Figs. 12-2 and 12-3). The surface layers of the epithelium may vary from a state in which it is nonkeratinized to one in which it is extremely well keratinized (Fig. 12-4). The base of the epithelium rests upon a well-defined lamina propria made up of dense bundles of collagen fibers. The basal cells may contain pigment (melanin). A submucosa is lacking. The remainder of the gingival tissue consists of bundles of connective tissue fibers (the gingival fibers) extending to the lamina propria, embedded in a tissue fluid ground substance. Also present are nerve fibers terminating in the epithelia as one of several kinds of sensory receptors and an adequate vascular and lymph supply. As in connective tissue found elsewhere in the body, cells usually associated with connective tissue, such as fibroblasts, macrophages, and white blood cells, are also present. On the surface of the free gingiva one may also observe in many instances a stippled appearance as well as minute folds apical to the interdental papillae.

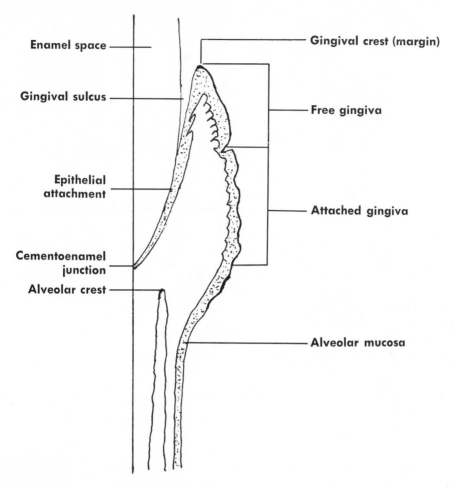

Fig. 12-1
A diagram illustrating structure of the gingiva.

FORMATION OF THE GINGIVA AND EPITHELIAL ATTACHMENT

When enamel is being formed, the four layers making up the enamel organ are compressed into a single layer—the *reduced enamel epithelium*—applied to the surface of the enamel. As the crown approaches the oral epithelium a perforation occurs, leaving a space through which the tooth protrudes. When the tip of the crown enters the oral cavity, it is covered by a horny pellicle, the *enamel cuticle;* all the components formerly applied to the crown are lost when the tooth enters the oral cavity. The events just described may be considered as the first step in the eruption of the tooth that is associated with the formation of the gingiva.

The second important step takes place as follows: It will be recalled that until this juncture only a small part of the crown has emerged into the oral cavity. If attention is now directed to part of the oral epithelium in contact with the emerging tooth, we observe that additional events have occurred, namely, (1) the proliferation of the stratum intermedium and (2) the union of this layer with the oral epithelium (the future gingiva) (Fig. 12-5). As the tooth continues to erupt the oral epithelium surrounding the surface of the tooth proliferates, accumulates several connective tissue bundles (the gingival fibers), adapts itself, and is firmly attached to the surface of the tooth by means of the gingival fibers and the epithelial attachment.

73

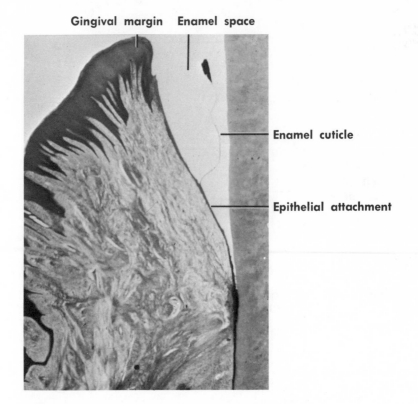

Gingival margin **Enamel space**

Enamel cuticle

Epithelial attachment

Fig. 12-2
Mesiodistal section of gingiva.

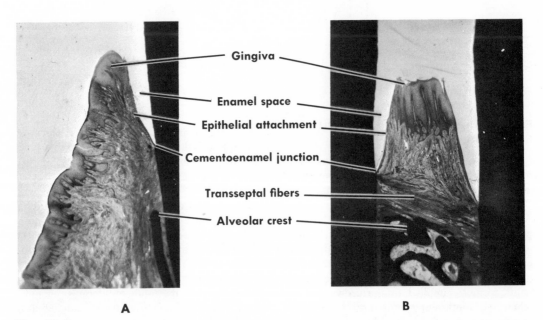

Gingiva

Enamel space

Epithelial attachment

Cementoenamel junction

Transseptal fibers

Alveolar crest

A

B

Fig. 12-3
Mesiodistal section of gingiva. A, Labiolingual section of gingiva. B, Mesiodistal section of gingiva (dental papilla).

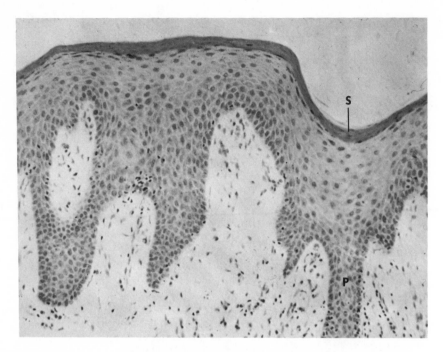

Fig. 12-4
Gingival mucosa showing surface layer, **S,** slightly keratinized; subjacent cells are thrown into pegs, **P.**

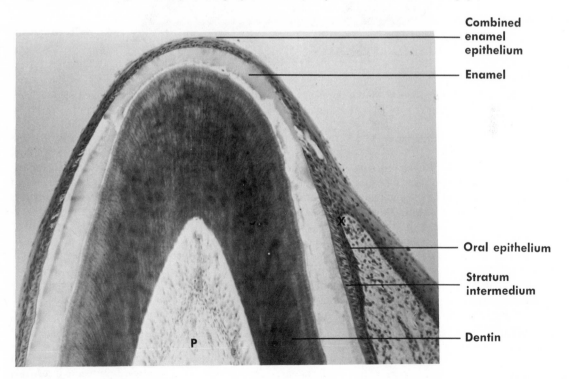

Fig. 12-5
Crown of tooth just prior to eruption, showing union of stratum intermedium with oral epithelium, **X. P,** pulp.
(From Bevelander, G.: Atlas of oral histology and embryology, Philadelphia, 1967, Lea and Febiger.)

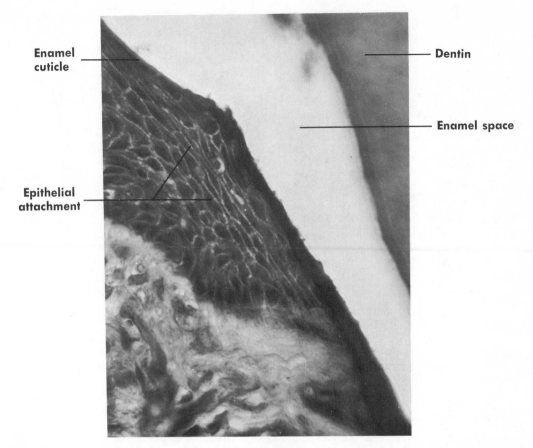

Enamel cuticle

Epithelial attachment

Dentin

Enamel space

Fig. 12-6

Detail of epithelial attachment. (From Bevelander, G.: Atlas of oral histology and embryology, Philadelphia, 1967, Lea and Febiger.)

The relation of this latter structure will be described.

The epithelial attachment (Fig. 12-6) is derived from the stratum intermedium. It originates at the level of the gingival sulcus, consists of from 10 to 15 cells in thickness, and tapers to one or two cells at its termination at the cementoenamel junction. This epithelium has several of the characteristics of stratified epithelia found elsewhere. The basal layer is cuboidal and rests upon an indistinct basal lamina. The more superficial cells are polygonal, while those near the surface of the tooth are squamous.

For many years the manner of gingival attachment has been confusing and the subject of many controversies. Several recent studies conducted at the electron microscope level have shown conclusively that the surface layer of the epithelial attachment is intimately attached to the surface of the tooth by means of hemidesmosomes located on the surface of those cells in contact with the tooth. Intervening between the cells and the enamel is often a layer or several layers of cuticle. Also of interest is the observation that mitotic activity and replacement occur in the cells of this epithelium, a fact which would lead one to expect that reattachment could occur following detachment. This is true in part; however, the favorable physiological environment needed for successful reattachment is not known and even if known would probably be difficult to achieve.

RETROGRESSIVE CHANGES

One of the most common modifications of the gingiva is a rootward movement of this structure known as gingival recession. This is accompanied by a downgrowth of the epithelial attachment. Recession occurs in varying degrees. It may progress to such a degree that the gingival crest occupies a position at or below the level of the cementoenamel junction. In this latter situation the cervical part of the tooth would be left unprotected. The presence of calculi, calcified masses located on the inner surface and encroaching on the gingiva proper, if not removed results in inflammation and atrophy of the gingiva.

In some instances there are several factors leading to retrogressive changes that result in the inflammation and loss of attachment which give rise to a so-called pocket. Whatever the etiological cause of retrogressive change may be, all tend to disrupt the normal anatomical relations and histological structure, giving rise to loss in normal function of the gingiva and attachment of the tooth.

13

ERUPTION AND SHEDDING

ERUPTION

The eruption of teeth is basically the result of growth, during which the crown and root are formed. This growth produces a tooth that begins to differentiate within the confines of the embryonic jaw. It results in a much elongated structure that, on completion of the crown, approximates the oral mucosa. In other words, growth results not only in the enlargement and elongation of the tooth but also in the tooth being positioned in the oral cavity. Hence, eruption, which may be considered as a final step in the growth of the tooth, consists of the extrusion of the crown into the oral cavity. Since the crown is virtually complete just prior to eruption, the process results then in the *occlusal movement* of the tooth (active eruption).

Several events precede or accompany eruption, and a review of these will help clarify this process. It will be recalled that in the enamel organ stage of tooth development the growing tooth is enclosed within a fibrous dental sac, which in turn lies enclosed within a bony crypt. Differentiation and growth result in the production of the mature tooth. Fibers derived from the dental sac become positioned in the root of the tooth and in the remodeling of bone that in this stage is known as the alveolus. During the occlusal growth and movement of the tooth considerable reorganization and repositioning of these two structures occur.

Important changes also occur in the tissues associated with the crown and oral mucosae. Just prior to eruption the crown is invested with the combined enamel epithelium. When the crown approaches and pierces the oral epithelium, a union of the oral epithelium and stratum intermedium occurs. The portion made up of the oral mucosa is modified to form the gingiva. The stratum intermedium on the cervical part of the crown is retained and is known as the epithelial attachment (Fig. 13-1).

When the tooth is erupting, the peridental fibers are not definitely oriented or firmly attached. This occurs later when the tooth comes into occlusion.

It will also be recalled that there are ten deciduous teeth and sixteen permanent teeth in each jaw. During early childhood the individual exhibits at first an incomplete and then a complete deciduous dentition. At 5 or 6 years of age loss of the deciduous anterior teeth begins to occur, and then the child has a mixed dentition. After loss of the deciduous teeth the permanent teeth erupt.

The permanent tooth germs in some instances give rise to succedaneous teeth; that is, they replace the deciduous dentition (Fig. 13-2). In those areas in which this does not occur the permanent tooth germs arise independently. The succedaneous tooth germs arise and develop very close to the root of the deciduous teeth.

At appropriate times, usually when the corresponding permanent tooth crown has fully developed, the root of the deciduous tooth undergoes almost complete resorption by osteoclastic activity. This process results in a loss of attachment, and the tooth is exfoliated (Fig. 13-3).

The eruption of the permanent teeth presents some problems not encountered by the eruption of the deciduous teeth. This results primarily from the fact that they develop in the jaw during the time the deciduous teeth are in their normal position and are not situated so that axial move-

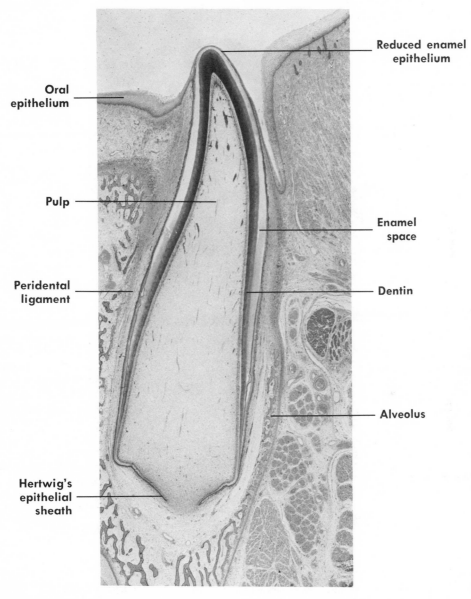

Oral epithelium

Pulp

Peridental ligament

Hertwig's epithelial sheath

Reduced enamel epithelium

Enamel space

Dentin

Alveolus

Fig. 13-1
Section of anterior tooth in stage of development just prior to eruption. (From Bevelander, G.: Atlas of oral histology and embryology, Philadelphia, 1967, Lea and Febiger.)

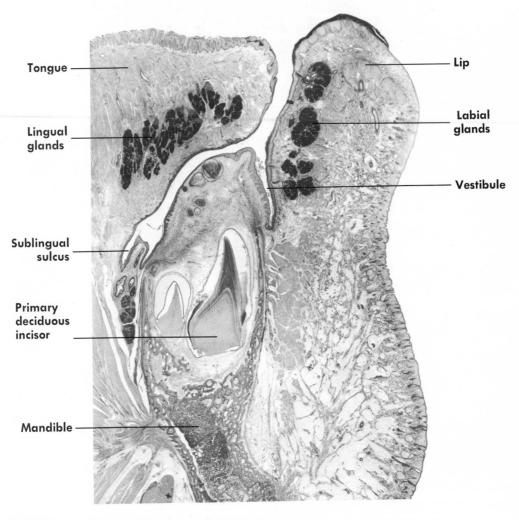

Tongue

Lingual
glands

Sublingual
sulcus

Primary
deciduous
incisor

Mandible

Lip

Labial
glands

Vestibule

Fig. 13-2

Sagittal section through lip and lower jaw of newborn infant, showing state of development and relations of teeth and associated structures. (Courtesy Dr. Sol Bernick, Los Angeles, Calif.; From Bevelander G.: Atlas of oral histology and embryology, Philadelphia, 1967, Lea and Febiger.)

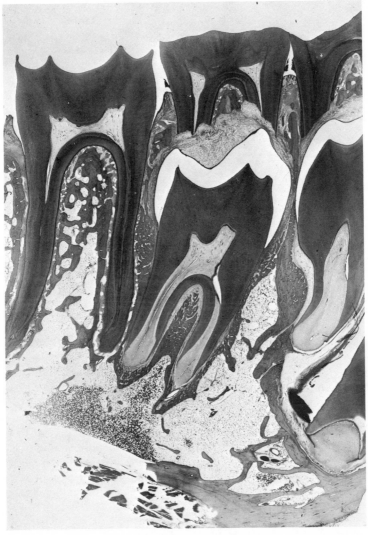

Fig. 13-3
Section through posterior region of lower jaw, showing teeth in stages of shedding and eruption. (From Bevelander G.: Atlas of oral histology and embryology, Philadelphia, 1967, Lea and Febiger.)

ment alone will bring them in a normal position in the dental arch. Hence, the permanent teeth must erupt not only in an occlusal direction to pierce the oral epithelium and protrude in the mouth but they must also assume a position with reference to the arch of the jaw, the space occupied by adjacent teeth, to assume normal occlusal contact with the opposing tooth. Accordingly, these teeth must and often do undergo several movements during eruption in addition to the axial movement necessary to bring the tooth into the proper alignment in the oral cavity.

SHEDDING

Shedding, or exfoliation, was mentioned briefly in the preceding paragraphs. At fairly regular and predictable times the crowns of the permanent teeth develop to their mature size, and at or just prior to this time osteoclastic activity of the root of the deciduous tooth occurs (Fig. 13-4). This process continues once it is initiated until most of the root is resorbed. In connection with this process the pulp is also resorbed, the peridental fibers are detached, and changes in the bony support of the tooth occur. Exfoliation of the tooth usually occurs

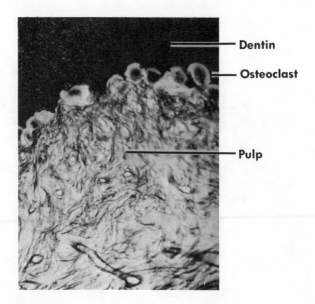

Fig. 13-4
Detail of root of deciduous tooth undergoing resorption.

unassisted, and as a rule, the crown of the succedaneous permanent tooth erupts in approximately the position occupied by the deciduous tooth shortly after exfoliation.

In a study of tooth eruption there are several factors that must be considered. As the root develops it causes the tooth to elongate. It is believed, however, that the apex of the root retains its same relative position during this process, and if this is true, it would account for movement of the crown of the tooth in an occlusal (incisal) direction.

As the crown continues to advance in the direction of the oral epithelium, there is a loss in the connective tissue and vascular elements in this region. When the crown meets the oral epithelium, a passive union between the stratum intermedium and the oral epithelium occurs. As the crown protrudes through the oral epithelium, that portion of the epithelium which surrounds the advancing crown is applied to the cervical portion of the crown as the epithelial attachment; the surrounding part of the epithelium becomes the gingivae.

As the tooth erupts the tissues that make up the developing peridental ligament are reoriented from a position in which most of the fibers are parallel to the long axis of the tooth to one in which they are more nearly at right angles. A certain amount of resorption of the alveolus also accompanies this process, together with subsequent rebuilding of the bony crypt.

In a study of the eruption of the deciduous teeth the relation of the permanent tooth germs is also of interest. At first these developing teeth are located on the lingual surface of the deciduous enamel organ. By the time the deciduous teeth have erupted the permanent tooth germs have been left behind and occupy a position near the apices of the deciduous anterior teeth and between the roots of the deciduous molars. From this position the permanent teeth erupt in an occlusal direction.

Shedding is the process whereby the deciduous teeth are eliminated to make room for the permanent teeth. This process is rather complicated, and many of the factors that are involved are incompletely understood.

Histological examination of the dental tissues that were made during this process reveal the following: (1) The root of the deciduous tooth undergoes rhythmic resorption; (2) the crown of the permanent tooth encroaches upon the root of the deciduous tooth; (3) it is believed that the proximity of the root and crown sets up a tissue tension, which in turn initiates or stimulates further resorption of the root of the deciduous tooth. One argument against this hypothesis, however, is the fact that sometimes the roots of deciduous teeth that do not, for some reason, have a succedaneous tooth also reabsorb.

82

14

PALATE AND TEMPOROMANDIBULAR JOINT

HARD PALATE

The epithelium of the hard palate (Fig. 14-1) is similar to that of the gingiva in that it possesses a cornified layer and a stratum granulosum. It is indented by elongated vascular papillae, which are responsible for the appearance of a pink color. A submucosa is present except in the region of the gingivae and in the midline area. The dense fibers of the submucosa are coarse and are arranged in a vertical direction. These fibers are firmly attached to the periosteum of the hard palate. The submucosa of the anterior third of the hard palate contains a considerable amount of adipose tissue and is accordingly known as the fatty zone. In the mucosa of the posterior two-thirds of the hard palate (Fig. 14-2) there are many mucous glands (the glandular zone). Occasionally, one may observe in the midline spherical or ovoid aggregation of epithelial cells, remnants of the early fusion of the palate. These structures are known as epithelial pearls.

SOFT PALATE

The soft palate (Fig. 14-3), a posterior continuation of the hard palate, is a musculotendinous structure. The mucous membrane of the oral surface consists of a nonkeratinized stratified squamous epithelium. There are relatively few short papillae present. The lamina propria contains scattered elastic fibers, and the loosely arranged submucosa contains many mucous glands. The epithelium characteristic of the oral surface continues for some distance around the border of the velum, where it appears as a pseudostratified ciliated columnar epithelium typical of the nasal tract.

TEMPOROMANDIBULAR JOINT

The temporomandibular joint (Fig. 14-4) is a diarthrosis which permits movement of the mandible. The important bony structures making up this joint are (1) the head of the condyle and (2) the mandibular fossa and articular tubercle of the temporal bone. A thick fibrous articular disc intervenes between the head of the mandible and the temporal bone. The disc separates the articular space into a lower portion, which intervenes between the head of the condyle and the lower margin of the disc, and an upper part, which separates the superior surfaces of the disc from the temporal bone. In the anterior region fibers of the external pterygoid muscle blend with the disc.

The head of the condyle consists internally of typical spongy bone. In young individuals the periphery of the condyle is made up of hyaline cartilage, which later in life is replaced by bone. The articulating surface of the condyle is invested with a layer of fibrocartilage.

The articular disc, as previously mentioned, consists of fibrocartilage. The superior aspect of the disc borders on the superior articular space, which in turn is in contact with the surface of the articular tubercle, which is covered with a dense layer of fibrocartilage as is the case for the head of the condyle.

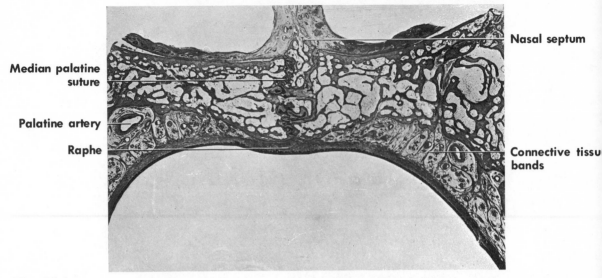

Median palatine suture

Nasal septum

Palatine artery

Raphe

Connective tissue bands

Fig. 14-1
Transverse section through hard palate. (From Pendleton, E. D.: J.A.D.A. **21:**488, 1934.)

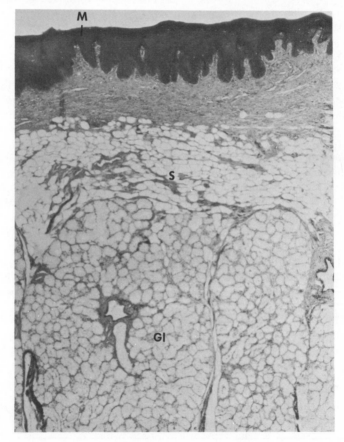

Fig. 14-2
Mucosa, **M**, and submucosa, **S**, of the hard palate. The submucosa contains numerous mucous glands, **Gl**, typical of the posterior two-thirds of the palate. (From Bevelander, G.: Atlas of oral histology and embryology, Philadelphia, 1967, Lea and Febiger.)

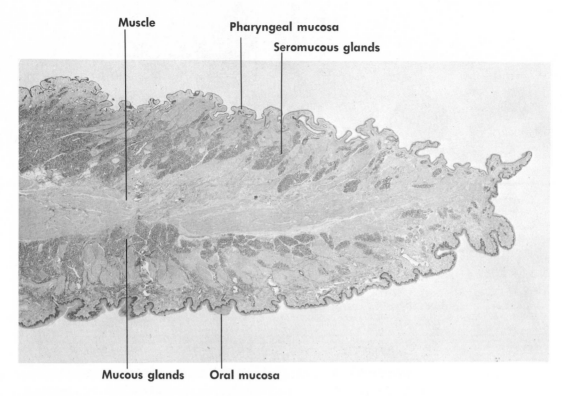

Muscle   Pharyngeal mucosa

Seromucous glands

Mucous glands   Oral mucosa

Fig. 14-3
Longitudinal section of the soft palate. (From Bevelander, G.: Atlas of oral histology and embryology, Philadelphia, 1967, Lea and Febiger.)

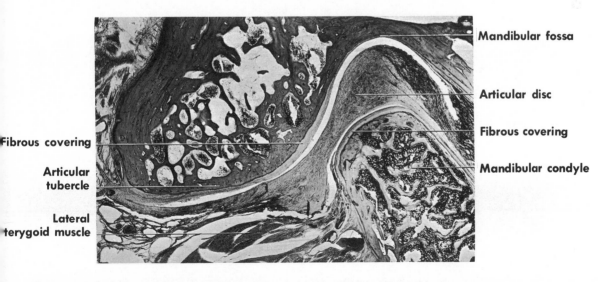

Mandibular fossa

Articular disc

Fibrous covering

Mandibular condyle

Fibrous covering

Articular tubercle

Lateral pterygoid muscle

Fig. 14-4
Sagittal section through temporomandibular joint of 28-year-old man. (Courtesy Dr. S. W. Chase, Western Reserve University, Cleveland, Ohio.)

INDEX TO PART TWO